W9-ASU-531

Rapid Access

GUIDE TO
PHYSICAL EXAMINATION

Rapid Access

GUIDE TO PHYSICAL EXAMINATION

DONALD W. NOVEY, M.D.

Instructor of Family Practice
Instructor of Medicine
Finch School of Medicine, Chicago Medical School
Attending Physician, Lutheran General Hospital
Park Ridge, Illinois
President, Medical Media Systems
Chicago, Illinois

Photography Produced by Medical Media Systems

http://www.medicalmediasystems.com

Director and Demonstrator: Donald W. Novey, M.D.
Photographer: Michael J. Gallagher
Medical Illustration: Christine Young

SECOND EDITION

M Mosby

St. Louis   Baltimore   Boston   Carlsbad
Chicago   Minneapolis   New York   Philadelphia   Portland
London   Milan   Sydney   Tokyo   Toronto

Publisher: Susie H. Baxter
Editor: Liz Fathman
Senior Developmental Editor: Laura C. Berendson
Project Manager: Patricia Tannian
Senior Production Editor: Melissa Mraz Lastarria
Book Design Manager: Gail Morey Hudson
Manufacturing Manager: Dave Graybill
Cover Design: Teresa Breckwoldt

SECOND EDITION
Copyright © 1998 by Mosby Inc.

Previous editions copyrighted 1988

Printed in the United States of America
Composition by Top Graphics
Printing/binding by R.R. Donnelley & Sons Company

Mosby–Year Book, Inc.
11830 Westline Industrial Drive
St. Louis, Missouri 63146

Library of Congress Cataloging in Publication Data

Novey, Donald.
    Rapid access guide to physical examination / Donald W. Novey;
photography produced by Medical Media Systems; director and
demonstrator, Donald W. Novey; photographer, Michael J. Gallagher;
medical illustration, Christine Young.—2nd ed.
        p.   cm.
    Includes index
    ISBN 0-323-00128-9
    1. Physical diagnosis—Atlases.   I. Title.
    [DNLM: 1. Physical Examination atlases.   2. Physical Examination
outlines.   WB 17 N942r 1998]
    RC76.N68   1998
    616.07′54—dc21
    DNLM/DLC
    for Library of Congress   98-3979
                                                                    CIP

98   99   00   01   02   /   9   8   7   6   5   4   3   2   1

To those who are willing to learn
the art of examination,
which, along with a kind and caring attitude,
is the secret to success in medicine.

and to Judy,

*my wonderful wife
and traveling companion through life.*

Preface

This is a book on technique. Its single-minded purpose is to clearly describe the precise methods used to perform most common examination techniques and to supply this information in an easily accessible manner.

The student or practitioner of the health professions often enters a situation where examination skills need to be learned or refreshed in a hurry. In an attempt to address that need, the emphasis in this book is not on the details of clinical pathology, but on organization of material and simplicity of presentation. In many cases, the technique is presented in a cinematographic form, with successive drawings showing the intricacies of the motion or technique involved. The book follows a very simple format, with text on the left-hand page and matching photographs or illustrations always on the right-hand page. In this way, any technique can be learned at a glance.

As an educator, I have tried to present each of the techniques in this book as graphically as possible, showing each one from the perspective of the examiner. This book is unique in its sole attention to examination technique. Its depth of technique description and use of over 750 photographs and illustrations makes it the most efficient text on this subject.

This book is suitable for any individuals who are learning or reviewing, or instructors who are teaching the art of history-taking and physical examination. A basic knowledge of anatomy and physiology is helpful but not required.

In this second edition, much of the text has been rewritten for clarity and accuracy, and the entire text has been reviewed and reformatted into a more readable style. Selected examples of abnormalities have been included for nearly every skill to illustrate the importance of each examination technique. (This text does not intend to describe the full range of abnormalities that can be seen during the examination.) By popular demand, two entirely new chapters have been added on the integrated screening examination and on the approach to the elderly patient. The retinal photograph section now includes color photos, and new illustrations have been added in several chapters. The entire selection of photographs has been resized and recropped for this more convenient spiral binding, allowing the book to be laid flat and studied while techniques are practiced.

This book may be used along with my videotape series, "Techniques of Physical Diagnosis—A Visual Approach," since the style follows closely. Several other publications have also been produced to assist the learner in recognizing abnormalities. These include the audiotape-textbook "The Guide to Heart Sounds—Normal and Abnormal" (CRC Press) for use in cardiac auscultation, the "Effective Retinal Diagnosis" videotape series for help in learning ophthalmoscopy, and "The Living Atlas of Medicine" videotape series for learning the art of disease recognition. This last series shows a wide variety of abnormal history and physical findings in common disorders, as demonstrated in actual patients. Its intent is to condense years of clinical experience into a few short programs. These and other programs can be reviewed in the website http://www.medicalmediasystems.com.

In an attempt to be gender-neutral, I have used both male and female models in this book. For practical reasons, I refer to "he" or "his" for the men and "she" or "her(s)" for the women. The gender neutrality of the examination techniques is implied.

I am very pleased to offer the second edition of this text for your use. Many, many students have learned their physical diagnosis skills using it. I hope this book will serve you well, and I welcome your comments to improve upon editions to come.

Donald W. Novey, M.D.

Acknowledgments

I wish to thank the people who helped turn this book into a reality. Michael Gallagher, the photographer, shot and printed the photographs with consistent excellence. Christine Young produced the many clearly understandable motion arrows and other illustrations. Both of these individuals worked long and hard to produce the large volume of original material presented here. Ms. Young also helped considerably with revisions for the second edition.

Other persons who contributed materials were Randall Bellows, M.D., who supplied the retinal and red reflex photographs, Michael Hawke, M.D., who supplied photographs of the ear canal, eardrum, and nasal turbinates, and Emily Littman, Ph.D., for her assistance with the mental status examination.

I am grateful to Evelyn V. Hess, M.D., for her contribution to the musculoskeletal examination.

Thanks also go to Stuart Oserman, M.D., Hymie Kavin, M.D., and George Geppert, M.D., for their feedback on the Integrated Physical Examination chapter. More thanks to Victoria Braund, M.D., Robert Moss, M.D., and William Rhoades, M.D., for their comments on the Approach to the Elderly Patient chapter.

The rewrite was executed entirely on my Micron laptop, which enabled me to take my office with me. The text was written in Word for Windows, and the extensive photograph database was managed with Microsoft Access. I thank my computer for not breaking down.

My final thanks goes to my wife Judy. (Judy Solari in the first edition!) Her support and expert help with the 750 photographs enabled this project to be completed on schedule.

Donald W. Novey, M.D.

Contents

1 How to Use This Book

TO LOCATE A SPECIFIC TECHNIQUE:
- Locate the appropriate organ system on the inside front cover.
- Follow the bar to the first page of that section.
- Find the desired technique in the Rapid Index. (If not listed, refer to the index at the end of the book.)

TO LEARN THE TECHNIQUE FOR AN ENTIRE ORGAN SYSTEM:
- Locate the appropriate organ system on the inside front cover.
- Follow the bar to the first page of that section. You will be led through the entire examination in proper sequence.

It's That Simple!

2 *Medical History Checklist*

The medical history generates most of the information needed to make a diagnosis. It also provides the opportunity to talk with your patient and begin the rapport-forming process. Learn it well. In the history-taking lies much of the art of medicine.

   I. IDENTIFYING INFORMATION (Basic Statistical Data)
   A. **Date the History Was Taken, Patient's Name, Medical Record Number, If Available.**
   B. **Age and Sex.**
   C. **Place of Birth.**
   D. **Marital Status.**
   E. **Current Occupation.**
   F. **(Optional) Race and Religion.**

   II. SOURCES.
   A. **Source of Information;** whether the information is from the patient, family, or friends.
   B. **Source of Referral;** who referred the patient.
   C. **Source of Patient's Usual Health Care.**

   III. CHIEF COMPLAINT.
   A. **A Short Statement,** in the patient's own words, that indicates the reason for requesting health care.
      1. It may be a statement of a current acute or chronic problem, or a request for routine screening.
   B. **Elicit with an Open-Ended Question:** "What brings you here?" or "What seems to be the trouble?"
      1. Elicit further information with "Anything else?"

   IV. HISTORY OF PRESENT ILLNESS.
   A. **A Detailed and Chronologic Account of the Patient's Current Problem.**
   B. **It Can Be Concisely Elicited by a Standard Series of Questions Called the Symptom Check List.***

---

*Adapted from Wasson J, et al: *The common symptom guide,* New York, 1992, McGraw Hill.

C. **To Speed the Questioning Process, It Is Helpful to Memorize the Letter Abbreviations: "A O L C R A R P C E".**

D. **The Letters Stand for:**
   1. A - Age, the patient's age.
   2. O - Onset of symptoms, detailed as:
      - C - events Coincidental with onset.
      - S - Similar events in the past.
      - S - Sudden or gradual onset.
      - D - Duration of symptom.
   3. L - Location of symptom (as well-defined anatomically as possible).
   4. C - Character of symptom (sharp, dull, aching, burning, etc.).
   5. R - Radiation of pain or sensation.
   6. A - Aggravating factors: "Is there anything you do that makes it worse?"
   7. R - Relieving factors: "Is there anything you do that makes it feel better?"
   8. P - Past treatment, detailed as:
      - W - When, where, and by whom.
      - S - Studies done and the results.
      - R - Results of past treatment.
      - D - Diagnosis.
   9. C - Course of symptom (getting better or worse).
   10. E - Effect on daily life (minor or interfering).

V. **PAST MEDICAL HISTORY (A Collection of Common Items of Information Not Related to Individual Organ Systems)**

A. **(Patient's) Opinion of General Health**

B. **Childhood Illness:**
   1. Measles, mumps, rubella, chickenpox.
   2. Diphtheria, pertussis.
   3. Rheumatic fever.

C. **Immunizations** (if they can remember).
   1. Ask in particular about last tetanus booster, which should be received every 10 years.

D. Adult Illnesses, significant past, chronic, or current (including psychiatric illness).
　　1. In addition, ask if the patient sees any other kinds of nontraditional health care providers, for acupuncture, homeopathy, etc.
E. Surgeries, inpatient or outpatient.
F. Injuries
　　1. Generally those requiring hospitalization or hospital care.
G. Hospitalizations.
　　1. Additional stays not described under injuries.
H. Allergies.
　　1. If asked alone, the patient often thinks of hay fever.
　　2. Is best to ask: "Any allergies to medications?"
I. Current Medications.
　　1. Prescription.
　　2. Nonprescription, including vitamins and oral contraceptives.
　　3. Home remedies, including herbal preparations. This information usually is not offered by the patient unless specifically asked.
　　4. If the list is extensive, record a survey of those taken within the past 24 hours.
　　　　▪ A useful approach is to ask the patient to bring all medicines with him/her to show you.
J. Habits.
　　1. Exercise history; type and frequency.
　　2. Substances:
　　　　▪ Tobacco: Ask if the patient smokes cigarettes.
　　　　　—If "yes," determine pack-year exposure by finding out the number of packs per day and for how many years. If the patient quit smoking, ask for how long and determine prior pack-year exposure.
　　　　　—If "no," ask about pipe smoking or tobacco chewing.
　　　　▪ Alcohol.
　　　　　—Do not simply inquire "Do you drink?" but "How much do you drink?"
　　　　　　—Determine volume and type of beverage.

- Caffeine.
  - —Ask type of drink (coffee, tea, soda, chocolate) and volume (in cups, bottles, or cans).
- Recreational drugs.
  - —Do not assume your patient does not use them.
  - —Ask simply: "Do you use any recreational drugs?"

3. Safety.
   - Does the patient wear seat belts?
   - Does the patient have smoke detectors in the home?

K. Sleep Patterns.
  1. Screen by asking if the patient has any problems with sleeping.
  2. If "yes," determine:
     - When the patient goes to bed and if he/she experiences any trouble falling asleep.
     - If there is frequent wakening during the night.
     - Any early-morning wakening (consistently earlier than usual).
     - Sleep disturbances often occur as part of major depressive disorders.

L. Diet.
  1. Determine any gross dietary deficiencies that could relate to the patient's current disorder.
     - Ask "Do you have any particular restrictions in your diet?" and "Are there any foods you can't or won't eat?"
  2. Elicit a 24-hour survey, beginning with yesterday morning.

VI. FAMILY HISTORY.

  A. Often Introduced with: "Now I would like to ask you about your family's health."
  B. In Most Cases, the History Is Concerned with Immediate Family consisting of parents, grandparents, siblings (brothers and sisters), and children.

C. **Begin with the Open-Ended Question:** "Any health problems in your family?"
   1. If a family member has a disorder, when the patient finishes, ask: "Anyone else with the same problem?"

D. **Then Get Specific:**
   1. "Are your parents still living?" If yes, continue with:
   2. "How old is your mother?"
      - "Any illnesses?"
   3. Repeat with father and grandparents.

E. **Finally, Ask the Standard List of Diseases,** omitting ones that were already mentioned.
   1. "Does anybody in your family have. . ." (ask each disease one at a time).
      - Diabetes, heart disease, high cholesterol, high blood pressure, stroke, kidney disease, cancer, arthritis, anemia, tuberculosis, glaucoma, gout, asthma, headaches, epilepsy, emotional illness
   2. Also ask about substance abuse (alcoholism, drug addiction) in family members.
   3. It is also quite useful to ask if anyone has had symptoms similar to those the patient is having now.
      - With unusual presentations, this often gives clues to an outcome.

VII. PSYCHOSOCIAL HISTORY

A. **The Basic Purpose Is to Answer Two Questions:**
   1. How is the patient's illness affecting his/her daily life?
   2. How will treatment affect his/her daily life?

B. **This Information Is Gained by Determining the Patient's:**
   1. Support system.
      - Home situation: alone or with family or friends?
      - Significant others: who can care for the patient in times of need?
   2. Geographic situation.
      - How far is the patient from the site of health care?
      - Can he/she get there easily?

3. Responsibilities.
   - How will short-term disability or absence affect his/her:
     —Occupation.
     —Family integrity/stability.
     —Family's support.
4. Daily life, best learned from description of a "typical day"

VIII. REVIEW OF SYSTEMS (A Comprehensive Review of all Organ Systems)
A. Question Technique.
1. Proceed from the general to the specific.
   - Begin with an open-ended question (but be ready to steer the patient back to the subject if he/she rambles).
   - Then get specific, asking each symptom or item listed one at a time.
2. Begin each list with: "Any problems with..."
   - Then string specific items together with "or" rather than "Do you have any problems with..."
     —This condenses the time needed to ask these fairly long lists.
   - Although the patient will often say "no" to the initial open-ended question, it is appropriate to follow up with the list.
3. Avoid leading questions.
   - These are questions worded in such a way that they lead the patient to a specific answer.
     —Such as: "Would you say this only happens to you when you lie down?"
     —Better to ask simply: "When does this happen?"
4. Learn (by practice) to ask sensitive and potentially embarrassing questions in a neutral and professional tone of voice.
   - By minimizing your own embarrassment, you minimize the patient's.

5. Follow the patient's lead, helping him/her to elaborate or continue. There are three methods:
   - Facilitation.
     —This encourages the patient to continue by using vocalizations such as "mmm-hmmm" or "go on . . ."
   - Reflection.
     —Repeating the last word or phrase the patient just said often triggers a release of more information on that subject.
   - Clarification.
     —Used, simply, when you are not sure what the patient is saying.
     —Say: "Tell me what you mean by . . ."

6. Avoid using medical jargon.
   - Convert medical terminology into plain English for the patient. If asked a question that uses an unfamiliar term, patients are more likely to reflexively say "no."

B. Organ Systems (Each begins with a sample open-ended question and is followed by the appropriate list of items.)

1. General.
   - "How is your health in general?"
   - Usual weight, recent weight change, fatigue, weakness, chills or fever, night sweats.

2. Skin.
   - "Any problems with your skin?"
   - Rashes, lumps, dryness, itching, color change (localized or within a mole), changes in hair or nails, skin care habits

3. Head.
   - (No suitable open-ended question.)
   - Headache, head injury.

4. Eyes.
   - "Any problems with your eyes?"

- Vision, change in visual fields, use of glasses or contact lenses, date of last eye examination, eye pain, redness, infection, excessive tearing, photophobia, double vision, glaucoma, cataracts, floaters, flashing lights.

5. Ears.
   - "Any problems with your ears?"
   - Hearing, use of hearing aid, tinnitus, vertigo (true spinning sensation), lightheadedness, earaches, infection, discharge.

6. Nose and sinuses.
   - "Any problems with your nose?"
   - Frequent colds, nasal stuffiness, hay fever, discharge, nosebleeds, sinus pain or infection.

7. Mouth and throat.
   - "Any problems with your mouth or throat?"
   - Condition of teeth and gums, use of dentures, last dental examination, bleeding gums, obvious lesions, sore tongue, frequent sore throat, hoarseness, dry mouth.

8. Neck.
   - "Any problems with your neck?"
   - Masses, swollen "glands," goiter, neck pain with movement or palpation.

9. Breasts.
   - In females: "Any problems with your breasts?"
     —In males: "Any problems with your chest or breasts?"
   - Lumps or dimpling, pain or tenderness, nipple discharge (color if present), does she do self-examination (frequency and at what time during cycle).

10. Respiratory.
    - "Any problems with your breathing?"
    - Cough, sputum production (if present, color and quantity), asthma, bronchitis, emphysema, hemoptysis, wheezing, pneumonia, tuberculo-

sis, pleurisy, last TB test (and result), last chest
film (and results).

11. Cardiac.
    - "Any problems with your heart?"
    - Heart trouble, dyspnea (if so, at rest or with ex-
      ertion), orthopnea, paroxysmal nocturnal dysp-
      nea, high blood pressure, rheumatic fever, heart
      murmurs, edema, chest pain, palpitations, past
      ECGs or other studies (and results).

12. Peripheral vascular.
    - "Any problems with your circulation?"
    - Varicose veins, thrombophlebitis ("blood
      clot"), cramping, intermittent claudication, rash
      or edema localized to legs or feet.

13. Gastrointestinal.
    - "Any problems with your stomach?"
    - Abdominal pain, heartburn, indigestion, trou-
      ble swallowing, appetite change, nausea, vom-
      iting, vomiting of blood, frequency of bowel
      movements, change in bowel habits, diarrhea
      or constipation, hemorrhoids, rectal bleeding
      or black tarry stools, food intolerances, exces-
      sive belching or passing of gas, jaundice, liver
      or gallbladder trouble, hepatitis.

14. Urinary.
    - "Any problems with your kidneys or bladder?"
    - Dysuria, usual pattern, excessive frequency,
      polyuria (excessive volume), nocturia, incon-
      tinence, dribbling, hematuria, urgency, hesi-
      tancy, infections, stones, prostate trouble,
      change in urine color or odor.

15. Male reproductive.
    - "Any problems with your penis or scrotum?"
    - Pain in penis, scrotum or testicles, testicular
      masses, history of venereal disease (and its
      treatment), hernias, frequency of (and any

physical difficulty with) intercourse, libido, sexual orientation (if relevant), hernia.

16. Female reproductive.
    - "Any problems with your female organs?"
    - Menstrual history: age at onset, frequency of menses, duration and amount of flow, date of last menstrual period, spotting, excessive flow, amenorrhea, dysmenorrhea, premenstrual tension, menopausal symptoms and date of onset, postmenopausal bleeding.
    - Obstetric history: prenatal course; complications; duration of pregnancy; problems with labor and delivery; condition, weight, and sex of infant(s); postpartum course; number of abortions, if any.
    - Additional: vaginal discharge (odor and color), pruritus, skin lesions, venereal disease (and its treatment), method of birth control, frequency of (and any physical difficulty or pain with) intercourse, libido, sexual orientation (if relevant), DES (diethylstilbestrol) exposure ("Did your mother take any hormones when she was pregnant with you?").

17. Musculoskeletal.
    - "Any problems with your muscles or joints?"
    - Joint pain, stiffness, swelling, redness or heat, muscle pain, cramping, swelling or tenderness to palpation, specific locations of symptom, limitation of motion, history of fractures, back pain, arthritis, gout.

18. Endocrine.
    - "Any problems with your glands or hormones?"
    - Hormone therapy, diabetes, polyuria, polydipsia, polyphagia, thyroid trouble, heat or cold intolerance, dryness of skin or hair, adrenal trouble, change in body hair.

19. Hematologic.
    - "Have you been told of any problems with your blood?"
    - Past diagnosis of disease, anemia, easy bruising or bleeding, blood type, past transfusion of blood or blood products, any reactions, lymph node enlargement.

20. Neurologic.
    - (No suitable open-ended question.)
    - Losses of consciousness, seizures, clumsiness, memory loss, tremors, tingling or numbness, localized weakness or paralysis.

21. Psychiatric.
    - "Now I would like to ask you a few questions about yourself."
    - Nervousness, tension, depression, subjective scale.
      —"Do you consider yourself a nervous person?"
      —"Are you under more stress lately?"
      —"Have you recently felt depressed?"
      —"On a scale of 1 to 10, with 10 meaning 'I feel great' and 1 meaning 'I feel terrible,' where are you today?"
      —This question combines mood, outlook, and physical comfort into a single index that reflects the patient's current assessment of his/her quality of life.

3 Vital Signs/General Assessment

15

I. VITAL SIGNS.

A. Temperature.

1. The undersurface of the tongue is warmest beneath the plexus of veins near the frenulum *(FIG. 3-1)*.

2. Prepare the thermometer:
   - If glass, shake the mercury down below 97° F.
   - If a digital thermometer, turn it on and place a plastic sheath over the probe.

3. Place the distal end under the tongue, near the base of the frenulum *(FIG. 3-2)*.

4. Leave the mercury thermometer in place for 3 minutes or, if digital, until the indicator signals completion (15 to 30 seconds).
   - After removal, read the mercury type quickly, since the mercury column will cool and shorten *(FIG. 3-3)*.
     —Turn the shaft of the thermometer until the silvery mercury column shows behind the degree markings.
     —The normal range of oral temperature is about 97.6° to 99° F.
   - The digital measurement can be read directly (and is often more accurate).

5. If using a tympanic thermometer, apply a disposable sheath and place into the ear canal. The unit beeps when the reading is done.
   - The tympanic reading represents "core" temperature, which is normally 99.6° F.
   - Watch for cerumen in the ear canal. This can artificially lower the reading.
   - When there is *any* doubt of the temperature taken by this method, repeat with another method.

6. Be aware of the normal circadian rhythm:
   - Body temperature is generally highest at 5:00 PM and lowest at 5:00 AM.

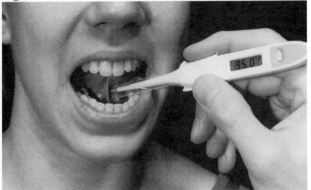
Fig. 3-1

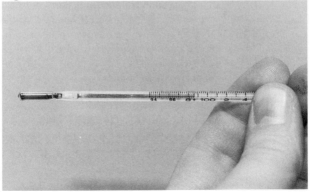
Fig. 3-2

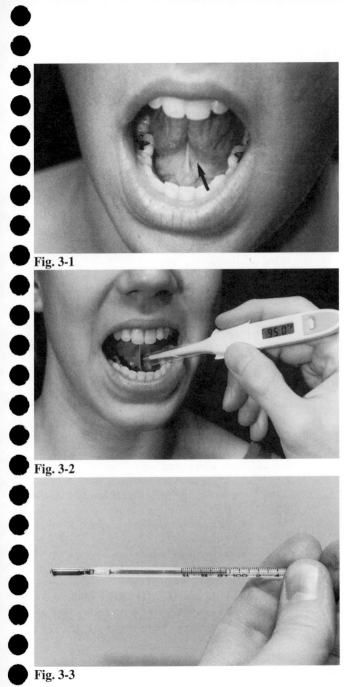
Fig. 3-3

- When interpreting the change in a patient's temperature, consider when the reading was taken, since
  elevation in the morning is more significant than the
  same amount of elevation in early evening.
- Also remember that temperature fluctuations are
  less in elderly patients or those with a decreased
  white cell count. Hot or cold beverages, or cigarette
  smoking can also alter the reading.

B. Pulse (Radial Artery Method).

1. Locate the radial pulse on the inner aspect of the radial
   bone. It is often easiest to palpate 1 or 2 cm proximal
   to the radial styloid.

2. Press the tips of two fingers into the natural groove
   (FIG. 3-4).
   - Pull them inward across the ventral wrist until the
     pulse is centered in the fingertips. Too firm a pres-
     sure occludes the pulse.
   - Count the pulse for 15 seconds and multiply by 4.
   - If the pulse is irregular, count for a full minute.
   - The range of normal pulse rates is 60 to 88 beats per
     minute, often slower in athletes.

3. Be aware of the normal respiratory variation (sinus arrhythmia), when the pulse rate increases with inspiration and slows with expiration.
   - This is pronounced in children and adolescents and
     fades with advancing adulthood *(FIG. 3-5).* At the
     onset of expiration, the slowing can be so pro-
     nounced that it may resemble a skipped beat.

4. If the pulse is grossly irregular:
   - Repeat your measurement using the carotid pulse
     (see Fig. 5-19).
   - If you are still unsure whether you are feeling every
     beat, check the apical pulse by listening over the
     cardiac apex with the stethoscope (see Fig. 5-25).

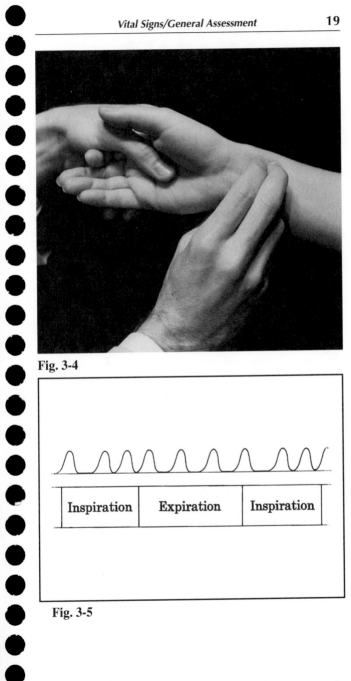

Fig. 3-4

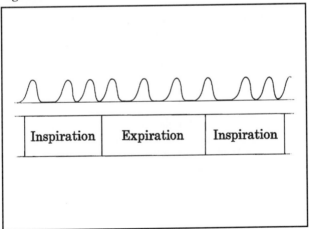

| Inspiration | Expiration | Inspiration |

Fig. 3-5

C. Respiratory Rate.

1. Two methods:
   - In an outpatient setting:
     —Discretely observe the movement of the patient's shoulders or abdomen. This is best done while your hand is still holding the patient's wrist after measuring the radial pulse.
     —When the patient is unaware you are watching his/her breathing, it is more likely to be his/her natural state.
   - In a heavily draped patient:
     —Listen to breath sounds with the stethoscope to determine the rate.

2. The range of normal respiratory rates is 12 to 20 breaths per minute, with occasional deep sighs.

D. Blood Pressure.

1. Palpate the brachial artery *(FIG. 3-6)*.
   - Press all four fingers near the insertion of the biceps tendon and move them until the artery is located.

2. Place the artery mark (or, if unmarked, the rubber tubing) over the pulse *(FIG. 3-7)*.

3. Before you wrap the cuff, see if it is the right size for the arm.
   - Many newer cuffs have fitting indicators *(FIG. 3-8)*.
     —The end of the cuff is the white index line and the middle of the cuff has range markings.
   - While wrapping the cuff, see if the index falls between the range marks.
     —If it does, it is the appropriate size.
     —If not, switch to the needed size.

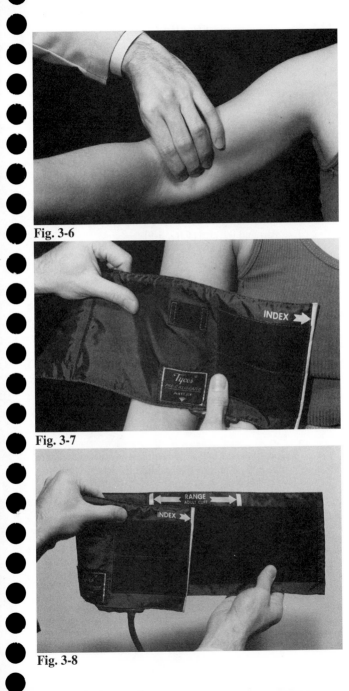

Fig. 3-6

Fig. 3-7

Fig. 3-8

4. Cuff sizes:
    - Large adult size - used for the obese arm.
    - Standard adult size - most often used.
    - Pediatric cuff - for the very slender arm.
    - A cuff too small for the arm produces a *falsely elevated* reading, whereas a cuff that is too large for the arm produces a *falsely lowered* reading.

5. Wrap the cuff snugly against the skin.
    - Keep the cuff one inch above the antecubital fossa.
    - Press the "index" end firmly against the skin and maintain pressure as you wrap the remaining cuff around the arm *(FIG. 3-9)*.
    - Once the Velcro catches, release your fingers from the edge and wrap the remaining cuff snugly around the arm *(FIG. 3-10)*.
      —Two fingers should just fit underneath the cuff.

6. Have the stethoscope earpieces in your ears and the chest piece set on the bell.

7. Support the arm at heart level.
    - Cradle his/her hand between your elbow and waist; this leaves both of your hands free.
    - Grasp the blood pressure bulb with one hand and palpate the radial pulse with the other *(FIG. 3-11)*.

8. Inflate the cuff until you can no longer feel the radial pulse, then pump up an additional 30 mmHg.

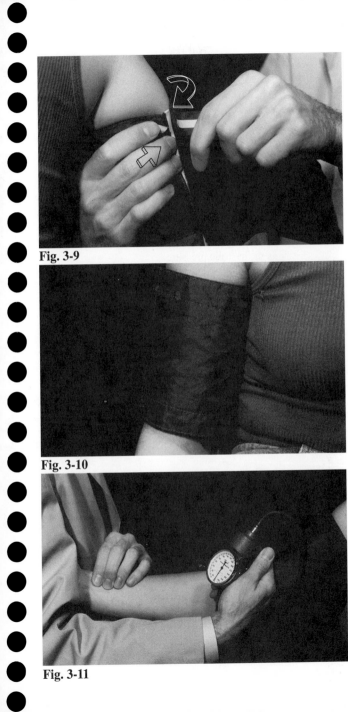

Fig. 3-9

Fig. 3-10

Fig. 3-11

9. Remove your hand from the radial pulse and place the stethoscope bell over the brachial artery *(FIG. 3-12).*
   - Grasp the valve release with the "bulb" hand and slowly open it; begin cuff deflation at about 3 mmHg per second.

10. Auscultation:
    - The very first beats will fade in and out with the respiratory cycle. (The systolic reading normally oscillates 2 to 3 mmHg.)
    - Note the presence of at least 2 consecutive beats as the systolic pressure.
    - Continue cuff deflation until the sounds muffle and disappear *(FIG. 3-13).*
      —Record this point of disappearance of sound as the diastolic pressure.
      —In some patients, the muffling takes longer to disappear. In this case, record the point of muffling and the point of disappearance separately (e.g., 120/80/44).

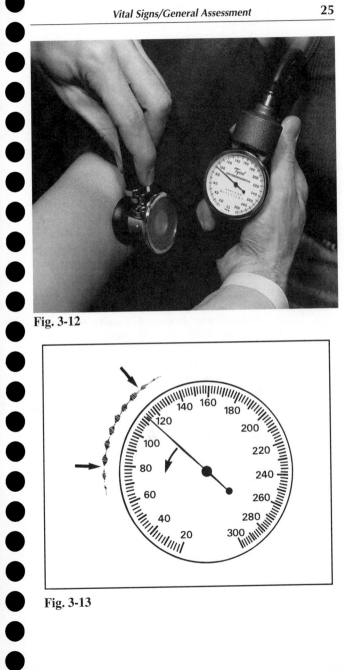

Fig. 3-12

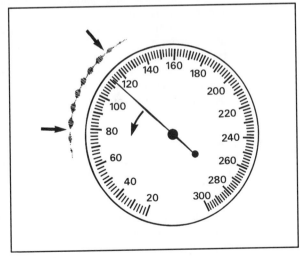

Fig. 3-13

11. Tips:
    - If pressure readings are taken more than twice in a row, deflate the cuff and elevate the arm for a few seconds to promote venous drainage.
    - The normal range of systolic pressures is 95 to 140 mmHg, with an average of 120 mmHg.
        —Normal diastolic range is from 60 to 90 mmHg, with an average of 80 mmHg.
    - Hypertension is defined as a persistent elevation greater than 140/90.
    - Some patients exhibit the "auscultatory gap," a silent area between systole and diastole seen most often with systolic hypertension.
        —Palpation of the radial pulse during inflation eliminates "landing" in the auscultatory gap and incorrectly determining the systolic pressure.
    - If the systolic pressure oscillates more than 15 mmHg from inspiration to expiration, this is called "pulsus paradoxus" and occurs with disorders such as severe airway obstruction or cardiac tamponade.
    - Hypertension is seldom diagnosed by a single reading (unless malignant).
        —Blood pressure may be elevated within 1 hour after smoking a cigarette and up to 12 hours after drinking alcohol.
        —If the pressure is elevated at the start of an exam, consider anxiety as the cause and repeat the reading at the end of the examination: it may be lower.

E. **Height and Weight** (Additional vital signs)
    1. For following changes in weight over time, attempt to use the same scale for each visit, and have the patient remove his/her shoes.

    2. Height is helpful to record on at least one visit. It is useful when calculating ideal body weight. In elderly patients, measure height at least once per year.

II. **GENERAL ASSESSMENT: An overall appraisal of features not inherent to a particular organ system.**

   A. **Appearance of Chronic Illness.**
      1. Manifested by pallor, emaciation, weakness, etc.

   B. **Apparent Age.**
      1. Are the physical appearance and health history in line with the physical age or more appropriate to an older or younger patient?

   C. **Body Type** (Average, tall and slender, or short and stocky).

   D. **Obvious Physical Defects or Deformations,** such as dwarfism or mongolism.

   E. **Posture and Gait** (Erect posture and springy gait or bent, difficult movement, use of cane or walker.)

   F. **Personal Hygiene and Dress** (This varies widely with different cultures.)

   G. **Odors** (Indicating certain pathologic states).
      1. Acetone (nail polish remover) breath: starvation or a diabetic in ketosis.

      2. Musty odor of severe liver disease.

      3. Urine/ammonia odor of uremia.

      4. Fetid odor of dental, pharyngeal, or bronchial infection.

4 *Head and Neck*

I. INSTRUMENTS AND MATERIALS NEEDED.

A. Ophthalmoscope, Otoscope with Speculae, Eye Chart.

B. 3 × 5 Inch Card, Pen or Pencil, Cotton-Tipped Applicators, Alcohol Swabs, Gauze Squares, Tongue Blades, Disposable Rubber Gloves.

C. A Room That Can Be Adequately Darkened.

D. Optional Items:
  1. Otoscope nasal (9mm) speculum or spring-loaded (Vienna) speculum and penlight.

  2. Pneumootoscopy bulb and tubing.

II. THE HEAD.

A. Sit Opposite the Patient with Your Eyes at the Same Level *(FIG. 4-1)*.

B. Begin Your Examination with the Face.

1. Let your first glance be a check for systemic diseases that show themselves in the face. Classic facies of disease include:
   - Startled stare of hyperthyroidism.
   - Puffy, tired face of hypothyroidism.
   - Moon facies of Cushing's syndrome.
   - Coarse facial features of acromegaly.
   - Immobile stare of parkinsonism.

2. Note:
   - Masses or edema. The earliest sign of edema is often eyelid puffiness.
   - Facial contours. Are they symmetric?
   - Facial expression, which reflects the patient's general feeling tone. Note expressions of happiness, sadness, anxiety, or anger.
   - Any involuntary movements or tics.

3. Talk with the patient.
   - Watch for any asymmetry of facial motion. Small degrees of paralysis will not show except with attempted expression.
   - Note especially a unilateral decrease in motion.

4. Have the patient look slightly away. Note:
   - The color and condition of the skin, including:
     —Its texture and presence of skin lesions.
     —Range of colors include cyanosis, pallor, jaundice, or pigmentation.
   - The amount of facial hair, especially at mustache and sideburn areas. In female patients, excessive hair in these locations often signals hirsutism.

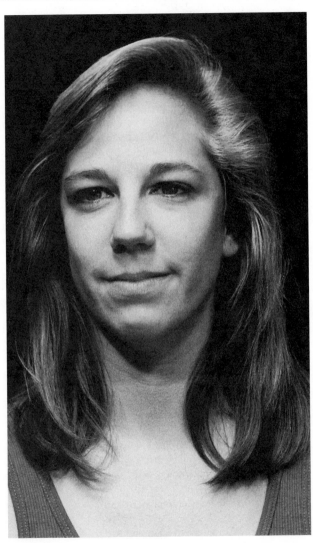

Fig. 4-1

C. Examine the Skull and Scalp (first, any wig or hair-piece must be removed).

1. Inspect the skull for its general size, shape, and contours. There is a wide range of normal skull morphology.

2. Note hair texture and quantity.
   - Pay attention to the pattern of hair loss, if any *(FIG. 4-2)*.
     —Male pattern baldness, with receding temples and apical thinning.
     —Female pattern baldness, with patchy, diffuse hair loss.
   - Ask about use of coloring or lubricating agents.
     —It is often difficult to tell true color and texture of hair. Dyes and bleaches make the hair coarser and drier.
     —If you are concerned with hair texture or color, simply ask the patient if this is the natural color.

3. Examine the scalp for skin lesions.
   - Have the patient bend her head slightly forward *(FIG. 4-3)*.
   - Inspect the skin by parting the hair in several places with your fingers. Note scaliness, lumps, or other skin lesions.
   - You must ask about a history of head trauma or surgery since the hair covers up many scars.

4. Palpate the scalp.
   - Use the palmar aspects of the fingertips.
   - Feel front to back with short sweeping motions *(FIG. 4-4)*.
   - Note lumps or tender areas.

5. Finally, palpate the temporal artery.
   - Feel anterior to the ear, from tragus to forehead. Rest your finger long enough to feel pulsations over the artery.
   - Feel for thickening or tenderness of the vessel *(FIG. 4-5)*. Palpate each side of the head.

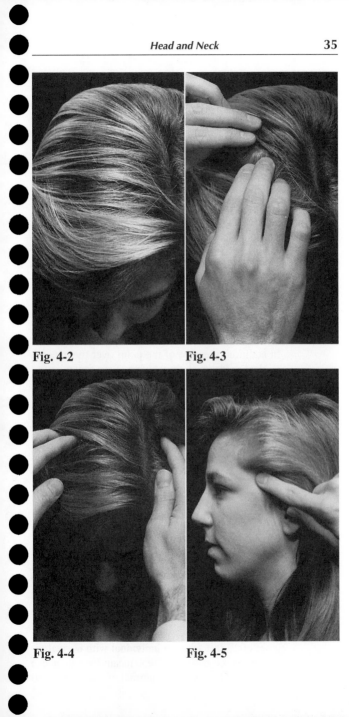

Fig. 4-2

Fig. 4-3

Fig. 4-4

Fig. 4-5

III. EXTERNAL EYE.

A. Visual Acuity (Considered the single most useful test of ocular function; it tests central vision and the optical media of the eye).

1. Position the patient 20 feet from a standard-sized eye chart.
   - The chart should be well illuminated.
   - The patient should wear corrective lenses unless they are used only for reading.
   - With elderly patients, allow them to wear their reading glasses. Use a pocket-sized eye chart card held 14 inches away.
   - Eye charts are available for illiterate patients that show numbers or "E's" in different positions. Eye charts for small children show simplified pictures, such as a dog or sailboat.

2. Have the patient cover one eye at a time with a card, not her fingers (because she can peek) *(FIG. 4-6)*. In addition, pressure of the palm over the eye can render the vision slightly blurred for a few minutes.
   - Be sure she keeps her head straight and does not look around the card.
   - Have her read the chart letters out loud. She should continue reading down until she can read only with difficulty.
   - Note the last line in which she can read more than half the letters *(FIG. 4-7)*.
   - If the patient cannot read the largest letters, move her closer to the chart until she can. Note distance.
   - Measure each eye separately, then both eyes together.

3. Record the visual acuity listed next to the line:
   - The numerator is the distance of the patient from the chart. The denominator is the distance from which a normal subject can read the line. The larger the denominator, the greater the refractive error.
   - For example, 20/40 vision means the patient can see at 20 feet what an individual with normal vision can see at 40 feet. 10/50 means the patient can see at 10 feet what the normal eye can see at 50 feet.

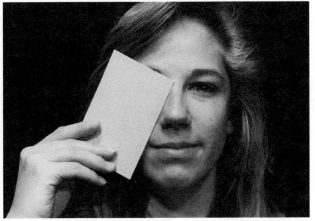

Fig. 4-6

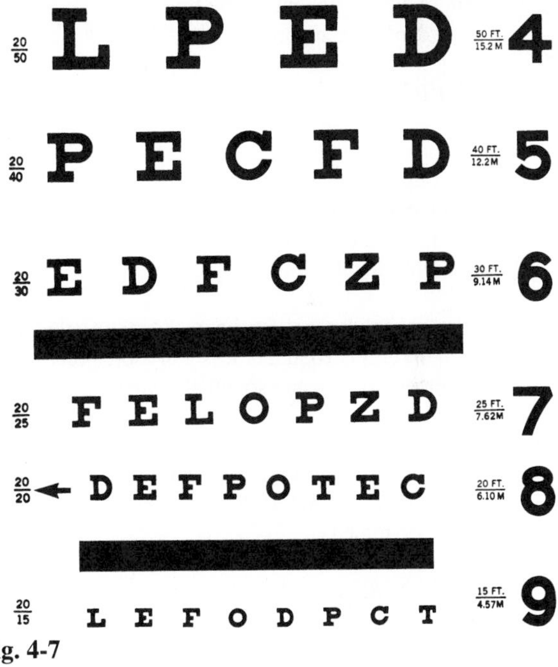

$\frac{20}{50}$ **L P E D** $\frac{50\ FT.}{15.2\ M}$ **4**

$\frac{20}{40}$ **P E C F D** $\frac{40\ FT.}{12.2\ M}$ **5**

$\frac{20}{30}$ **E D F C Z P** $\frac{30\ FT.}{9.14\ M}$ **6**

$\frac{20}{25}$ **F E L O P Z D** $\frac{25\ FT.}{7.62\ M}$ **7**

$\frac{20}{20}$ ← **D E F P O T E C** $\frac{20\ FT.}{6.10\ M}$ **8**

$\frac{20}{15}$ **L E F O D P C T** $\frac{15\ FT.}{4.57\ M}$ **9**

Fig. 4-7

4. If no chart is available, compare her vision to yours using any nearby printed material *(FIG. 4-8)*.

5. If she cannot read any lettering:
   - See if she can count fingers held twelve inches away *(FIG. 4-9)*.
   - Or see hand motion
   - Or tell light from dark. This is tested by turning the examination room light on and off, or by shining a light into the patient's eye.

6. Visual field testing is described in Chapter 12, Neurologic Examination.

B. **Compare the Two Eyes for Prominence** *(FIG. 4-10)*.
   1. If there is any question of bulging, especially unilaterally, tilt the patient's head forward.
      - Compare each cornea to the lid below: see if one or both corneas bulge far beyond the lid margins *(FIG. 4-11)*.

   2. If one or both eyes seem to bulge:
      - Roughly measure the distance from the angle of the eye to the corneal apex, using a pocket ruler. View the eye from the lateral side *(FIG. 4-12)*. Sight directly from the ruler to the cornea.

   3. The normal distance from cornea to the angle (palpebral fissure) is 16 mm or less. For more precise measurement, obtain an exophthalmometer.

C. **Eyelids.**
   1. The examination sequence can be remembered by the mnemonic "SIMPLE."
      - S—Symmetry
      - I—Inflammation
      - M—Masses
      - P—Position
      - L—Lashes
      - E—Edema

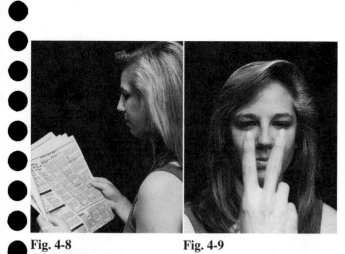

Fig. 4-8   Fig. 4-9

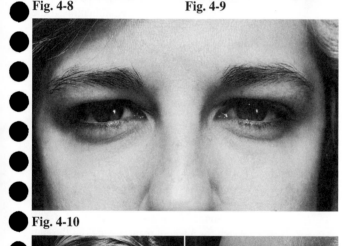

Fig. 4-10

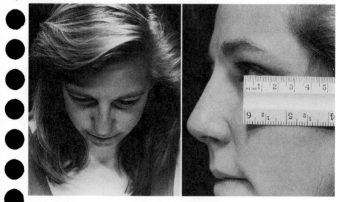

Fig. 4-11   Fig. 4-12

2. First note symmetry of the lids.
   - Is the distance between upper and lower lids equal in both eyes *(FIG. 4-13)?*
   - See if the patient can close her eyes completely. The lids should press together tightly enough to nearly engulf the lashes *(FIG. 4-14).*

3. Note any inflammation or masses, especially at the lid margins *(FIG. 4-15).*
   - Note redness or scaling of the skin.
   - If a mass is seen, palpate it by running a finger gently across the lid surface *(FIG. 4-16).*
     —For any portion of the eye examination, if the eye appears reddened, wear protective gloves before palpation. It is very easy to contract an eye infection.
   - Examine the lacrimal ducts; only the openings, or puncta, are normally visible as a small opening on each medial upper and lower lid margins.
     —If the patient complains of increased tearing, check for lacrimal duct obstruction.
       • If this area is swollen, palpate gently for tenderness; this would be a distended lacrimal sac.
       • Then press your index finger onto this area or over the medial inferior orbital rim and gently milk your finger toward the eye *(FIG. 4-17).* Watch for material regurgitating out through the lower punctum.
   - If an enlarged lacrimal gland is seen or suspected:
     —Have the patient look down and medially.
     —Lift the upper lid and look for the lacrimal gland *(FIG. 4-18).*
       • It is located in the upper and lateral recesses of the lid.
       • A small portion of the gland, yellow-pink in color, is normally visible.

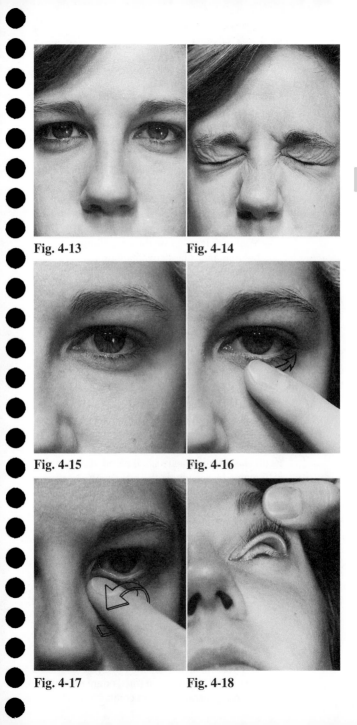

Fig. 4-13

Fig. 4-14

Fig. 4-15

Fig. 4-16

Fig. 4-17

Fig. 4-18

4. Note the position of the lids.
   - Note drooping or retraction (where sclera shows above the iris) *(FIG. 4-19)*.
     —The upper lid usually rests about half way between the limbus (periphery of cornea) and the pupil.
     —The lower lid margin rests just at or below the limbus.
   - Note any visible sclera above or below the iris.
     —Visible sclera above the iris can indicate the lid retraction of hyperthyroidism.
     —Visible sclera below the iris, along with eye bulging, indicates exophthalmos.
   - See if the lower lid turns out or in.
5. Inspect the lashes, which should be evenly distributed along the lid margins.
   - Tweezing and makeup can obscure the normal appearance of the lashes.
   - Also note the eyebrows for quantity and distribution of hair. Note any lateral thinning, which can occur with thyroid disease.
6. Note edema of the lids. This shows as a thickening of the upper lids or puffiness on or below the lower lids.

D. **Examine the Conjunctiva,** a continuous sheet of epithelium from globe to lids.
   1. The bulbar conjunctiva shows the white sclera beneath and contains many small blood vessels.
      - Examine by separating the lids widely. Never apply pressure on the globe when attempting to separate the lids. Instead, hold the lids against the rim of the bony orbit *(FIG. 4-20)*.
      - Check for inflammation and masses on the lateral and medial sclera *(FIGS. 4-21* and *4-22)*.
        —Note scleral color:
          • Fatty deposits can have a yellow hue and can be mistaken for jaundice.
          • In dark-skinned patients, pigmented areas may show as small dark spots or patches near the limbus.
        —Note conjunctival redness:
          • If present, do the inflamed vessels concentrate near the limbus, as in iritis, or are the vessels more generalized, as in conjunctivitis?

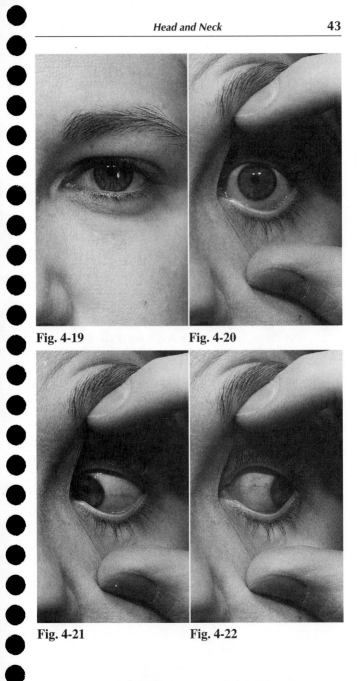

Fig. 4-19

Fig. 4-20

Fig. 4-21

Fig. 4-22

2. The palpebral conjunctiva.
   - Check under the lower lids *(FIG. 4-23).*
     —Have the patient look up.
     —Depress both lower lids with your thumbs.
     —Note color and presence of any lesions.
       - Severe anemia may show as marked pallor.
       - You may see faint yellow vertical striations under either lid. These are the oil-producing meibomian glands.
   - Check under the upper lids.
     —Place your thumb on the superior orbital rim *(FIG. 4-24).*
     —Have the patient look down as you retract the lid up and outward.

E. Inspect the Cornea and Iris.

1. Cornea.
   - Inspect the surface by moving an otoscope or penlight up and down from the side. The light should reflect as a pinpoint bright dot *(FIG. 4-25).*
     —Note any cloudiness or opacities. Normally, the cornea should be smooth, transparent, and shiny.
     —A surface defect causes the dot of reflected light to be grainy or irregular.
   - You may see a corneal arcus in elderly persons.
     —This is seen as a full or partial gray or white ring around the edge of the cornea. It is not medically significant in this age group. In patients under age 40, it may signal hypercholesterolemia.
   - Inspect the curve of the cornea.
     —Have the patient look down. You will see the contour of the cornea as outlined by the curve of the lower lid.
     —The normal cornea shows a gentle curve. In keratoconus, a conical shape to the cornea, the lower lid clearly outlines a rounded triangular shape.

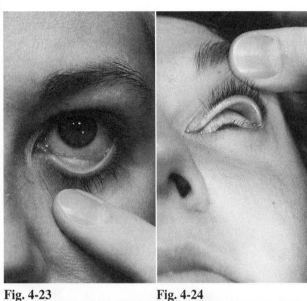

Fig. 4-23   Fig. 4-24

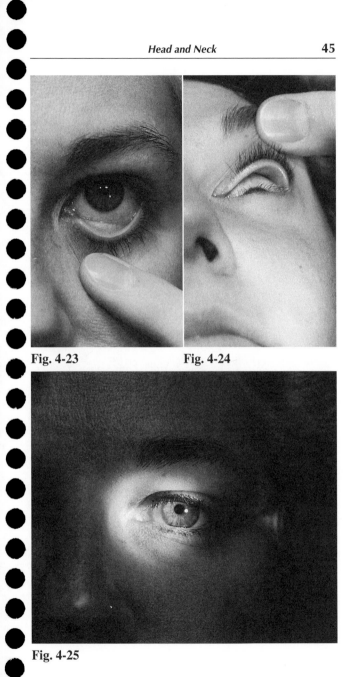

Fig. 4-25

- To check for a narrow corneal angle.
  - —Shine a light obliquely across each eye. It normally illuminates the entire iris.
  - —When the corneal angle is narrow (because of a shallow anterior chamber):
    - You will see a crescent-shaped shadow on the side of the iris *away* from the light *(FIG. 4-26).*
    - This indicates an anatomic predisposition for narrow-angle glaucoma and is important if planning to use dilating eyedrops (see page 58).

2. Iris
   - Inspect for its shape, color, nodules, or vascularity.
     - —Patients with prior cataract surgery often have an iridectomy scar, a black slit near its outer edge.
     - —In these patients, the lens is surgically absent, called *aphakia.* Without the lens for support, the iris often flutters with each movement of the eye.
   - Observe the pupils *(FIG. 4-27),* which should be round and symmetric.
     - —The pupils are normally slightly unequal in 5% of normal individuals, but inequality of pupil size should initially be viewed with suspicion.
       - Because many drugs can alter pupil size, remember to ask about medications the patient is using, particularly eye drops.
     - —Pupils tend to be normally smaller in infants, the elderly, and in hyperopic (far-sighted) individuals.
     - —Pupils tend to be normally slightly dilated in persons with myopia (near-sightedness) or lighter-colored irises.

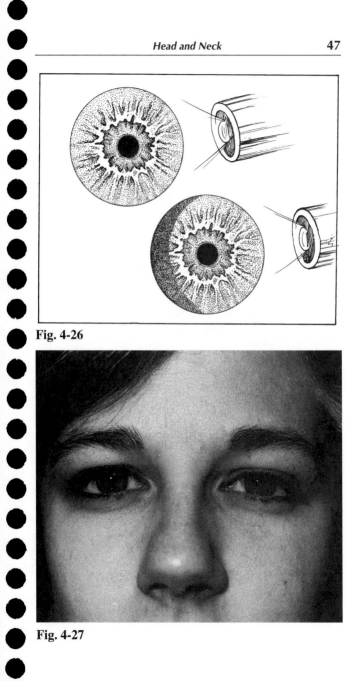

Fig. 4-26

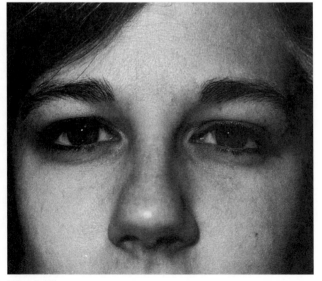

Fig. 4-27

F. Check Pupillary Responses.

1. Accommodation (near reflex).
   - Darken the room slightly.
   - Place your finger or a pencil 12 inches from the bridge of the patient's nose. Ask the patient to stare past the pencil at the wall behind you *(FIG. 4-28)*.
   - Then, have her focus on the pencil.
   - Independent of light, the pupils will constrict and the eyes will converge *(FIG. 4-29)*.

2. Response to light.
   - Darken the room slightly.
   - Have the light source to one side of the patient's head *(FIG. 4-30)*. If the patient watches the light, her pupils will constrict from a "near reflex" response and not because of the light stimulus itself.
   - Flash the light in one eye using a swivel motion; leave it on the eye a long time to allow full constriction *(FIG. 4-31)*.
   - Note:
     —The direct response: constriction in the eye stimulated.
     —The consensual response: constriction in the opposite eye.
   - Follow this with the *swinging flashlight test.* Have the patient look straight ahead, then shine the light back and forth from one eye to the other.
     —This helps compare the light sensitivity of each eye. For example, with an optic nerve defect, when the light shines on the involved eye, both pupils dilate.
   - Use a bright light source and a completely darkened room before deciding the response is absent.
     —Absence of the light response indicates neural disease, including disorders of the retina.
     —Cataracts never completely obliterate light perception.

3. Both accommodation and light responses are normally present, but their speed of constriction varies; response time is markedly slowed in the elderly.
   - With the *Argyll Robertson pupil,* a finding of neurosyphilis, the pupils constrict to accommodation but not to light.

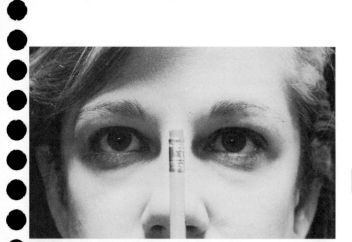
Fig. 4-28

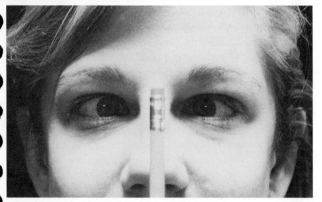
Fig. 4-29

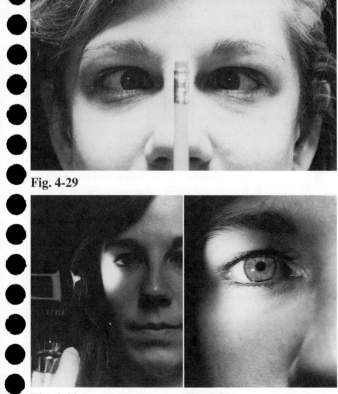
Fig. 4-30   Fig. 4-31

G. Extraocular Motion (This can be tested in three ways.)

    1. Note symmetry of gaze.

- Aim a light source about two feet from the patient, directly in front. Hold the light distant enough to prevent convergence of gaze *(FIG. 4-32)*.

  —Ask the patient to stare at the light.

- The dot of reflected light should be in the same location on each cornea, usually near the center of each pupil.

  —When one eye does not look directly at the light, the reflected dot of light moves to the side opposite the deviation. For example, if the eye deviates medially, the reflection appears more laterally placed than in the other eye.

  —You can approximate the angle of deviation by noting the position of the reflection. Each millimeter of displaced reflection represents about seven degrees of ocular deviation.

    2. Check the six cardinal positions of gaze.

- First, a review of the six basic directions of extraocular motion and the muscles involved: *(FIG. 4-33)*

  —(1) Lateral gaze: lateral rectus muscle.

  —(2) Medial gaze: medial rectus.

  —(3) Gaze up and out: superior rectus.

  —(4) Gaze down and in: superior oblique.

  —(5) Gaze up and in: inferior oblique.

  —(6) Gaze down and out: inferior rectus.

- As a reminder of cranial nerve innervation, use the following mnemonic: "SO_4 LR_6, remainder 3." This states that:

  —The superior oblique muscle is innervated by cranial nerve IV (trochlear).

  —The lateral rectus muscle is innervated by cranial nerve VI (abducens).

  —The remaining extraocular muscles are innervated by cranial nerve III (oculomotor).

  —Familiarity with these innervations will assist you in determining the neurologic deficit when testing extraocular motion.

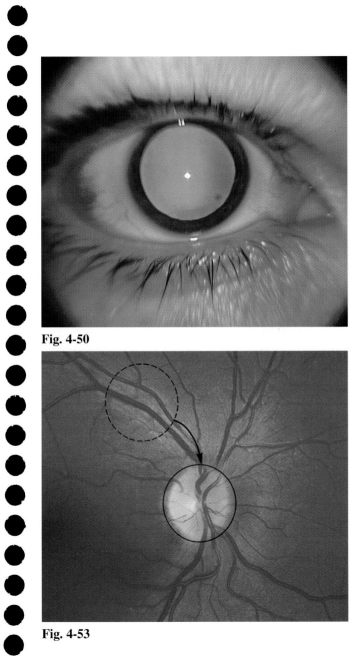

Fig. 4-50

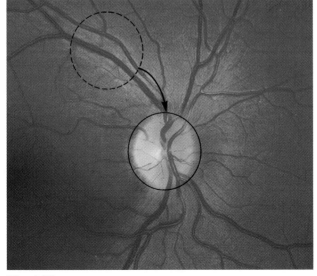

Fig. 4-53

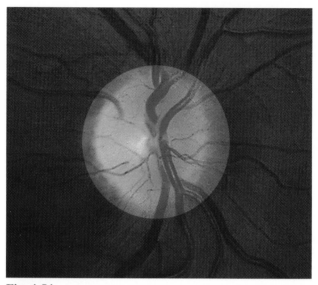

Fig. 4-54

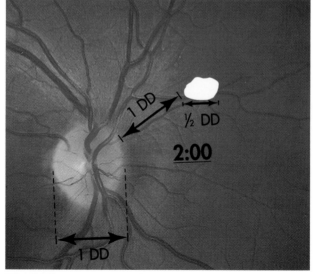

Fig. 4-55

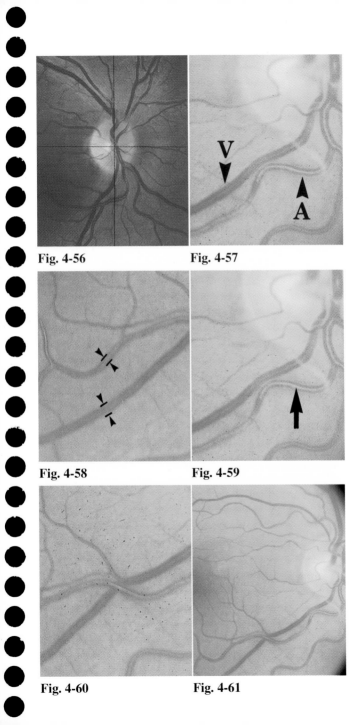

Fig. 4-56

Fig. 4-57

Fig. 4-58

Fig. 4-59

Fig. 4-60

Fig. 4-61

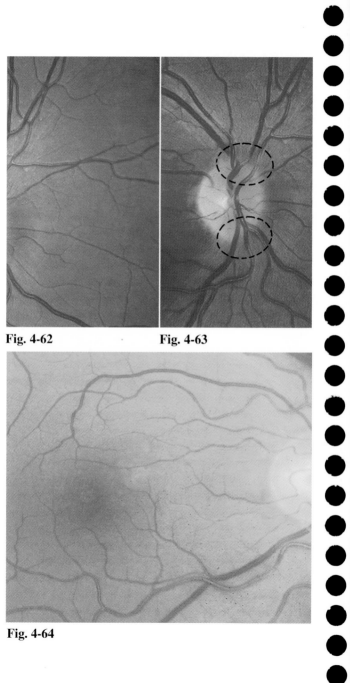

Fig. 4-62   Fig. 4-63

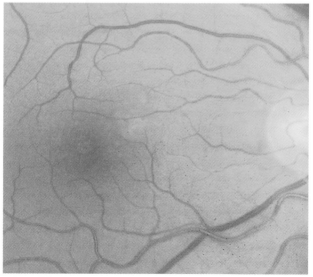

Fig. 4-64

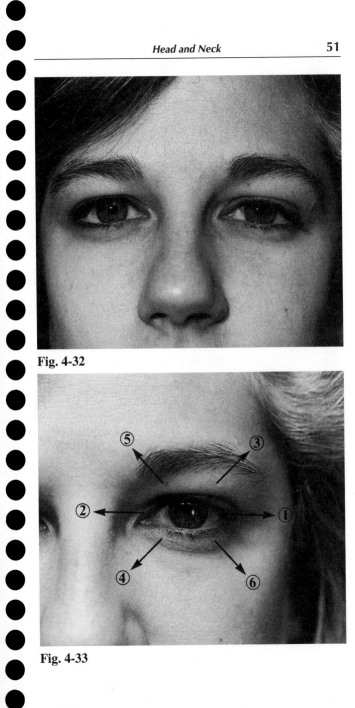

Fig. 4-32

Fig. 4-33

- Place your finger or a pencil 12 inches from the bridge of the nose. Ask the patient to follow you with her eyes, but without turning her head. If head turning does occur, place your hand on top of the head for gentle restraint.
  —In an elderly person, hold the test object further away, since near vision often requires corrective lenses.
- Trace the six directions, coming back to the center after each motion (*FIGS 4-34* through *4-39*). With downward gaze, you may wish to hold the patient's upper lids open to better see the eyes.
  —Some clinicians prefer to draw a large "H" in the air to test the six directions of gaze.
  —Watch for normal synchrony of eye motion. This is called conjugate gaze.
  —Carry the eyes to the extremes of gaze, to exaggerate any muscle weakness.
  —Watch for nystagmus, particularly with upward or lateral gaze.
    • When the patient is looking far to the side, you will see normal end-positional nystagmus. This is a rapid shift of the eye toward the direction of gaze followed by a slow drift away. This motion cycles repeatedly as long as the gaze is held in that position.
    • Pathologic nystagmus occurs when it is seen in the region of full binocular vision (not just at the periphery.) It produces a rapid component (the rapid shift of the eye) in the same direction regardless of which direction the eyes are looking.
    • Describe nystagmus in the direction of the *fast* component.

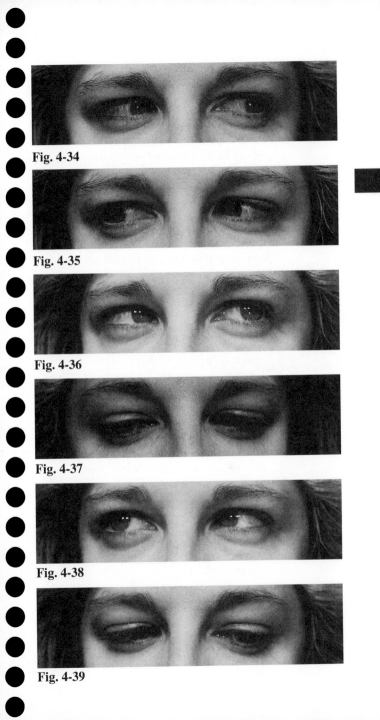

Fig. 4-34

Fig. 4-35

Fig. 4-36

Fig. 4-37

Fig. 4-38

Fig. 4-39

- Finish by checking for lid lag. Placing the test object in the midline, moving it first up and then quickly down (*FIGS. 4-40* and *4-41*).
  —Normally, the upper lid covers the top of the iris and lowers as quickly as the eye moves.
  —With lid lag, the upper lid will delay for a moment in its lowering to follow the eye. This is a sign of hyperthyroidism.

3. To bring out a mild eye deviation, use the cover test. (This can detect minor deviations as small as five degrees.)
   - Have the patient look at a specific point, such as the bridge of your nose (*FIG. 4-42*).
   - Cover one of her eyes with a card. As you do this, watch the other eye (*FIG. 4-43*).
     —Normally, the uncovered eye will not move at all.
     —If it moves, it was not straight before the other one was covered.
   - Then cover the opposite eye and repeat.
   - Typically, in cases of long-standing strabismus (deviated eye), one eye has become dominant, with the other eye deviated medially or laterally. When the dominant eye is covered, the less dominant eye snaps to the midline position.

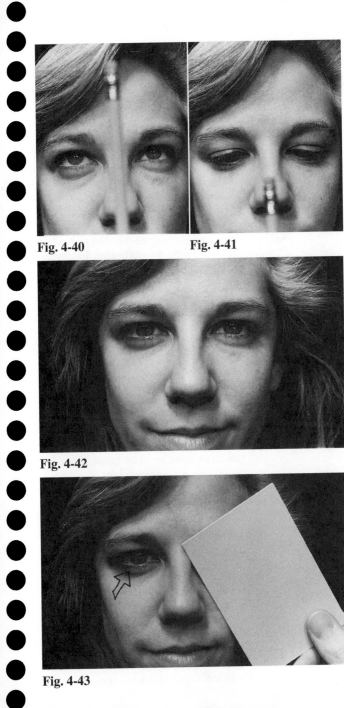

Fig. 4-40   Fig. 4-41

Fig. 4-42

Fig. 4-43

IV. INTERNAL EYE

A. Requires the Use of the Ophthalmoscope

1. Description of the instrument: *(FIG. 4-44)*
   - Has a set of 22 lenses (varies with model):
     —Eleven convex (positive diopters, black numbers), used for viewing more anterior structures of the eye.
     —One "plano" (zero diopters, number "0"), used to begin the examination.
     —Ten concave (negative diopters, red numbers), for focusing on the retina.
   - The lenses permit focusing on different parts of the patient's eye and adjustment, in part, for the patient's or your refractive error *(FIG. 4-45)*.
   - Many models have a small wheel that selects filters that modify the light beam *(FIG. 4-46)*. There are settings for:
     —(1) Wide round circle - recommended for most routine use.
     —(2) Small round circle - used if excessive pupillary constriction occurs.
     —(3) A grid (resembling a rifle-sight) - for following the size of a lesion over time.
     —(4) A narrow slit (optional) - to identify protruding retinal lesions.
     —(5) 4000k color temperature filter - a gray filter that produces most accurate color of tissues; also useful for light-sensitive eyes.
     —(6) A green (red-free) filter - used to highlight hemorrhages, microaneurysms, or other vascular changes on the retinal surface. It causes red-colored structures to appear dark brown.
     —(Optional) a cobalt-blue filter - used to illuminate the cornea during fluorescein eye examination, when looking for corneal abrasions.
   - The top of the battery cylinder has a rheostat for controlling the light intensity. Use maximum brightness unless the patient cannot tolerate it *(FIG. 4-47)*.
     —Remember that if the light source is dimmed, its color becomes more orange-red, and makes color recognition of retinal structures more difficult.

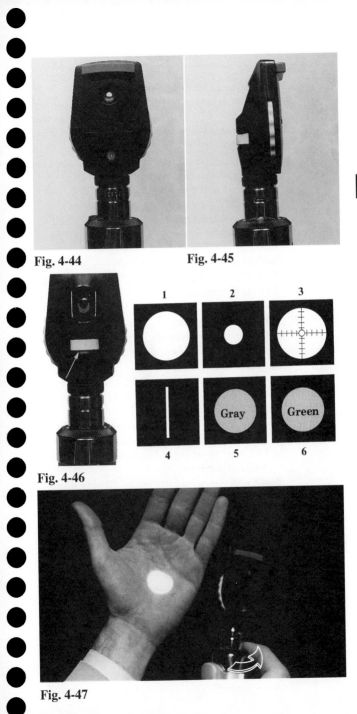

Fig. 4-44

Fig. 4-45

Fig. 4-46

Fig. 4-47

2. Holding the ophthalmoscope.
   - Have your index finger on the lens wheel and thumb on the light source *(FIG. 4-48).* (This way you can adjust both refraction and brightness while you are looking.)
   - Use the 'right-hand rule.'
     —To view the patient's right eye:
       • Stand to the patient's right side.
       • Hold the scope in your right hand.
       • Look through the scope with your right eye.
       • Have the patient look over your right shoulder at a defined point.
     —To view the patient's left eye:
       • Stand to the patient's left side and use your left hand and eye.

3. Preparation for viewing.
   - You can usually view the retina without dilating the pupils, unless you need an accurate inspection of the macula.
     —Dilating eyedrops (mydriatics) may be used *only* if you are sure the patient does not have glaucoma.
     —As a general rule, avoid dilating drops in hyperopic (farsighted) Caucasian individuals over age 40. This group is at highest risk of acute angle closure glaucoma.
     —In addition, avoid the use of dilating drops in patients with head injury or coma, in whom a dilated pupil can signal brain injury.
     —The usual medication is 0.5% tropicamide alone or followed by 10% phenylephrine HCL.
   - The patient's corrective lenses can be removed unless she has a high degree of astigmatism or refractive error. The examiner can also remove his/her glasses unless also having a high degree of refractive error or astigmatism.
   - Darken the room (but not completely dark). In complete darkness, the patient cannot fixate and her eyes will wander.
   - Inform the patient she may blink as needed during the examination.

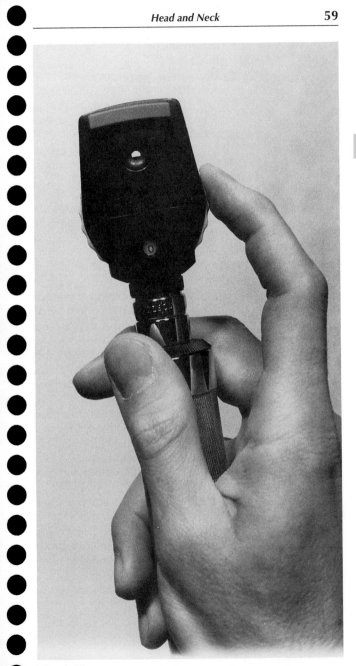

Fig. 4-48

4. Viewing the red response.
   - Method:
     - —Place your thumb on the patient's brow, to act as a bumper *(FIG. 4-49)*. If the patient blinks too often, gently elevate her upper lid. (If you retract the upper lid too much, the eye becomes irritated, causing even more blinking.)
     - —Ask the patient to stare past you at the opposite wall. Shine your ophthalmoscope light at a point on the wall where she should fixate.
     - —Turn the lens wheel to "zero."
     - —Stand about one foot away from the patient and about 15 degrees to the side. This will bring the beam of light into the region of the optic disc and is least irritating for the patient.
     - —Examine the pupil through the ophthalmoscope.
   - Result:
     - —The beam of light passes through the transparent media of the eye. From external to internal, these structures consist of the cornea, anterior chamber, lens, and vitreous humor.
     - —If this optical axis is clear, the light will reflect off the retina with a clear orange-red color. You will see this glow shining back through the pupil *(FIG. 4-50)*.
   - If the red response is decreased, turn the lens wheel to obtain a more detailed view of the opacity.
     - —A +15 through +20 setting allows focusing onto the cornea, anterior chamber, or lens.
     - —A +4 through +10 setting allows focusing on the vitreous.
     - —The most common cause of decreased transparency is a cataract. Focus your lens wheel on this opacity and see if it is denser centrally (nuclear cataract) or peripherally (cortical cataract). If a cataract is present, it will often interfere with your ability to visualize the retina.
     - —Afterward, return to zero diopters to focus on the retina.

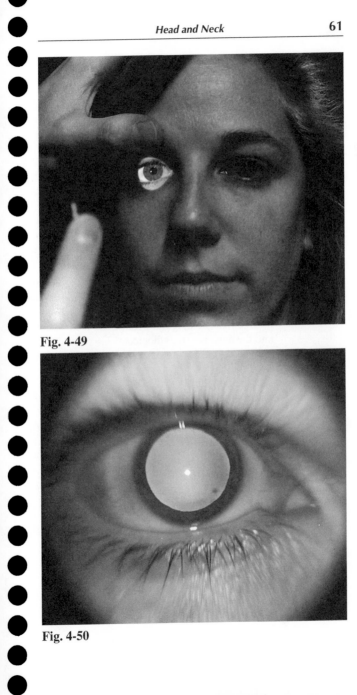

Fig. 4-49

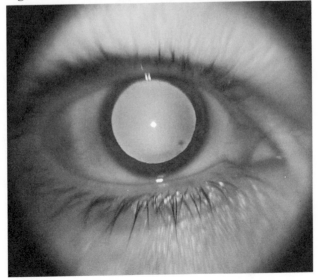

Fig. 4-50

5. Begin to view the retina.
   ▪ Move your eye and scope closer to the patient *(FIG. 4-51)*. Keep both eyes open and relaxed.
     —Stay at the same 15 degree angle. This will keep the optic disc in your line of sight.
     —Sandwich the scope between your thumb and forehead or glasses *(FIG. 4-52)*.
       • The ophthalmoscope head has a rubber bumper to prevent scratching of eyeglasses.
       • Your thumb prevents the scope from touching the cornea.
       • Keep the viewing aperture exactly in front of your eye.
       • Corneal reflection can be minimized by moving the scope very slightly to one side or the other. Attempt to focus *past* the reflection onto the retina.
   ▪ Bring the retina into focus by rotating the lens wheel.
     —In myopics (nearsighted) rotate the lens wheel into the negative (red) diopters.
     —In hyperopics (farsighted) rotate into the positive (black) diopters.
   ▪ Locate the optic disc *(FIG. 4-53,* also see color insert after p. 50*)*.
     —Often, a vessel is seen first.
     —Follow the vessel branches backwards. The vessel branches converge onto the disc much as the branches of a tree converge to the trunk.
     —When shifting your gaze on the retina, move the scope and your head as a unit, pivoting around the pupil. In this way, the light beam stays centered through the pupil.
     —The disc is the least light-sensitive portion of the retina. Technically, it is the *blind spot.* Use this time to fine-tune your focus of the retina. It is the least irritating part of funduscopy for the patient.

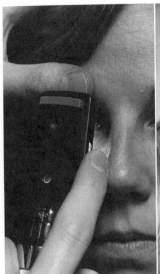

Fig. 4-51

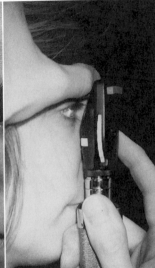

Fig. 4-52

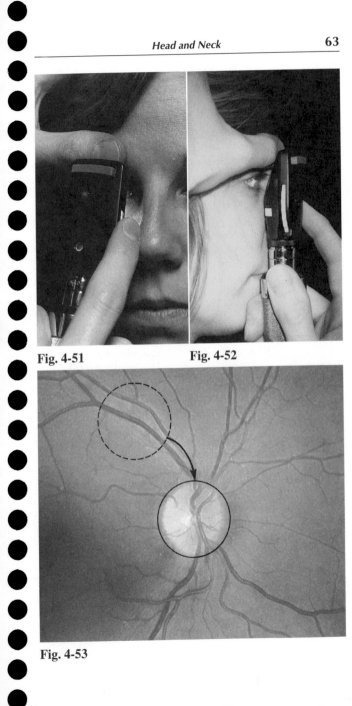

Fig. 4-53

6. Inspect the disc *(FIG. 4-54)*.
   - The disc is a creamy yellow or pink in color. It is round or vertically oval and is slightly darker on its nasal side.
   - Note the distinctness of its margins. The nasal border is normally less distinct than the temporal border.
   - You will often see thin white or pigmented crescents at the disc margin, especially at its temporal border.
   - The optic disc is used as a standard of measurement on the retina. Its size is referred to as a "disc-diameter" (DD).
     - The size and distance of a lesion from the disc is defined in disc diameters *(FIG. 4-55)*.
     - The position of a lesion is more precisely defined by imagining the retina to be the face of a clock with the disc at its center. Note the location of the lesion by its clock position.
   - Note the cup to disc ratio.
     - The optic cup is visible in about 50% of patients. It shows as a lighter area in the center of the disc. Its horizontal diameter is normally 0.4 the size of the disc or less.
     - An increase in cup size suggests glaucoma.
       - There are some normal variations in cup size that can mimic glaucoma.
       - Horizontal elongation of the cup is common in African-Americans, with a cup to disc ratio up to 0.7.
       - Vertical elongation of the cup is more commonly pathologic.
     - Whenever an enlarged optic cup is seen, evaluate for glaucoma with a check of intraocular pressure.

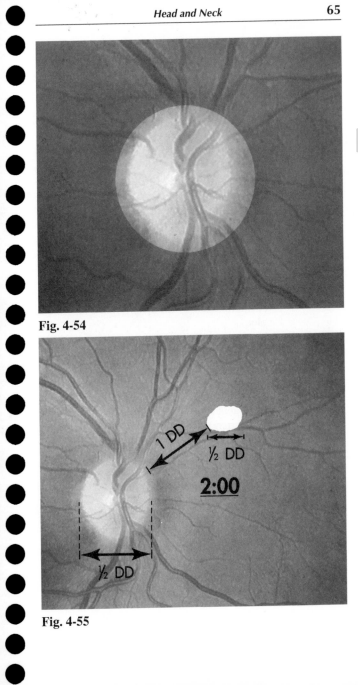

Fig. 4-54

Fig. 4-55

7. Begin tracing vessels.
   - Choose one branch at a time and follow it outward.
   - There are usually four sets of vessels, named for the quadrant each occupies *(FIG. 4-56):*
     —Superior nasal, superior temporal.
     —Inferior nasal, inferior temporal.
   - Note the following vessel characteristics:
     —Distinguish arterioles from venules. Arterioles are brighter red and have a distinct light reflection; venules are slightly larger and darker in color *(FIG. 4-57).*
     —Estimate the A:V ratio *(FIG. 4-58).* This is the thickness of the arteriole compared to its parallel venule. The normal ratio is 2:3 and is best measured 1 or 2 DDs from the disc.
     —Note the arteriolar light reflection seen as the thin white streak in the center of the arteriole *(FIG. 4-59).* It should be about one quarter the width of the arteriole and is normally bright and white in color.
       • Note any widening of the streak or a yellowing in color. This can occur with arteriosclerosis of aging or from long-standing hypertension.
     —Observe the arteriovenous intersections (crossings) *(FIG. 4-60).* These are most accurately assessed about two disc-diameters from the disc.
       • The arterioles and venules normally cross and intertwine each other, with no change in the size or course of either vessel at these crossings.
       • In long-standing hypertension, AV nicking can occur, with the venule seeming to disappear on either side of the arteriole.
     —Follow the vessels peripherally and note the regular decrease in caliber. Watch for segmental narrowing of the arterioles, a finding in hypertension.
     —Note any vessel tortuosity *(FIG. 4-61).*

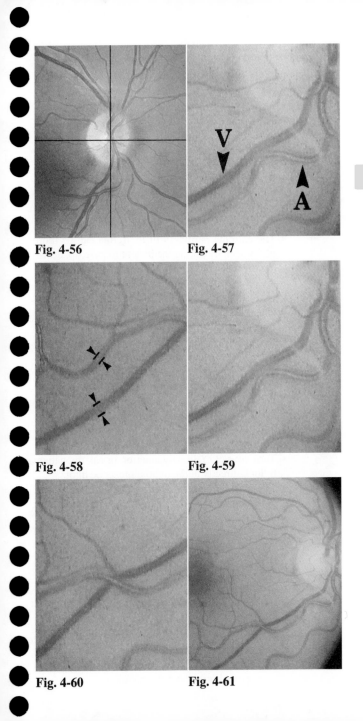

Fig. 4-56

Fig. 4-57

Fig. 4-58

Fig. 4-59

Fig. 4-60

Fig. 4-61

8. Inspect the retinal background, the area between vessels *(FIG. 4-62)*.
   - Its granular orange color will lighten or darken according to skin or hair color. In dark-skinned individuals, the background can even appear tigroid, with irregular stripes of light and dark color.
   - Note any focal areas of hyperpigmentation or hypopigmentation.
   - If lesions are seen on the background, note their size (in disc diameters), shape, color, and distribution.
   - The extreme periphery of the retina can be more easily seen by asking the patient to gaze up, down, out, or in. For example, to see the superior pole of the retina, ask the patient to look up.
9. Check venous pulsations *(FIG. 4-63)*.
   - Observe the venules where they emerge or cross over the disc margin.
   - You can usually see at least one vein pulsating (dilating with cardiac systole).
   - The presence of spontaneous venous pulsations usually indicates that intracranial pressure is normal.
10. Finally, view the macula *(FIG. 4-64)*. (This is usually performed last since it is uncomfortable for the patient.)
    - Turn your gaze directly anterior, or ask the patient to look directly at the ophthalmoscope light.
    - The macula is about two disc-diameters temporal to the disc and is a round, brownish area of pigment one disc-diameter wide.
      —It is surrounded by retinal vessels trailing toward it but is free of visible vessels itself.
      —It is shaped like a shallow dish. You might see a shimmer of light reflecting around its rim.
      —In its center, look for a minute glistening spot, the *foveal pit reflex*. This is a reflection from the fovea centralis, the area of highest visual acuity.
      - Absence of the foveal pit reflex can indicate flattening of the macula, a sign of macular edema. This always needs to be verified by an ophthalmologist's examination.

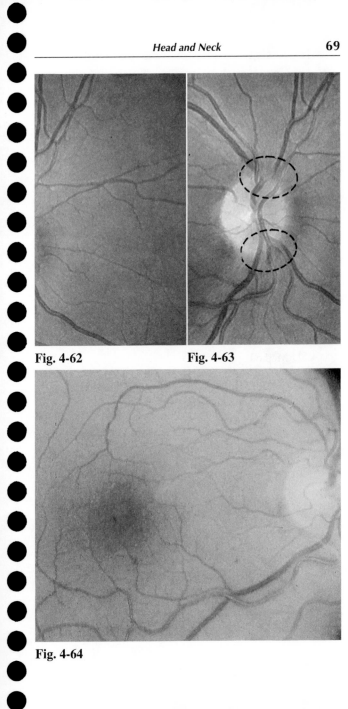

Fig. 4-62   Fig. 4-63

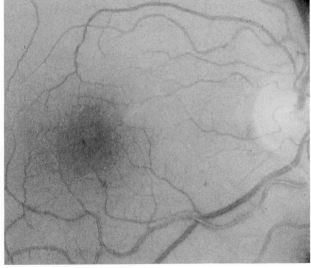

Fig. 4-64

V. ADDITIONAL HEAD AND EYE TESTS (Used if abnormalities are seen or suspected.)

A. Cranial Auscultation.

1. Used when a cerebral artery aneurysm or arteriovenous fistula is suspected. (In these situations, a patient may even complain of a distant humming sensation in the head.)

2. Use the bell of the stethoscope.
   - Place it over:
     —Each temple area *(FIG. 4-65)*.
     —Each closed eye (gently) *(FIG. 4-66)*.
   - Listen for a bruit (a cyclic "whooshing" sound). Normally, none are present.

B. Eyelid Eversion.

1. Used to more thoroughly examine the upper palpebral conjunctiva.

2. Method:
   - Explain the entire procedure to the patient before you begin. Reassure the patient during the procedure and move gently but deliberately.
   - Ask the patient to look downward but still keep her eye slightly open. This prevents contraction of the orbicularis oculi muscle, which would prevent free motion of the lid.
   - Gently grasp the upper lashes and lift them slightly away from the eye *(FIG. 4-67)*. Do not pull on the lashes, since this causes reflexive eyelid spasm.
   - Place the tip of a cotton-tipped applicator about 1 cm above the lid margin, at the upper tarsal border *(FIG. 4-68)*.

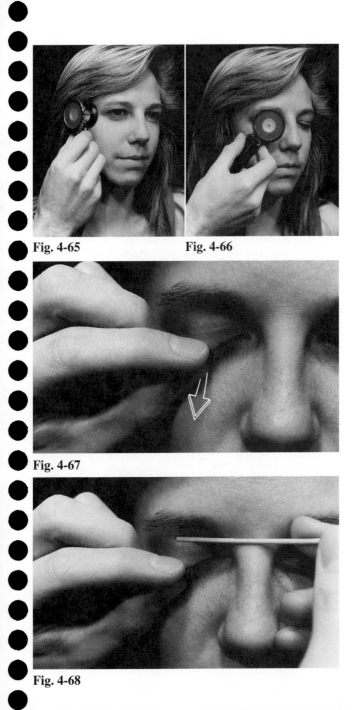

Fig. 4-65

Fig. 4-66

Fig. 4-67

Fig. 4-68

- Now, while still holding the lashes, push gently downward with the applicator tip *(FIG. 4-69).*
    —Push on the lid, not onto the eyeball. This will evert the upper eyelid.
- Hold the lashes against the upper orbital ridge (not against the eyeball) *(FIG. 4-70).*
    —Inspect for inflammation or foreign bodies.
    —Because the upper lid is normally concave, eversion causes a vertical fold to appear on the nasal side. It is not to be mistaken for a mass.
- To end:
    —Again pull the lashes slightly away from the eye.
    —Ask the patient to look up and blink. The lid will return easily to its normal position.

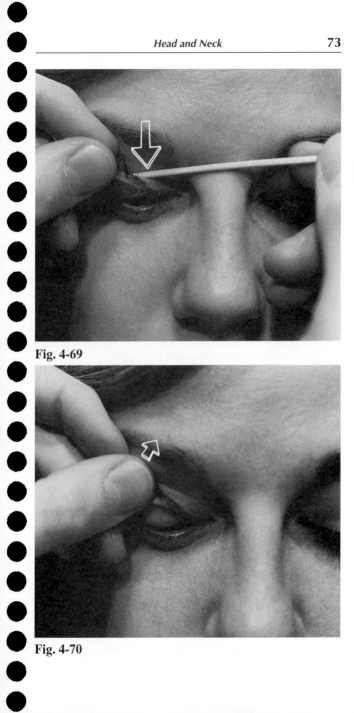

Fig. 4-69

Fig. 4-70

VI. EAR.

A. External Ear.

1. Note symmetry of the ears for position and size *(FIG. 4-71)*.

2. Then examine each ear separately *(FIG. 4-72)*.
   - Is the helix smooth and round?
   - Check the rim of the auricle for nodules.
   - If the ear lobe is pierced, check for nodules or scaliness near the hole.
     —Scaliness here is common with nickel dermatitis, because nickel is common in many jewelry alloys.
   - Note any discharge from the canal, and its color.
   - Check behind the ear for nodules or scaliness *(FIG. 4-73)*.
     —This is a common location for the scaling of seborrheic dermatitis or the soft bulging of sebaceous cysts.

3. If the patient complains of ear pain, gently move the helix up and down and, in addition, press on the tragus.
   - When either of these two maneuvers elicit tenderness, it signals otitis externa, an inflammation of the external auditory canal.

4. Further examination requires the use of the otoscope.

B. Internal Ear.

1. Use of the otoscope.
   - Make sure the otoscope batteries are fresh. A bright white light is needed to see the true color of the eardrum.
   - Attach a speculum, using the largest one that will enter *(FIG. 4-74)*. The speculum is needed to separate the flexible walls of the outer portion of the canal.
   - If possible, use disposable speculae. Otherwise, clean the speculum before and after each use.
   - Hold the otoscope in one of two ways:
     —With the battery cylinder uppermost *(FIG. 4-75)*. This allows you to brace the scope against the patient's head and is a most useful position for stabilizing a moving patient (e.g., a child).
     —In a vertical position with the otoscope head uppermost *(FIG. 4-76)*. This usually feels more comfortable and is the more common position.

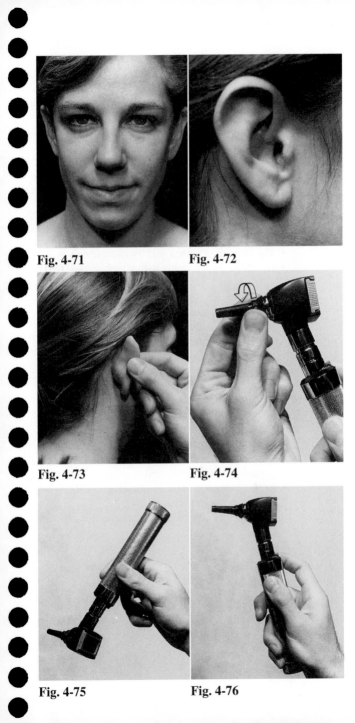

Fig. 4-71

Fig. 4-72

Fig. 4-73

Fig. 4-74

Fig. 4-75

Fig. 4-76

2. Entering the ear canal.
   - Anatomy:
     —The external auditory canal is about 1 inch long.
     —It is supported in its outer one third by cartilage and in its inner two thirds by bone.
     —The skin over the bony canal is thin and *extremely* sensitive.
     —In adults, the canal curves down and forward from auricle to eardrum. In infants and small children, the canal tends to be more directly horizontal.
   - Tilt the patient's head slightly away from you.
   - Grasp the auricle gently with your free hand *(FIG. 4-77).*
     —Use the thumb and forefinger, stabilize the head with the remaining fingers.
     —In adults, pull the auricle slightly up and backwards to straighten the external canal.
       • In small children, pulling the helix slightly down and outward is sufficient.
   - Watch yourself insert the speculum. Then look through the speculum and guide it further in, using a slightly down and forward direction *(FIG. 4-78).* Never blindly insert the speculum into the ear.
     —The most common error beginners make is to insert the speculum too deeply. This may cause pain and can hinder further examination.
   - Examine the skin of the external canal *(FIG. 4-79).*
     —Note the normal hair and wax.
       • Wax may be golden and viscous, or dark and scaly.
       • If excessive wax is present, removal should be supervised by an experienced clinician.
     —Note inflammation or exudate on the skin. Also note foreign bodies or osteomas (bony outgrowths) in the canal.
       • If the canal is inflamed or swollen, proceed *cautiously,* as external otitis renders the canal quite tender.
   - Then focus further back at the eardrum itself.

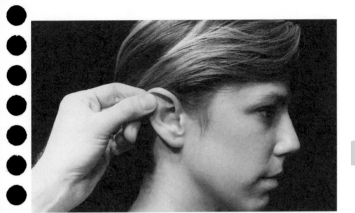
Fig. 4-77

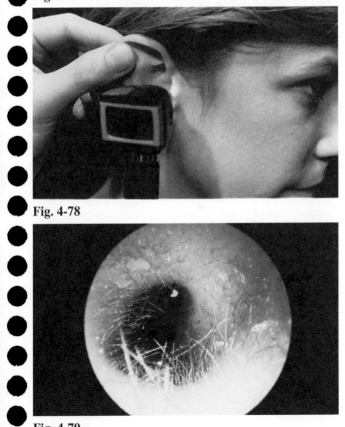
Fig. 4-78

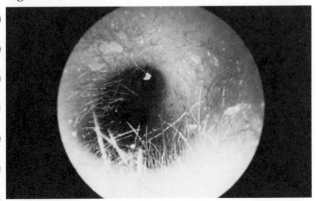
Fig. 4-79

3. Examine the eardrum.
   - Orientation: *(FIG. 4-80)*
     —The drum is positioned obliquely in respect to
       the ear canal. (The anterior-inferior quadrant is
       usually the most distant from the examiner.) Be-
       cause of this, the drum appears tilted.
     —The drum is arbitrarily divided into quadrants
       (FIG. 4-81).
       • The long process of the malleus forms the
         vertical (although tilted) axis.
       • A line perpendicular to this, through the drum
         center, forms the four quadrants.
       • They are anterior superior and inferior, and
         posterior superior and inferior.
   - Observe features of the drum:
     —Note its color. It is normally a translucent pearly
       gray.
     —Note its shape.
       • It is normally slightly concave.
       • Its center is pulled inward by one of the ossi-
         cles, the malleus.
       • The majority of the drum (except the very top
         portion) is taut and is called the pars tensa.
     —Note the landmarks on the drum.

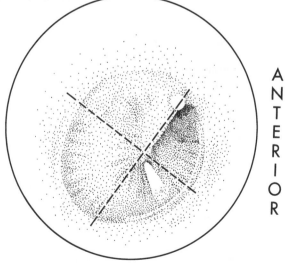

Fig. 4-80

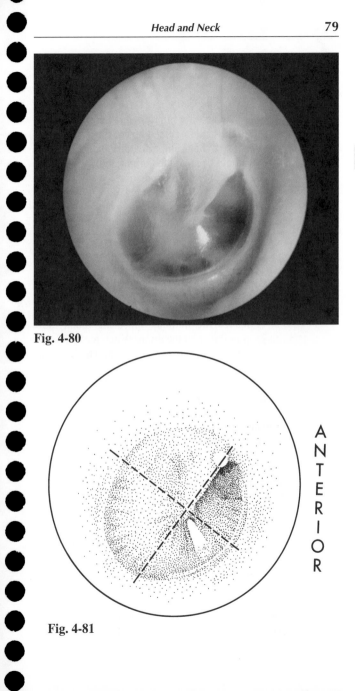

ANTERIOR

Fig. 4-81

4. Landmarks of the eardrum *(FIG. 4-82).* (You will need to move your scope around to see the entire drum.)

- ▪ (1) The light reflection, seen as a triangular cone of light in the anterior inferior quadrant *(FIG. 4-83).*
- ▪ (2) The reflection extends from the periphery to the center of the drum, called the *umbo.*
  - —It should be sharp and bright; dulling of the reflection implies inflammation.
- ▪ (3) The malleus appears as a white line extending down and backwards from top to umbo. Its surface may also be covered by blood vessels, mimicking inflammation.
  - —Note whether the drum is:
    - • Bulging—caused by infection and often accompanied by a decrease in the light reflex and change in drum color.
    - • Retracted—where the drum pulls inward and leaves the malleus appearing much more prominent on the drum. Watch for bubbles or a fluid level behind the drum, which can occur with serous otitis media.
- ▪ (4) Its short process is a tiny white knob projecting outward near the rim. The drum folds over the short process forming the anterior and posterior malleolar folds above it.
- ▪ (5) The pars flaccida, a more relaxed portion of the drum, lies above the short process and between the two folds.
- ▪ (6) Then view the annulus—(a fibrous ring that surrounds the drum except at the pars flaccida. It appears whiter and denser than the rest of the drum.
  - —Look here for perforations, since they typically occur near this rim.
  - —The base of the drum is sometimes obscured by the floor of the external canal.

C. Hearing Tests, including the Rinne and Weber tests, are reviewed in Chapter 12, Neurologic Examination.

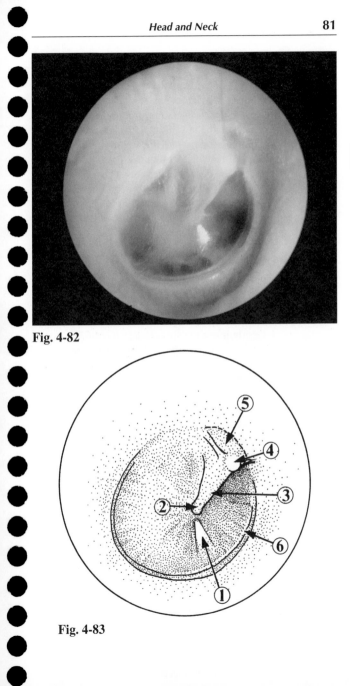

Fig. 4-82

Fig. 4-83

VII. NOSE.

    A. External Nose.

        1. Inspect the nose from the front *(FIG. 4-84)*.
- Note any deviation in size, shape, or color.
- Note the smooth contour from bridge to tip.

        2. Then check the nose from the side *(FIG. 4-85)*.

        3. Palpation is only done in cases of nasal pain or a history of recent facial trauma.

        4. To see if the nasal cavities are patent:
- Have the patient breath through one nostril at a time. One side is normally more patent than the other, although this alternates during the day *(FIG. 4-86)*.

    B. Internal Nose.

        1. Speculum examination.
- Tilt the patient's head slightly back. Keep your left hand on the top of her head to reposition her as needed.
- Gently insert the speculum *(FIG. 4-87)*.

    —Use the otoscope with the largest ear speculum, or use a short broad nasal speculum attachment.

    —Insert the speculum into the lateral side of the nose; avoid touching the nasal septum, as it is very sensitive.
- As an alternate method, hold the otoscope with thumb and forefinger, handle tipped upward. Brace the knuckles of the same hand lightly against the patient's cheek. This allows a dexterous pencil-grip of the scope.

- Examine the septum.

    —Transilluminate the septum by aiming the light at the septum and look into the other nostril.
- A septal perforation will show a spot of white light shining through. An intact septum will show a smooth pink glow.

    —Inspect its shape through the speculum.
- The septum is rarely straight. Its irregularity usually causes no disturbance unless severe.
- Note any crusting or dried blood on the septum. It often correlates with the source of a recent nosebleed.

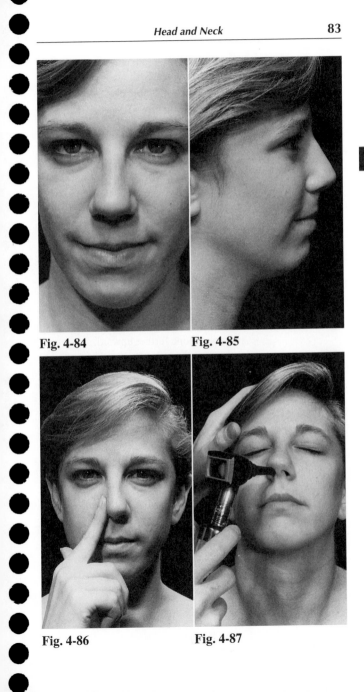

Fig. 4-84

Fig. 4-85

Fig. 4-86

Fig. 4-87

- Staying clear of the septum, ease the speculum further in, aiming posteriorly and upward to visualize the turbinates.
  —The inferior turbinate (1) is usually visible *(FIG. 4-88)*.
    - It lies like a finger along the lower lateral wall of the nose. When it swells, it causes the sensation of nasal congestion.
    - Its color, as are all the turbinates, is normally redder than the oral mucosa. It is often mistaken by beginners as being inflamed.
    - If discharge is present, note its color.
    - Note the size of the nasal airway, seen as a black space between turbinate and septum. The size of the airway often correlates with the patient's subjective sensation of nasal congestion.
  —Focus further back to see the middle turbinate (2).
    - Aim your scope further upward.
    - Look under the turbinate for polyps or sinus drainage. Milky discharge from near the middle turbinate is highly suggestive of sinusitis, when symptoms are present.
  —The superior turbinate is not usually visible.

2. An alternate method *(FIG. 4-89)*.
   - Use a spring-loaded (Vienna-type) nasal speculum with a pocket flashlight or headlamp.
   - Tip the patient's head slightly back.
   - Hold the speculum in your left hand. Stabilize it with your index finger on the side of the nose.
   - Open the speculum blades vertically to avoid pressure on the nasal septum. Open the blades as widely as patient comfort allows.

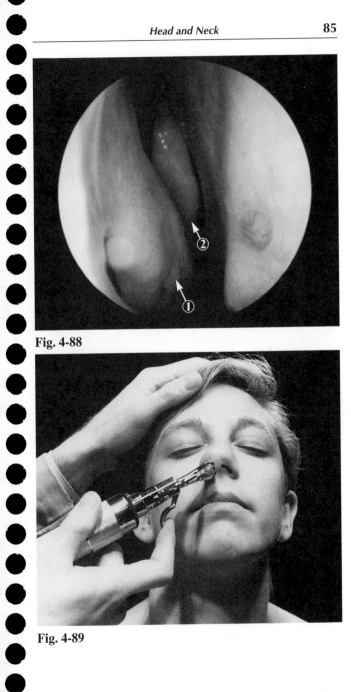

Fig. 4-88

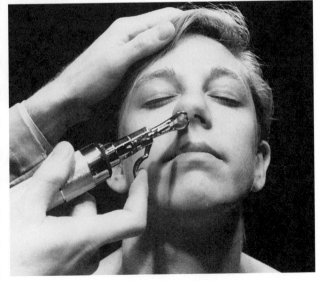

Fig. 4-89

C. **Palpate the Paranasal Sinus Areas for Tenderness.**
   1. There are four sinus areas: frontal, maxillary, eth-
      moidal, and sphenoidal.
      ▪ Only the frontal and maxillary are accessible to
        physical examination.
      ▪ In normal subjects, firm pressure does not cause
        tenderness. The presence of tenderness is sug-
        gestive of sinusitis.

   2. Palpate the frontal sinuses.
      ▪ Press the thumbs upward from deep under the
        orbital ridge *(FIG. 4-90)*. Avoid pressure onto
        the eyes.

   3. Palpate the maxillary sinuses.
      ▪ Press upward with the thumbs on each zygo-
        matic arch *(FIG. 4-91)*.

   4. You can also percuss over each sinus area for sim-
      ilar symptoms *(FIG. 4-92)*.
      ▪ Some clinicians prefer to lay a finger over each
        sinus area and use two-handed percussion, sim-
        ilar to percussing the chest.

VIII. **THROAT (mouth and pharynx; examined from
      front to back).**
   A. **Observe Mobility of the Jaw (see *Fig 11-2*).**
      1. Have the patient open and close her mouth.
         ▪ Note the extent of opening and any shift in align-
           ment of the teeth during motion. Use the mid-
           line between the upper and lower central incisors
           as a guide to alignment.

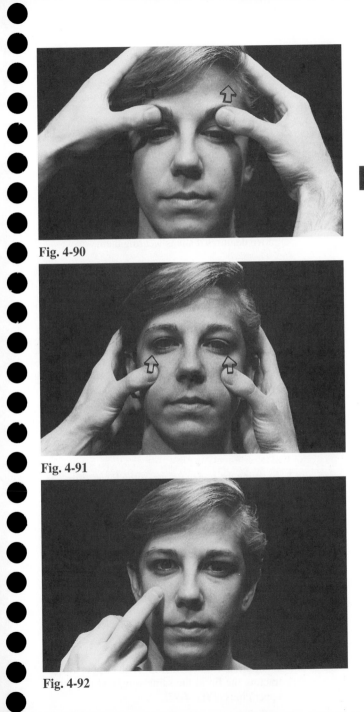

Fig. 4-90

Fig. 4-91

Fig. 4-92

    2. Palpate the temporomandibular joint.
- Place your index finger in front of the tragus of each ear *(FIG. 4-93)*.
- Press into the joint space as she opens and closes her mouth *(FIG. 4-94)*.
- Feel for tenderness, crepitus, or asymmetry of motion; pain here is often referred to the patient's ear.

    3. To examine further, use the otoscope or a pocket flashlight to illuminate, and have the patient remove dentures if she is wearing them.

B. Examine the Lips and Gums.

    1. Note the color and condition of the skin:
- On the lips (note skin dryness, cracking or lumps) *(FIG. 4-95)*.
- At the *vermilion* border (for vesicles or ulcerations).
  —This is a common location for herpes simplex.
- And at the *angle* of the lip (for fissuring).
- Palpate any suspicious areas for induration.
  —A whitening or heavy scaling of the lower lip can signal actinic cheilitis, a premalignant lesion. Induration in this same area can signal the presence of lip carcinoma.

    2. Examine the undersurface of the lower lip.
- Patient's mouth should be relaxed and partially open. Pull the lip down with two fingers or tongueblades *(FIG. 4-96)*.
- Note color, texture, and moisture, including the gutter between lip and gums. The mucosa should be wet and smooth.

    3. Check the lower gums for any inflammation, swelling, or recession. Normally it rises smoothly between the teeth and is light pink. Note any bleeding or gum hypertrophy.

    4. Examine the undersurface of the upper lip (retracting the lip in the same way) and inspect the upper gums *(FIG. 4-97)*.

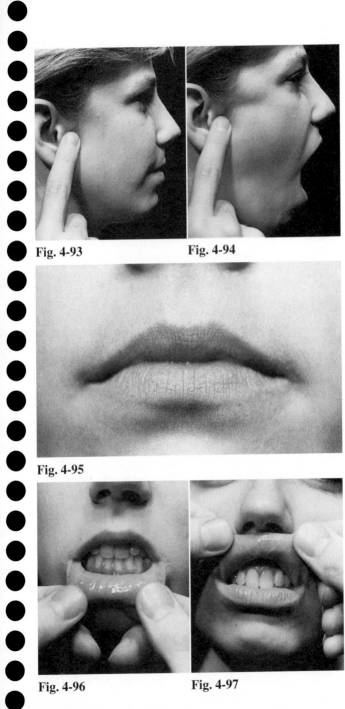

Fig. 4-93

Fig. 4-94

Fig. 4-95

Fig. 4-96

Fig. 4-97

C. Check the Teeth and Lateral Gum Tissue.

1. Have the patient's mouth partially open.

2. Retract the lip and cheek with a tongue blade.
   - Check each tooth one at a time through each dental arch *(FIG. 4-98)*. Assess for the yellow-brown discoloration or erosion of dental caries.
   - You may wish to use a dental mirror as a retractor to observe less accessible surfaces.
     —With the increased use of smokeless tobacco, particularly among adolescent males, pay close attention to any white or reddened areas between lip and gums, or between the cheek and lower gums. These can signal early oral carcinoma or its precursor.

3. This screening is no substitute for a complete dental examination. It will, however, show the gross problems that may need attention.

D. Examine the Buccal Mucosa.

1. Use the tongue blade to pull the lateral lip to one side *(FIG. 4-99)*.

2. Note the color and texture of the mucosa.
   - Dark-skinned patients often have patches of pigment here, as well as on the gums.
   - You may also see thin yellow sebaceous glands under the mucosal surface.

3. Pull the cheek further away.
   Note on the cheek mucosa:
     —(1) The parotid (Stensen's) duct, a small mound located behind the upper second molar.
     —(2) The bite line, visible as a white line of thickened mucosa between the occlusal surfaces of the molars.
       • A prominent bite line can signal bruxism, a tendency to grind the teeth.

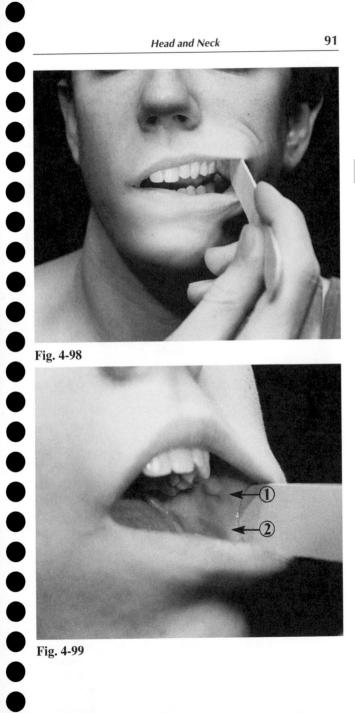

Fig. 4-98

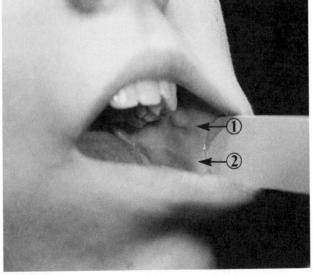

Fig. 4-99

E. **Inspect the Tongue** *(FIG. 4-100)* (have the patient extend her tongue).

1. Note its color and normal velvety surface.
   - The smooth texture is caused by the predominant filiform papillae (taste buds).
   - Small red dots (fungiform papillae) are visible throughout the surface, especially at the sides and tip.
   - The large circumvallate papillae form an inverted V at the posterior tongue.
   - Also note any tremor, ulcers, or deviation.

2. Inspect the sides and bottom of the tongue.
   - Malignancies are more likely to develop here than on the upper surface *(FIG. 4-101).*
   - The undersurface is normally smooth.
     —Watch for white or reddened patches that can indicate a premalignant lesion or early oral carcinoma.
     —You can often see dilated veins here, especially in the elderly.
     —Oral candidiasis appears as cottage-cheese–like exudate on the tongue, cheeks, or palate.

3. Inspect the floor of the mouth, a high-risk area for oral malignancies *(FIG. 4-102).*
   - Note submandibular (Wharton's) ducts (1), seen as small openings on either side of frenulum.
   - Note the fold over the sublingual gland (2), visible as a V-shaped ridge pointing anteriorly at base of the tongue.

4. (Optional) Palpate the tongue (used especially for male patients, those over age 50, or with heavy exposure to tobacco or alcohol).
   - Wear disposable rubber gloves.
   - Wrap a 4-inch square of gauze around the tip of the tongue, to maintain traction.
   - Pull the tongue gently to your right. You can now see the more posterior edge.
   - Palpate each side with one finger, feeling for induration *(FIG. 4-103).*
   - If any areas of whiteness, redness, or induration are seen during any part of the oral examination, pay special attention to lymph node exam since oral cancer spreads first to local lymph nodes.

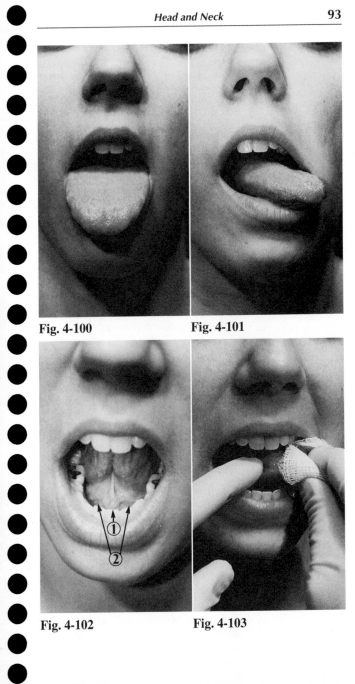

Fig. 4-100

Fig. 4-101

Fig. 4-102

Fig. 4-103

F. Examine the Pharynx.

1. Hold a tongue blade like a chopstick. This will provide enough leverage to apply pressure *(FIG. 4-104)*.

2. First examine the palate *(FIG. 4-105)*. (Tilt the patient's head back slightly.)

   - The hard palate is normally white, and the soft palate is pink. Look for petechaie at the junction of hard and soft palate.

   - Make a mental note of breath odor: sometimes diagnostic (heavy alcohol use, ketoacidosis).

3. Then try to visualize the posterior pharyngeal wall *(FIG. 4-106)*.

   - If not completely visible:

     —Gently press the tongue blade onto the middle third of the tongue. If the blade is too anterior, the tongue will mound up and obscure the pharynx; if too posterior, the patient will gag.

     —Have the patient say a prolonged "ah. . . ." This should further depress the tongue and raise the uvula.

     —As an alternate maneuver, ask the patient to "pant like a puppy dog" (and demonstrate this). Although it sounds humorous, it is remarkably effective in raising the soft palate, lowering the tongue, and suppressing the gag response.

   - Observe the following structures:

     —(1) The uvula; it should rise in the midline when the patient vocalizes (cranial nerve X).

     —(2) The posterior pharyngeal wall, with its small translucent red islands of lymphoid tissue.

       • Note any *post-nasal drip* flowing down the posterior wall, and its color.

     —(3) The palatine pillars, anterior and posterior

     —(4) The tonsil (which lies between the pillars). It is normally the same color as the surrounding oral mucosa. Note any enlargement, redness, exudate or ulcerations.

       • If exudate is present, note whether it is pinpoint, patchy, or confluent. Exudate in viral or streptococcal pharyngitis tends to be patchy, whereas exudate in infectious mononucleosis or diphtheria tends to be more confluent.

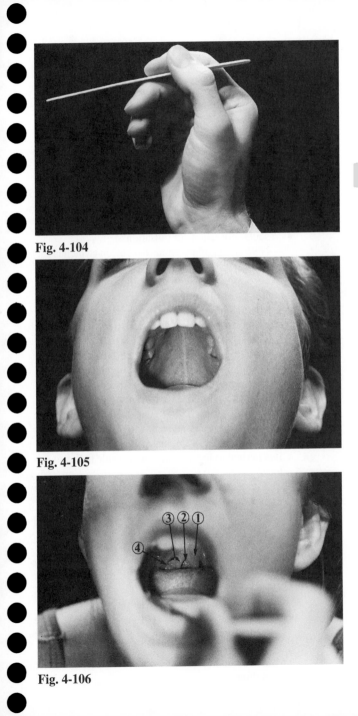

Fig. 4-104

Fig. 4-105

Fig. 4-106

IX. NECK.
   A. Briefly Inspect for Symmetry or Visible Masses.
      1. Use oblique lighting to highlight subtle neck structures
         (FIG 4-107).
      2. Note the following:
         ▪ The thyroid cartilage (1) and sternomastoid muscles
           (2), as landmarks for palpation.
         ▪ Local swellings in the neck, particularly:
           —Over the parotid glands.
           —Over regional lymph nodes.
           —Under the mandible.
         ▪ Vascular dilatations or pulsations.
           —Note any jugular venous distension (which is fur-
           ther described in Chapter 5, The Heart).
         ▪ Scars of previous neck or thyroid surgery.
   B. Palpate for Lymph Nodes.
      1. The examination requires a systemic approach:
         ▪ Feel for the following characteristics:
           —Node size, shape, and tenderness.
           —Mobility, consistency, and delimitation (whether
           modes are separate or matted together).
         ▪ Palpate lightly with one or two fingers.
           —Use a circular or to-and-fro motion.
           —Position her head with your free hand to keep the
           opposing muscles relaxed. You may wish to flex her
           neck slightly toward the side you are examining.
         ▪ It is normal to feel small, soft movable nodes in any
           location.
           —If nodes are enlarged or tender, reexamine the area
           they drain.
      2. Palpate the nodes in order: (turn the patient's head to
         one side)
         ▪ First, *preauricular* nodes *(FIG. 4-108).*
           —Press on the tragus and milk anteriorly.
           —If palpable, the nodes will slide under your finger.
         ▪ Then *post-auricular* nodes *(FIG. 4-109).*
           —Palpate on or under the mastoid process.
         ▪ *Occipital* nodes *(FIG. 4-110).*
           —Palpate at the base of the skull, lateral to the thick
           bands of muscle.
           —When finished, turn the patient's head back to the
           midline.

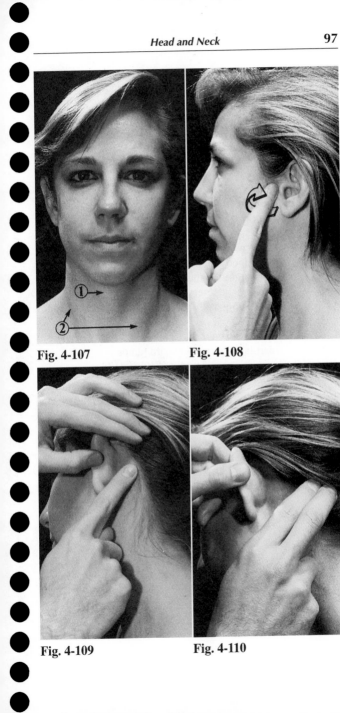

Fig. 4-107

Fig. 4-108

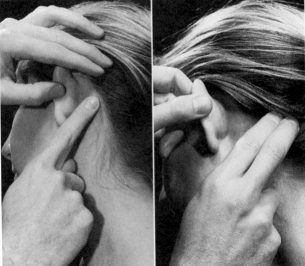

Fig. 4-109

Fig. 4-110

- *Submental* nodes *(FIG. 4-111)*.
  —Reach your flexed index finger under the chin and milk forward.
  —The finger will compress the node against the ramus of the mandible.
- *Submandibular* nodes *(FIG. 4-112)*.
  —Feel halfway back to the angle of the jaw.
  —Use the same technique as for submental nodes.
- *Anterior cervical* nodes *(FIG. 4-113)*.
  —Feel anterior to and over the sternomastoid muscle throughout its whole length. The uppermost nodes are the *tonsillar* nodes, which typically enlarge with a tonsillar infection. Below these are the superficial cervical nodes, which overlie the sternomastoid muscle.
  —The carotid artery lies in the same location as the tonsillar nodes. The artery will pulsate; the nodes will not.
  —Do not mistake the hyoid bone, above the thyroid cartilage, for a stony hard tumor.
- Posterior cervical nodes *(FIG. 4-114)*.
  —Feel posterior to the sternomastoid muscle in the same manner as for anterior cervical nodes.
- Deep cervical chain *(FIG. 4-115)*.
  —Encircle the sternomastoid muscle with your thumb and fingers.
  —Feel deeply with an up-and-down motion.
- Supraclavicular nodes *(FIG. 4-116)*.
  —Reach across with your opposite hand and feel deeply in the groove behind the clavicle.
  —You will normally feel bands of the platysmus muscle. Do not mistake these for enlarged nodes.

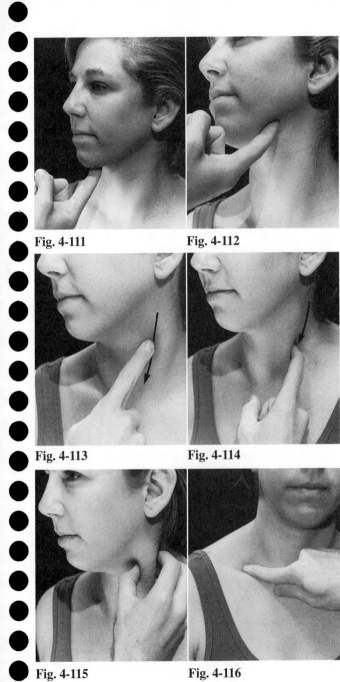

Fig. 4-111

Fig. 4-112

Fig. 4-113

Fig. 4-114

Fig. 4-115

Fig. 4-116

C. Examine the Thyroid Gland.

1. Anatomy: *(FIG. 4-117)*
   - The gland is butterfly-shaped. Its two lobes are joined at their lower third by the isthmus.
     —The lobes are irregular and conical in shape.
     —Each lobe is about 5 cm long and 3 cm thick.
     —The lobes wrap posteriorly around the trachea.
   - The lateral portion of each lobe is covered by sternomastoid muscle.
     —The lobes are normally soft and barely palpable.
   - Above the gland is the cricoid cartilage.
     —Its distinct lower edge serves as a landmark from which to locate the gland.

2. Inspect the gland *(FIG. 4-118)*.
   - Have the patient's neck slightly extended.
     —This is especially important if the patient is obese or has a short neck.
   - To highlight the gland, use tangential lighting. A normally-sized gland is often just barely visible.
   - Give the patient a cup of water and watch the gland as she swallows.
     —The gland will rise with each swallow.
     —The right lobe is normally slightly larger than the left.
     —Both lobes are more prominent in females than in males. In addition, pregnancy will cause a normal slight increase in thyroid size.
   - Watch for unusual bulging of thyroid tissue in the midline or behind the sternomastoid muscle *(FIG. 4-119)*.
     —Any mass that moves with swallowing is likely to be within or adherent to the thyroid gland.
     —If enlargement is seen, note whether it is generalized, as with a goiter, or localized, as with a thyroid nodule or cyst.

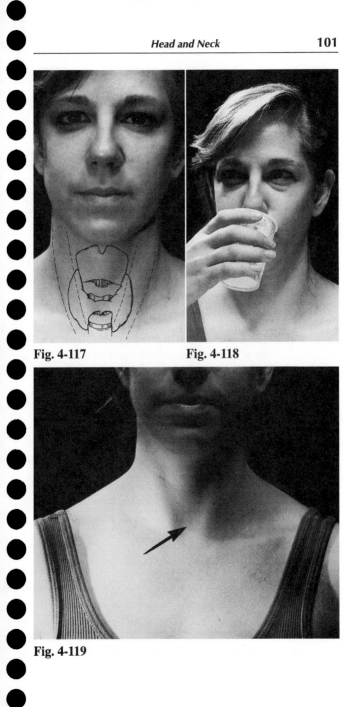

Fig. 4-117

Fig. 4-118

Fig. 4-119

3. Palpate the gland.
   ▪ Palpation is more easily done from behind.
     —Slightly extend the patient's neck.
     —Rest your thumbs on the base of the patient's neck *(FIG. 4-120)* and reach your fingers in front.
     —Locate the cricoid cartilage *(FIG. 4-121)*. The gland usually lies about 1cm below.
   ▪ Palpate the isthmus *(FIG. 4-122)*.
     —Slide your finger upward in short milking motions from the sternal notch. You will feel the isthmus pop across your fingers. Note its thickness.
     —Then have the patient swallow and feel the soft isthmus rise between your fingers.
   ▪ Palpate the lobes.
     —The patient should keep the cup of water. She will need it for repeated swallowing.
     —Tilt the patient's head toward the side you are examining.
     —To feel for the medial portion of each lobe: brace the trachea with one hand and palpate the lobe with the other *(FIG. 4-123)*.
       • Reach your fingers between the sternomastoid and trachea, at the level of the isthmus. Feel again as the patient swallows. Note size, consistency, tenderness, and any nodules.
     —To feel for the main and lateral portion of each lobe: use one hand to deviate the trachea toward the examining hand.
       • Encircle the sternomastoid with the examining hand with fingers in front and thumb behind the muscle *(FIG. 4-124)*.
       • Have the patient swallow again to facilitate palpation of the entire lobe.
       • This technique is particularly useful for significant gland enlargement.
     —If you feel nothing, simply slide both sets of fingers gently up and down below the level of the cricoid cartilage as the patient swallows.
       • The normal thyroid is often barely felt as a soft fusiform swelling around the trachea.

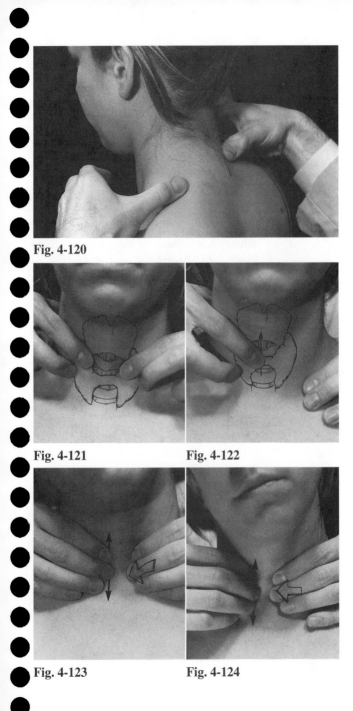

Fig. 4-120

Fig. 4-121

Fig. 4-122

Fig. 4-123

Fig. 4-124

- Palpation from the anterior approach. (This is not as easy for beginners).
  —Palpate the isthmus as before, using the index finger *(FIG. 4-125)*.
  —Then brace the trachea with one thumb and feel the medial portion of the lobe with the other thumb and fingers *(FIG. 4-126)*. Have the patient swallow.
  —Palpate the main portion of each lobe.
    • Deviate the trachea with one thumb.
    • Encircle the sternomastoid muscle with the examining hand, thumb in front, fingers behind the muscle *(FIG. 4-127)*.
    • Have the patient swallow again.
- If the gland is enlarged or has a nodule, listen over each lobe with the stethoscope bell for a possible bruit.
  —The presence of a thyroid bruit strongly suggests hyperthyroidism.

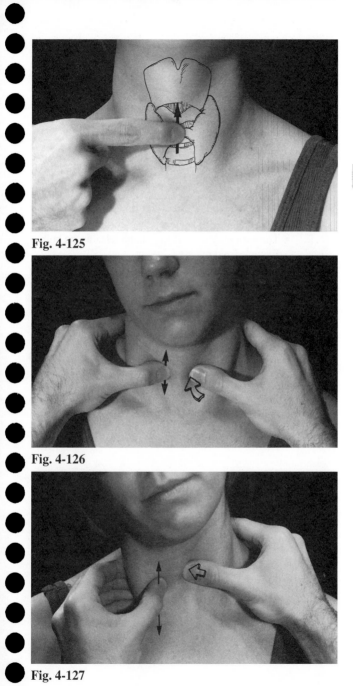

Fig. 4-125

Fig. 4-126

Fig. 4-127

X. ADDITIONAL TESTS (Used if abnormalities are seen or suspected.)

A. **Pneumootoscopy:** to assess eardrum mobility

1. Attach a rubber bulb and tubing to the otoscope *(FIG. 4-128)*.

2. Insert the speculum firmly enough to produce an air seal *(FIG. 4-129)*. Gently squeeze and release the bulb.

3. This exerts pressure against the eardrum.
   - The normal drum will retract and relax as the bulb is squeezed and released.
     —Typically, you will see the most motion as you release the bulb. This causes the drum to momentarily move toward you. If overt motion is not seen, watch for a flicker of the light reflection.
   - A decrease in motion suggests middle ear fluid, adhesions, or an open perforation.
   - An increase in motion will occur over a large healed perforation, since the healed eardrum is thinner.

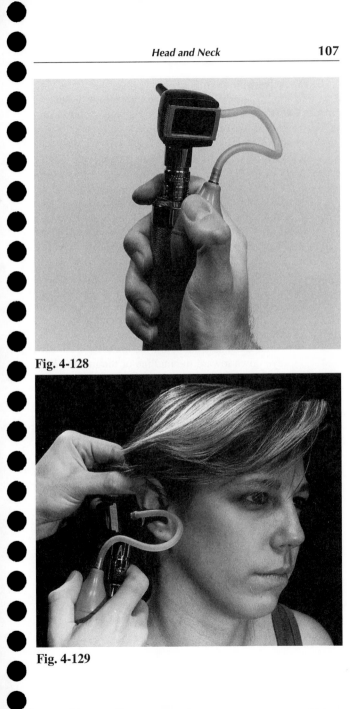

Fig. 4-128

Fig. 4-129

B. **Sinus Transillumination.**
   1. Used when sinus tenderness or drainage is present.
      - The test requires a strong light source and a completely darkened room.

   2. Transilluminate the frontal sinus (use a transilluminator attachment).
      - Place the light source firmly under the superior orbital rim, close to the nose *(FIG. 4-130)*.
      - Shield the light with your hand.
      - Watch for a dim red glow on the forehead (on the same side). The light is passing through the air-filled frontal sinus.
      - Check the other side.

   3. Transilluminate the maxillary sinus.
      - Have the patient's head tilted back and mouth open. Be sure to remove upper dentures.
      - Shine the light from below the inner aspect of each eye down toward the midline of the mouth *(FIG. 4-131)*.
      - Watch for a similar red glow on the hard palate. The light is passing through the air-filled maxillary sinus.

   4. The test is most useful when:
      - There is a clear asymmetry of transillumination, especially if one sinus transilluminates and the other one does not.
      - There are other signs of sinus disease, such as:
        —Sinus area pain or tenderness.
        —Purulent nasal discharge, particularly if originating near the middle turbinate.
        —Maxillary tooth pain (maxillary sinusitis).

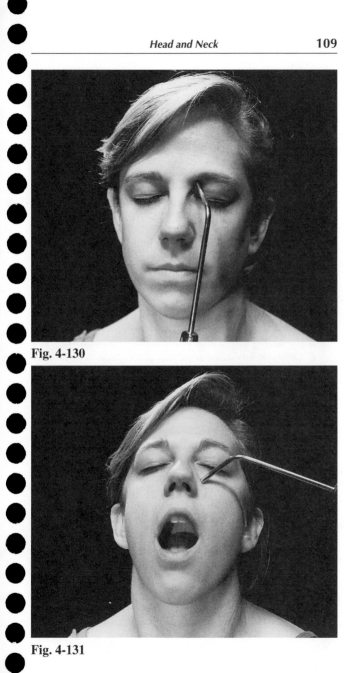

Fig. 4-130

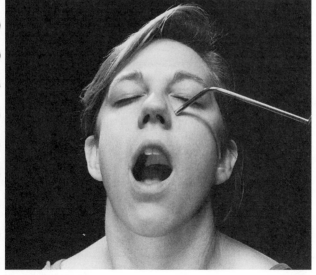

Fig. 4-131

5 *The Heart*

I. **TOPOGRAPHIC ANATOMY.** These lines and landmarks assist the caregiver in locating areas for examination and in documenting the location of findings.

   A. **Reference Lines** (see *Fig. 8-1*).
      1. Anterior: the *midsternal* and *midclavicular* lines.
      2. Lateral: the *anterior* and *midaxillary* lines.

   B. **Bony Landmarks** *(FIG. 5-1)*.
      1. *Sternal notch:* marks the junction of sternum and clavicles.
      2. *Sternal angle:* marks the junction of sternum and second rib.
      3. Below this is the *second interspace* and other interspaces are counted down from it. Document the location of findings as the intersection of reference lines and interspaces.
      4. *Xiphoid process* marks the junction of sternum and inferior costal margin.

   C. **Surface Projections** *(FIG. 5-2)*.
      1. The junction between left and right heart is not directly anterior but is rotated to the left.
      2. Most of the anterior cardiac surface is right ventricle, which lies substernally. The right atrium occupies a small area on the right, and the left ventricle occupies a small area on the left.
      3. The base is the junction between heart and great vessels; it lies just below the sternal angle.
      4. The apex, the tip of the left ventricle, extends to the midclavicular line in about the fifth interspace.

   D. **Four Auscultation Areas,** which overlap somewhat:
      1. Mitral: near the apex *(FIG. 5-3)*.
      2. Tricuspid: near sternum and fifth interspace.
      3. Pulmonic: near sternum and second or third interspaces but can be higher or lower.
      4. Aortic: anywhere from right second interspace (often the loudest) to the apex.

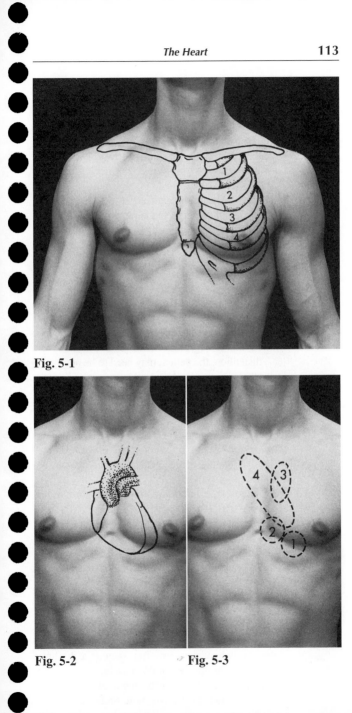

Fig. 5-1

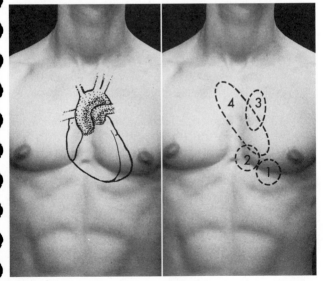

Fig. 5-2   Fig. 5-3

II. INSPECTION.
A. Jugular Venous Pressure (JVP).
1. Position the patient.
   - Elevate the patient from horizontal so the jugular vein shows an oscillating level of distention or pulsations. Make sure the patient's head is supported to relax the neck muscles. The neck and upper chest should be exposed.
   - Tip the head slightly away from the side being viewed, with the neck in the same plane as the thorax, and use tangential lighting to increase shadows. If no oblique lighting is available, use a pocket penlight.
   - If the JVP is high, near the angle of the jaw, raise the patient nearer to the upright position.
   - If the JVP is low and no neck vein distention can be seen, lower the patient until nearly supine.
     —Most patients are examined at an angle between 30 and 45 degrees from horizontal. With severe distention, the patient may need to be nearly upright.
     —Make a mental note of the angle of elevation of the head of the bed or examination table. This angle will be used when recording your findings.
2. Locate the *sternal angle,* felt as a horizontal ridge within 5 cm of the sternal notch *(FIG. 5-4).*
   - This landmark is about 5 cm above the right atrium in the supine position.
3. Then focus your attention above the right clavicle *(FIG. 5-5).*
   - The external jugular vein (1) appears as a slightly distended column with the top showing a small up-and-down oscillation.
     —To confirm its location, compress the vein just above the clavicle; it will distend *(FIG. 5-6).*
     —Then remove the finger and watch it fall to its natural level.
   - The internal jugular vein (2) is located beneath the sternomastoid muscle, but its pulsations transmit to the skin where they are often seen as a rhythmic movement at the base of the muscle.
   - When visible, the measurement of the internal jugular venous pressure is more accurate.

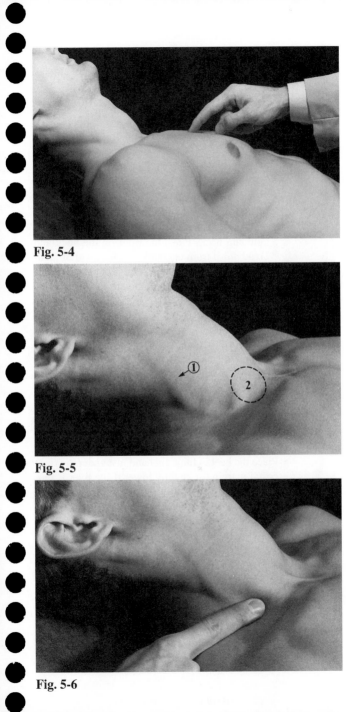

Fig. 5-4

Fig. 5-5

Fig. 5-6

4. Locate the highest level of pulsations in either area (internal vein if visible).
   - Measure the *vertical* distance from this point to the sternal angle.
     —If the distention rises *above* the sternal angle, hold a horizontal marker from the top of the visible distention over to and above the sternum. Place the ruler on the sternal angle and read *up* to the level of the pencil *(FIG. 5-7)*.
     —If the distention ends *below* the sternal angle, hold a horizontal marker between the sternal angle and neck. Place the ruler on the neck and read *down* from the marker to the level of jugular venous distention *(FIG. 5-8)*.
   - Record the distance in centimeters above or below the sternal angle and the angle of inclination. (For example, jugular venous pressure is 5 cm above the sternal angle at 45 degrees.)
     —The level will normally fall slightly with inspiration and rise again with expiration. Over 3 cm of distention above the sternal angle is considered elevated.

5. Hepatojugular reflux (used if right ventricular failure is suspected).
   - Position the patient as if measuring for JVP.
   - Place the heel of the right hand just under the right costal margin (or slightly lower if the liver is tender) *(FIG. 5-9)*.
   - Press in for 15 to 30 seconds. During pressure, make sure the patient breathes normally, since straining falsely elevates the JVP.
   - With right ventricular failure, the vertical rise in JVP will exceed 1 cm and will remain elevated as long as abdominal pressure is maintained. In healthy subjects, neck vein distention will last only a few seconds *(FIG. 5-10)*.

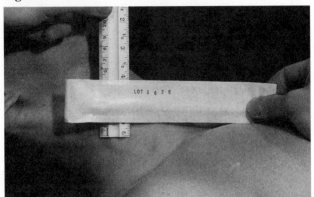

Fig. 5-7

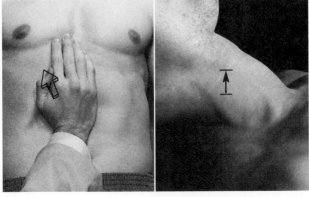

Fig. 5-8

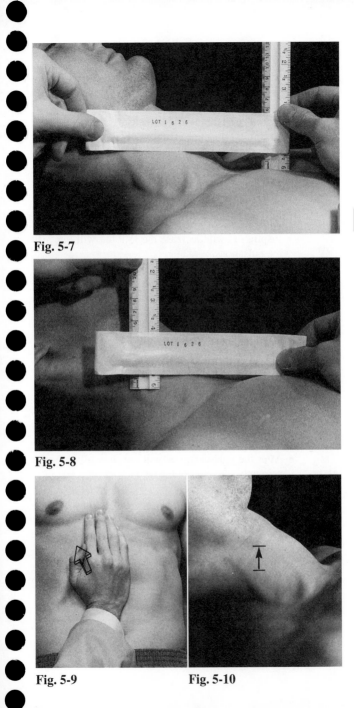

Fig. 5-9   **Fig. 5-10**

B. Observe Venous Pulsations. These pulsations do not originate from the venous system itself, but reflect changing pressures in the right atrium.

　　1. Position the patient as for measurement of JVP. A pocket flashlight aimed tangentially can produce shadows, making the pulsations more visible.

　　　　▪ Watch the pulsations at the base of the sternomastoid muscle.

　　　　▪ The right internal jugular vein provides a slightly more direct channel from the right atrium compared to the left-sided vein.

　　　　▪ Inspiration will decrease the JVP but will magnify the pulsations.

　　2. You can more easily interpret the pulsations by auscultating the heart while you are observing.

　　3. With the unaided eye, you can see two episodes of rising and falling *(FIG. 5-11).*

　　　　▪ The a wave and x descent. The a wave is the highest part of the total pulsation, which occurs just before S_1. The x descent occurs just after S_1 and is simultaneous with the carotid pulse.

　　　　▪ The v wave and y descent. The v wave is a brief flutter in the vein just after S_2. The y descent reflects the fall in right atrial pressure.

　　　　▪ After the y descent, you will see slow filling of the vein until the onset of the next a wave

　　4. Note the intensity of each wave and the speed of its collapse.

　　5. Remember that the jugular is a *double* pulsation, whereas the carotid is *single*. In addition, the venous pulsation will decrease with upright position or inspiration, and will increase with the Valsalva maneuver. It is not firmly palpable. The carotid pulse is unaffected by the above maneuvers and is easily palpable.

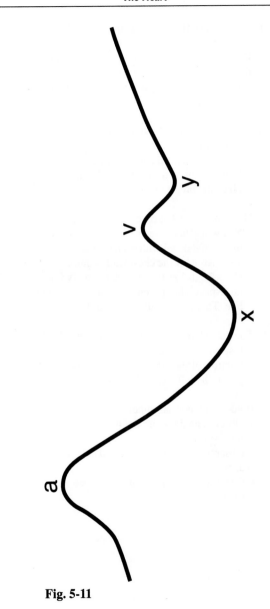

Fig. 5-11

C. **Then Observe the Apical Impulse,** the lowest and most lateral impulse on the chest wall *(FIG. 5-12).*

1. Position the patient so light bounces tangentially off the skin, using a lamp or window light.
   - If the patient is dyspneic, have him slightly raised rather than supine.

2. Stand at the patient's right side.
   - You may wish to crouch down so shadows become more pronounced and the pulsation is more visible.
   - In a patient with pendulous breasts, have her displace the breast up and left.

3. Note size and location of the impulse.
   - You will actually see a small area, 2 cm or less, moving up and down with each heartbeat. The impulse is less distinct if the chest wall is muscular or obese.
   - Describe its location, which normally is near the fifth interspace about 2 cm medial to the midclavicular line. This varies with body build.

4. Then check for other movement *(FIG. 5-13).*
   - Inspect above the apex, medially (where a slight retraction often moves in synchrony with the apex) and at the left sternal border.

5. If no left precordial impulses can be seen:
   - Observe again while the patient holds his breath in full expiration.
   - Observe with the patient rolled onto his left side (this alters location).
   - Check the right precordium in case there is dextrocardia.

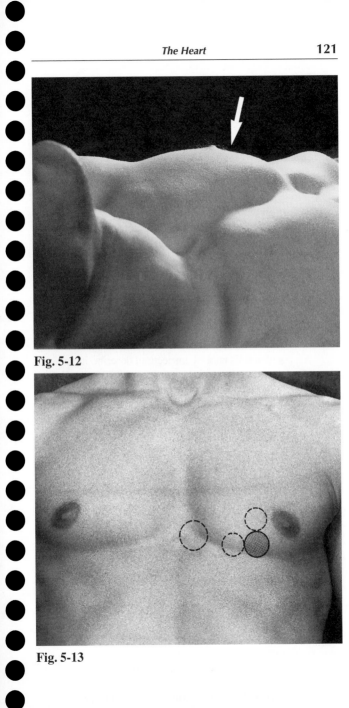

Fig. 5-12

Fig. 5-13

III. PALPATION.

A. Begin Palpation with the Apical Impulse.

1. Position the patient as for inspection.

2. Position your fingers: *(FIG. 5-14)*
   - If you can see the apical impulse, place the tip of your middle finger in the interspace over it.
   - If you cannot see it, place your finger in the average apex location (usually the fifth interspace just medial to the midclavicular line, or slightly above or below).
   - Then place your index fingertip one interspace above and ring finger one interspace below the apical impulse. You are now feeling in 3 interspaces.

3. Rest your hand flat and assess the impulse. It may take a few seconds to "tune in" to the faint sensation. It is felt as a brief tap.
   - Describe the size in interspaces felt as a single impulse; one is normal, two or three is enlarged.
   - Describe the intensity as normal or forceful.
   - If not located by inspection, describe its location as centimeters lateral to the midclavicular line, or interspaces below the fifth intercostal space.
   - If you cannot feel the impulse, try these maneuvers:
     —Roll the patient about 45 degrees toward the left lateral decubitus position. As before, this intensifies the impulse, but invalidates its location.
   - Have the patient exhale fully and stop breathing for a few seconds.

4. You can estimate the duration of the apical impulse more easily by watching the motion of the stethoscope as you listen over the apical impulse.
   - It is normally a brief outward motion *(FIG. 5-15)*.
   - It begins with S_1 and lasts a third or half of systole. A sustained lift, lasting more than two thirds of systole, suggests left ventricular dilatation or hypertrophy.

5. As a general rule, enlargement of the apical impulse indicates left ventricular dilatation, as in congestive heart failure. In these situations, the apical impulse may also shift laterally. A mediastinal shift can also move the apical impulse laterally. A downward shift of the impulse toward the xiphoid process often occurs with chronic obstructive pulmonary disease.

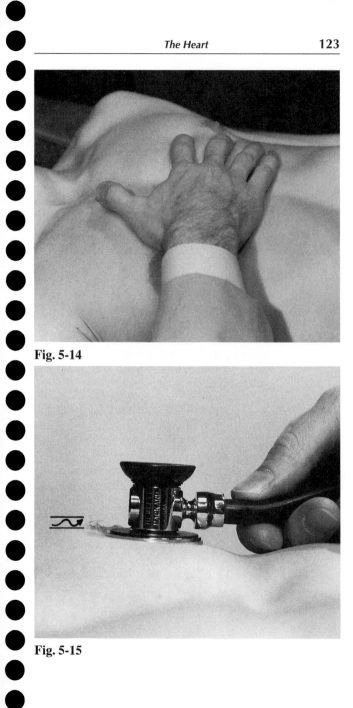

Fig. 5-14

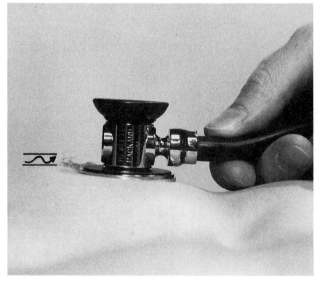

Fig. 5-15

B. **Palpate Over the Entire Precordium for Other Impulses or Vibratory Thrill.**
  1. *Impulses* are brief thrusts against the examining fingers occurring in synchrony with the cardiac cycle. Feel for these with the fingertips of three fingers.
  2. *Vibratory thrill* is a palpable vibratory sensation that resembles the feeling of placing your hand over the throat of a purring cat. Feel for vibratory thrill with the base of the fingers, since joints are better equipped to sense vibration.
  3. Palpate in order: *(FIG. 5-16)*
     - The sternoclavicular joints and upper sternum; you will normally feel little or no pulsation.
     - Second right interspace and sternal border (the *aortic* area); if a thrill is felt here, as from aortic stenosis, see if it transmits into the carotid arteries.
     - Second left interspace and sternal border (the *pulmonic* area). Pulsations here overlie the pulmonary artery and may be palpable normally in children, thin-chested individuals, or after exertion. Pulmonary hypertension may make these pulsations more apparent.
     - Left lower sternal border (*tricuspid* area); one can normally feel a slight pulsation in a child or thin individual. Feel here for a sustained impulse called a *heave* or *lift,* which can indicate right ventricular dilatation. Such an impulse can also expand to include the right lower sternal border.
     - Apical area, usually the same location as the point of maximum impulse (PMI), unless other nearby impulses are prominent. This is the *mitral* area. Pathologic third (S_3) and fourth (S_4) heart sounds may be more easily felt here than heard. A third heart sound will produce a double impulse sensation of S_2, the second heart sound. A fourth heart sound will produce a double impulse sensation of S_1, the first heart sound.
  4. Then slip the fingertips under the right costal margin *(FIG. 5-17)* near the xiphoid process. Push up and in as the patient deeply inhales. This will move the fingers away from the aortic pulsation and closer to the right ventricle. An impulse here can signify right ventricular enlargement.

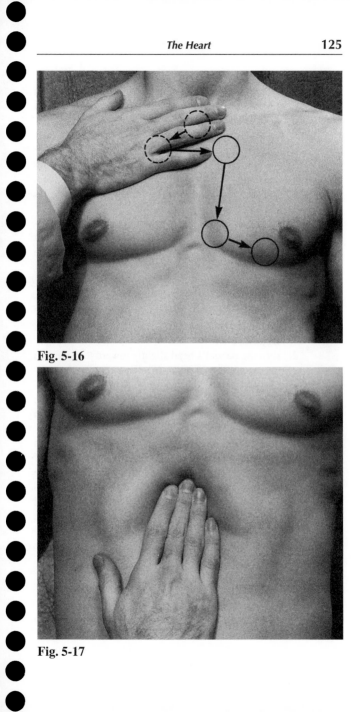

Fig. 5-16

Fig. 5-17

5. A note on vibratory thrill:
   - This is the palpable component of a loud, harsh heart murmur. It can signal the need for careful auscultation.
   - More sensation of vibration is produced by a low-pitched murmur than a high-pitched one.
   - When a thrill is heard, describe its location, timing in cardiac cycle, and any radiation of the vibration.
   - A murmur accompanied by a palpable thrill is more likely to be pathologic.
   - Pericardial friction rubs can sometimes be palpated, though they are usually found easiest by auscultation. If a pericardial effusion develops, the rub disappears.

C. **Palpate the Carotid Artery.**
   1. It is advisable to auscultate the carotids for bruit before you palpate (see *Fig. 5-21*). Do not palpate the carotid if you hear a bruit, since it can cause further occlusion.
   2. Turn the patient's head slightly toward the side you are examining *(FIG. 5-18)*. This relaxes the sternomastoid muscle.
   3. Stay below the tip of the thyroid cartilage. The carotid sinus is near this point and pressure on it can cause a reflex drop in pulse rate or blood pressure.
   4. Orient yourself by palpating the thyroid notch with the tip of your index finger. Then, place the pads of two fingers below that level on the flat side-surface of the thyroid cartilage. Push your fingers gently into the neck; your fingertips will encounter the carotid pulsation in its location between the trachea and sternomastoid muscle. Palpate one side at a time *(FIG. 5-19)*.
   5. Note pulse rate and regularity. Also note:
      - The rate of rise: accelerated or delayed (it is normally rapid).
      - The peak intensity or presence of a double peak.
      - The rate of fall; smooth or stepwise (it normally collapses more slowly).

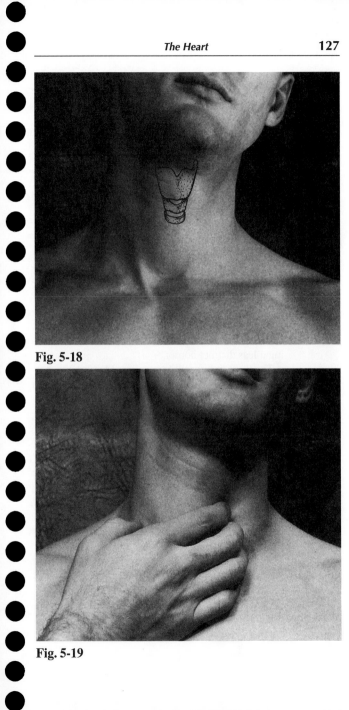

Fig. 5-18

Fig. 5-19

6. Then note any palpable vibration. Remember: any carotid bruit or thrill should prompt a recheck of the right upper sternal border for transmission of an aortic valve murmur.

7. Examine the other side, turning the patient's head accordingly.

IV. PERCUSSION *(FIG. 5-20)*.

A. The Right and Left Hand Technique of Percussion Is Reviewed in Chapter 6, Thorax and Lungs.

B. Locate the Lateral Heart Border:

1. Stand to the patient's right side.

2. Percuss in one-inch intervals from anterior axillary line to sternum in the third, fourth, and fifth interspaces. Note the change in percussion note from resonance to dullness.

3. It is best to have the patient hold his breath in mid-expiration during each of the three percussion runs. Otherwise, the heart moves with breathing, producing a less distinct border.

- The three points will form a line. Measure this border directly from the midsternum. In this way, you can compare measurement directly to a posterior-anterior chest roentgenogram.

C. Percussion of the Heart Is Considered Optional.

1. Chest radiographs allow the most accurate determination of size.

2. Inspection and palpation locate the apex and gauge left ventricular dilatation.

3. Right ventricular enlargement is usually substernal and is not usually accessible by percussion.

D. Use Percussion to Outline the Left Lateral Heart Border.

1. This is most useful when the apical impulse cannot be seen or palpated, such as in cases of pericardial effusion.

2. It can also be used as a confirmatory test of left ventricular dilatation, which shifts the lateral heart border, along with the apical impulse, more to the left.

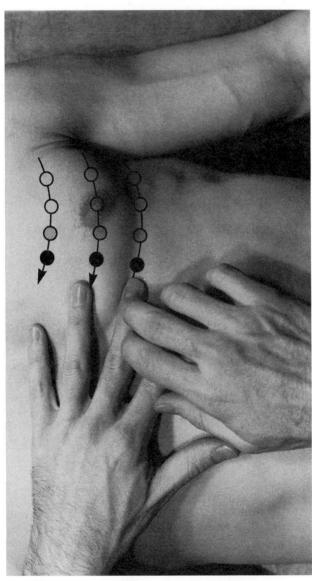

Fig. 5-20

V. AUSCULTATION.

A. Begin with the Carotids.

1. Place the stethoscope bell lightly over each carotid artery *(FIG. 5-21)*.

2. Listen while the patient holds his breath for bruits or a transmitted murmur. Remember that any carotid bruit or thrill should prompt a recheck of the right upper sternal border for transmission of an aortic murmur.

B. Prepare for Cardiac Auscultation.

1. Prepare the patient.
   - Heart sounds are best heard with the room quiet and the patient warm and comfortable. Faint heart sounds cannot be heard in a room full of mechanical noise or talking.
   - Have the anterior chest region ready to undrape for auscultation. Never auscultate through clothing, since it can diminish the heart tones and add artificial crackling or rustling sounds.

2. Prepare the stethoscope *(FIG. 5-22)*.
   - The earpieces should be large enough to fit snugly into the ears to block out room noise. They should aim down and forward to fit the external ear canal, and they should be under enough spring tension to stay comfortably in place.
   - The tubing should be thick and short; optimal length is one foot. Longer tubing is definitely more convenient, but the increased length dampens the sound proportionately.
   - The chest pieces (there are commonly two) vary in their function.
     - The diaphragm: *(FIG. 5-23)* accentuates high-frequency sounds. It should be pressed firmly against the skin during auscultation.
     - The bell: *(FIG. 5-24)* should be pressed just enough to form an air seal with the skin. If greater pressure is applied, the skin under the bell becomes taut and acts as a diaphragm, blocking the low-frequency sounds you need to hear.

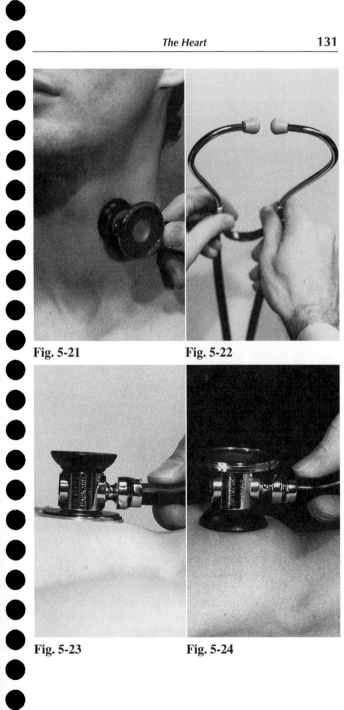

Fig. 5-21

Fig. 5-22

Fig. 5-23

Fig. 5-24

3. Prepare yourself.
   - Be comfortable. Sit if necessary. If you lean over the patient, your concentration will be on your back, not on the heart tones.
   - Examine from the patient's right side.
   - Feel free to close your eyes while listening. This will enable you to concentrate on the heart sounds.
   - Take your time. There is a normal "tuning-in" period when the scope is first applied to the chest. The longer you listen, the more you will hear.

C. **Start By Placing the Diaphragm Firmly Over the Apex** *(FIG. 5-25).*
   1. If you cannot tell which tone is S_1, synchronize it with the carotid pulse. S_1 just barely precedes the carotid pulsation.
      - Another method is to start at the aortic area, where S_2 is loudest, and use it as a guide to timing S_1 and other sounds.
      - Heart sounds are fainter in patients with increased chest wall fat or muscle, or with pulmonary emphysema.

   2. Note the rate.
      - Record in beats per minute. If quite regular, count for 15 seconds and multiply by four. If the rate is unusually slow, fast, or irregular; count for a full minute.

   3. See if the rhythm is regular or irregular. If irregular, try to identify a pattern:
      - Is it predictably irregular, such as in premature beats with a regular rhythm?
      - Does the rate vary consistently with respiration? In normal respiratory variation, also called *sinus arrhythmia,* the pulse rate slightly increases during inspiration and decreases during expiration
      - Or is it totally irregular, as in *atrial fibrillation* or *atrial flutter* with varying block?

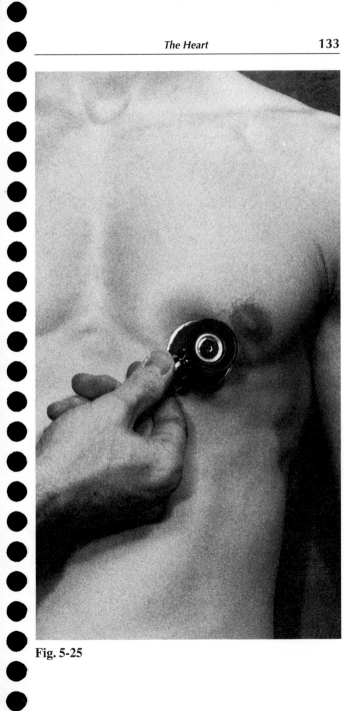

Fig. 5-25

4. Then inch your way through the four auscultation areas; mitral, tricuspid, pulmonic, and aortic *(FIG. 5-26)*.
   - Note the intensity of S_1 and S_2. Normally, S_1 is louder than S_2 when listening at the apex, and softer than S_2 when listening at the base *(FIG. 5-27)*.
   - Their amplitude at any one position should remain stable.

5. Note splitting of: *(FIG. 5-28)*
   - S_1: normally heard at the left lower sternal border (tricuspid area) during expiration.
   - S_2: normally heard at the left upper sternal border (pulmonic area) during quiet inspiration. In youthful patients, a narrow split may persist into expiration.

6. As you inch, focus your attention selectively for each component in the cardiac cycle *(FIG. 5-29)*.
   - Listen for extra heart sounds in systole, then in diastole, ignoring all murmurs.
   - Then listen for murmurs, first in systole and then in diastole, ignoring any extra heart sounds (clicks or thumps).
   - When learning the cardiac examination, it is best to:
     —First learn how to record the murmur with all its characteristics (see page 142).
     —Then integrate these findings with those obtained through inspection and palpation.

7. Then switch to the bell *(FIG. 5-30)*.
   - Press lightly again and inch your way through the four auscultation areas *(FIG. 5-31)*.
   - Listen especially for low-pitched murmurs and diastolic filling sounds (S_3 and S_4).

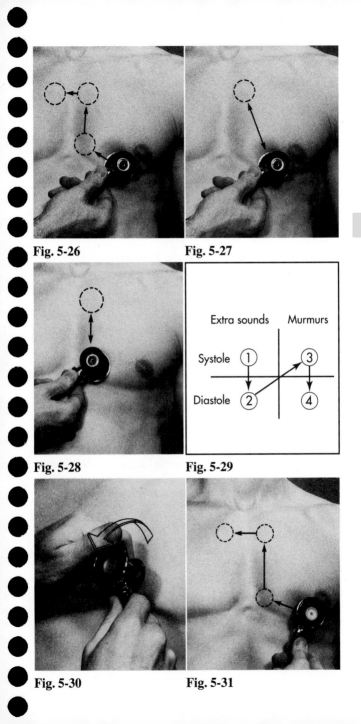

Fig. 5-26

Fig. 5-27

Fig. 5-28

Fig. 5-29

Fig. 5-30

Fig. 5-31

VI. ADDITIONAL TESTS. These are used when abnormalities are heard or suspected. Again, if you suspect an abnormality, take your time in listening. Be sure of what you are hearing.

   A. To Bring Out a Left-Sided S_3 or S_4, or mitral valve murmur (especially mitral stenosis):

      1. Position the patient onto his left side *(FIG. 5-32)*. This allows the cardiac apex to fall closer to the chest wall.

      2. Listen over the apex with the bell.

   B. To Bring Out Aortic and Pulmonary Murmurs or Extra Sounds, have the patient sit up and lean slightly forward *(FIG. 5-33)*.

      1. Listen over the base with the diaphragm. This allows the cardiac base to fall closer to the anterior chest wall (the sitting position often decreases a benign pulmonic flow murmur).

      2. Then have the patient fully exhale and hold it: listening here accentuates aortic murmurs, especially in aortic regurgitation.

   C. Another Maneuver Is Changes with Breathing.

      1. A deep inspiration increases right heart filling and so accentuates right-sided extra sounds and murmurs.

         ▪ Listen over the tricuspid and pulmonic areas.

      2. Left-sided sounds will decrease during inspiration, but to a lesser degree.

         ▪ Listen over the mitral and aortic areas.

      3. Expiration causes the reverse, again affecting right-sided sounds more than left.

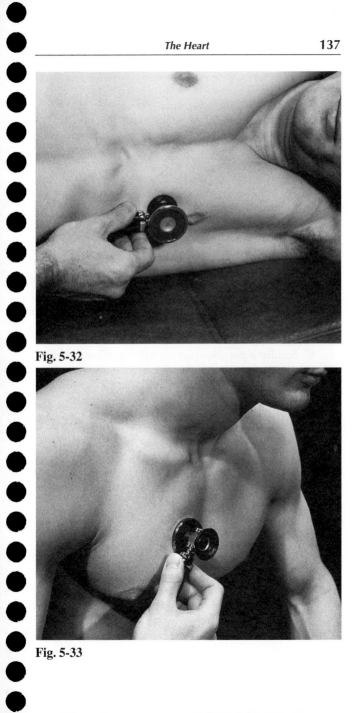

Fig. 5-32

Fig. 5-33

D. Valsalva Maneuver. WARNING! Do not perform on a patient with known coronary or cerebrovascular disease or with a cardiac arrhythmia.

1. Listen during strain: *(FIG. 5-34)*
   - Have the patient take a deep breath and bear down against a closed glottis. Hold no longer than 8 to 10 seconds.
   - This causes a decrease in systemic venous return, causing a decrease first in right, then left heart filling.
   - As stroke volume decreases, blood pressure may fall and cause a compensatory rise in pulse rate.

2. And release:
   - The release causes increased filling of the right heart, then the left, and is known as "overshoot."
   - The alteration in filling affects each side's extra sounds and murmurs accordingly.

E. Sudden Squatting. (similar warning as listed above)

1. Stand to the patient's right side and slightly in front.
   - Face the patient, place the stethoscope on his chest, and be ready to squat down.
   - Ask the patient to squat and go down with him *(FIG. 5-35)*.
     —As an alternate method, sit in a chair facing the patient. Reach up with your stethoscope when he is standing, then keep the stethoscope on the skin as he squats in front of you.

2. This allows you to listen immediately after the change in position.
   - Squatting increases venous return and system resistance. This increases stroke volume, left ventricular size and arterial pressure. Most murmurs increase with this maneuver except for those of hypertrophic cardiomyopathy and mitral valve prolapse, which may decrease.

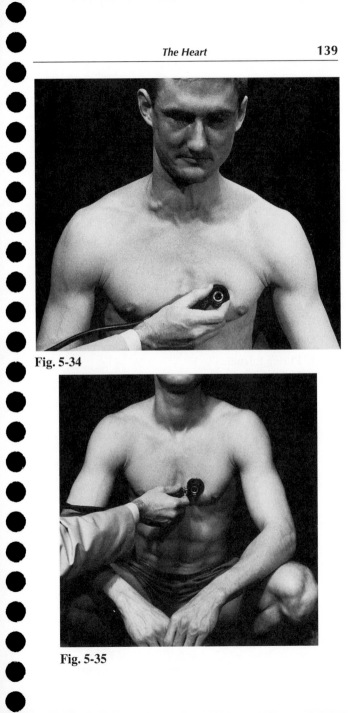

Fig. 5-34

Fig. 5-35

F. Other Maneuvers:

1. Passive leg raising, which increases systemic venous return. This affects right-sided events then, several beats later, left-sided events.

2. Postural change: this has two variations.
   - Lying down from sitting or standing has the same effect as passive leg raise.
   - Sitting or standing after lying down has the *opposite* effect.
     —It is especially useful to tell a physiologic S_2 split, which narrows with the upright position, from a fixed S_2 split, which does not.

3. Isometric exercises (same warning as Valsalva, page 138).
   - Have patient squeeze a calibrated handgrip device and sustain the grip for 30 to 40 seconds while you listen *(FIG. 5-36).* Instruct the patient not to strain (Valsalva) while squeezing.
   - This has an effect similar to sudden squatting.

G. Pitting Edema.

1. Press *gently* onto the:
   - Lower anterior tibia or medial malleolus, or dorsum of foot *(FIG. 5-37)* (if the patient has been standing or sitting).
   - In the normal subject, no pitting results *(FIG. 5-38).*
     —With disease, the finger will sink into the edematous skin, leaving a depression called *pitting.*

2. Sacrum (if the patient has been supine).
   - If pitting edema is truly present, the finger will sink into the skin.

3. Record pitting by measuring the depth of the depression in millimeters.

H. Related Areas to Examine.

1. Blood pressure. See Chapter 1, Vital Signs.

2. Peripheral pulses.

3. Color of face and nailbeds (looking for cyanosis), clubbing of digits. See Chapter 6, Thorax and Lungs.

4. Auscultate the chest for crackles of congestive heart failure. See Chapter 6, Thorax and Lungs.

5. Enlargement of liver or spleen. See Chapter 8, The Abdomen.

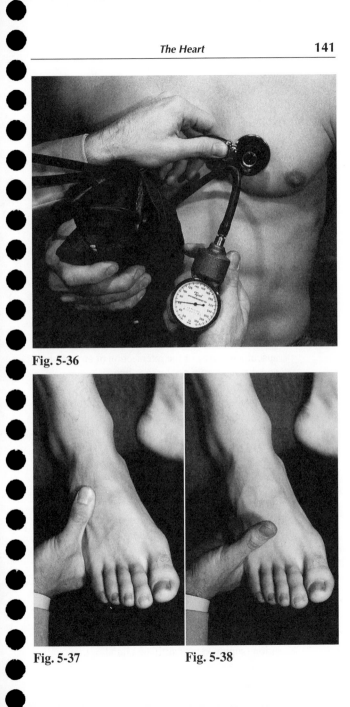

Fig. 5-36

Fig. 5-37   Fig. 5-38

I. **Finally, Whenever You Hear a Murmur, Record These Characteristics:**
   1. Its intensity.
      - Graded 1 through 6.
        —1 is intermittently audible. It is usually masked by normal hospital room noise.
        —2 is normally faintly audible.
        —3 is medium intensity, without a vibratory thrill.
        —4 is medium intensity with a vibratory thrill.
        —5 is the loudest murmur heard with the stethoscope in contact with the chest wall.
        —6 is audible with the stethoscope lifted slightly off the chest.
   2. Its pitch and quality.
      - Pitch is described as high, medium, or low.
      - Quality is described as harsh, blowing, rumbling, or musical.
   3. Its location of maximal intensity. Describe it as an auscultation area or the intersection of an interspace and distance from a reference line.
   4. Its radiation *(FIG. 5-39)*.
      - Move the stethoscope around the location of maximal intensity.
      - See in which direction, if any, the murmur maintains its tone and much of its intensity (e.g., aortic stenosis radiating to the carotid arteries).
        —In locations besides radiation, the murmur quickly muffles.
   5. Its timing *(FIG. 5-40)*.
      - Systolic or diastolic.
      - Early, mid, or late (1, 2, and 3).
      - Or holosystolic, lasting throughout systole (4).
   6. Also define the change in intensity of the murmur:
      - Crescendo: gradually gets louder (5).
      - Decrescendo: gradually gets softer (6).
      - And diamond-shaped, also called crescendo-decrescendo or ejection murmur (7).
   7. And finally, any change with respiration or body position (supine versus sitting or standing).

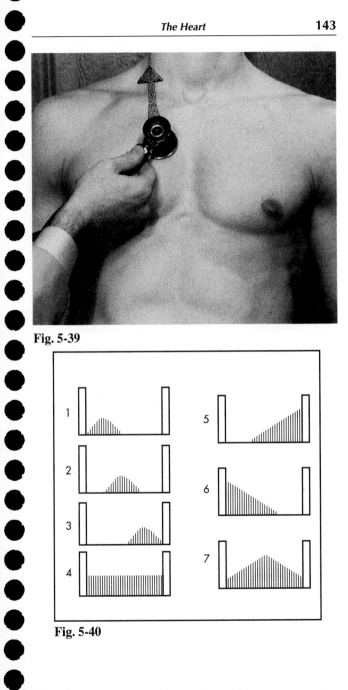

Fig. 5-39

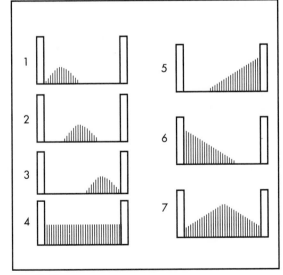

Fig. 5-40

6 *Thorax and Lungs*

I. TOPOGRAPHIC ANATOMY.

A. Reference Lines.

1. Anteriorly:
   - The midsternal line, from xiphoid process to pubic ramus *(see Fig. 8-1)*.
   - The midclavicular lines, from midclavicle to inguinal ligament.
2. Laterally: *(see Fig. 8-2)*
   - The anterior axillary line extends downward from the anterior axillary fold.
   - The midaxillary line descends from the midaxilla.
   - The posterior axillary line extends downward from the posterior axillary fold.
3. Posteriorly: *(FIG. 6-1)*
   - The midspinal and midscapular lines.
   - The intrascapular and infrascapular areas.
4. Describe findings relative to these lines.

B. Lung Borders–as if seen through the skin.

1. Anteriorly: *(FIG. 6-2)*
   - The apices rise about 3 cm above the inner clavicle.
   - The medial borders are nearly fused until the fourth interspace where left border is displaced by heart.
   - The lung and pleural borders move between the sixth and ninth ribs in the midclavicular line (MCL).
   - The sternal angle or fourth thoracic spine mark the bifurcation of the trachea.
     —The second rib joins the sternal angle, and interspaces can be counted from this point.
   - The right middle lobe is mostly accessible anteriorly, and is centered behind the right fifth interspace.
2. Laterally: *(FIG. 6-3)*
   - The lung and pleural borders move between the eighth and eleventh ribs in the midaxillary line.
   - The oblique (major) fissure extends from the third thoracic spine diagonally downward to the sixth rib in the MCL.
   - Right minor fissure extends horizontal near fourth rib.
   - The oblique and minor fissures outline the borders of the right middle lobe.
3. Posteriorly: *(FIG. 6-4)*
   - The lung border expands from the tenth rib to the twelfth, the pleural gutter.
   - Note most of the posterior lung field is lower lobe.

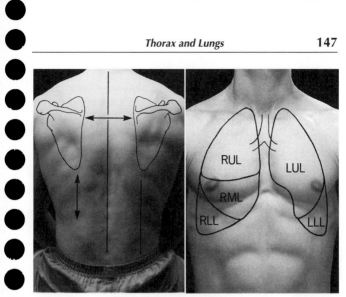

Fig. 6-1

Fig. 6-2

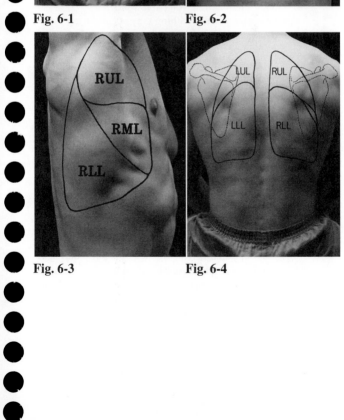

Fig. 6-3

Fig. 6-4

II. INSPECTION

  A. **Check for Related Signs of Pulmonary Disease (the patient does not need to be fully undressed at this point)** *(FIG. 6-5).*

  1. Facial expression.
     - Anxiety or restlessness (think: hypoxia) and drowsiness (think: CO_2 narcosis).

  2. Changes in color.
     - Cyanosis: seen first in the nailbeds, especially near the lunula, then periorally or in the tongue.
     - Facial flushing: seen on the nose, malar prominences, and earlobes (think: polycythemia from hypoxia).

  3. Jugular venous distention: is it constant or occurring only with expiration.

  4. Pursed lip breathing (on expiration).
     - Open-mouthed breathing may occur during severe dyspnea since it requires less work (think: COPD).

  5. Clubbing of digits *(FIG. 6-6).*
     - Produces spoon-shaped nails and drumstick-shaped distal phalanges; the base of the nail will sink under finger pressure.
     - In congenital clubbing, the nail shape is altered but the nailbed is firm.
     - Clubbing not specific to pulmonary diseases alone.

  B. **Note Breathing Pattern:**

  1. Note the respiratory rate.
     - This is best performed discretely, since the rate is more accurate when the patient is unaware of being observed.
     - This portion may be performed during vital signs, as follows:
       —After you finish taking the radial pulse during vital signs, leave your hand on the pulse and discretely move your gaze to the patient's abdomen or shoulders and count the respiratory rate over 15 seconds, then multiply by four.

  2. Note ease and regularity.
     - Watch for an interruption to inspiration followed by a grunt or cough; usually caused by pleuritic pain.

  3. Note audible breathing.
     - Even at close proximity, the patient's breathing is *normally* barely audible.

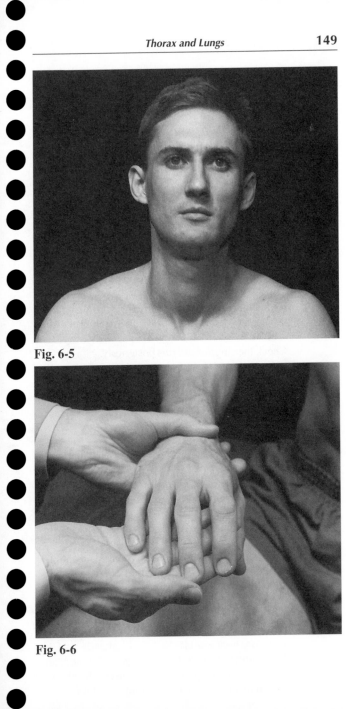

Fig. 6-5

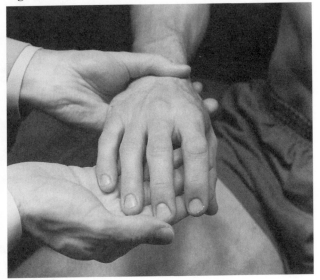

Fig. 6-6

- Listen for wheezing, stridor, grunting, or cough.
4. Further examination requires chest to be bared. Portions may be draped when inspection is completed.

C. Observe the Bony Thorax.

1. For sternal elevation or depression *(FIG. 6-7)*.
   - Sternal elevation indicates pectus carinatum
   - Sternal depression indicates pectus excavatum
2. For symmetry of rib motion.
   - Best seen viewing the chest from about a 6-foot distance. Note full or restricted expansion.
   - If asymmetry is suspected, observe again during deep inspiration.
3. For motion of the costal angle.
   - It is normally about 90 degrees and widens with inspiration *(FIG. 6-8)*.
   - Paradoxical motion (narrowing with inspiration) occurs with diaphragmatic depression from hyperinflation.
4. Check the slope of the ribs posteriorly.
   - Are they angled 45 degrees to the spine (normal) or fixed horizontally (obstructive lung disease) *(FIG. 6-9)*.
   - Do the ribs move separately with inspiration or as a single unit.
5. Is there barrel-chesting?
   - Compare the anterior-posterior distance to the lateral *(FIG. 6-10)*.
   - Normally, the anterior to lateral ratio is 1:2 to 5:7.
   - Barrel-chesting produces a ratio near 1:1.

D. See if the Patient Uses Accessory Neck Muscles During Inspiration *(FIG. 6-11)*.

1. Visible as a tightening of the sternomastoid and strap muscles of the neck, or as a transient hollowing behind the clavicles with inspiration.
   - Also seen as an elevation of the clavicles with inspiration.
2. Patient may assume a posture that aids the effect of accessory neck muscles.
   - Patient sits upright, leaning slightly forward, arms are straight and propped onto knees, chair seat, or examination table (think: asthma or COPD).

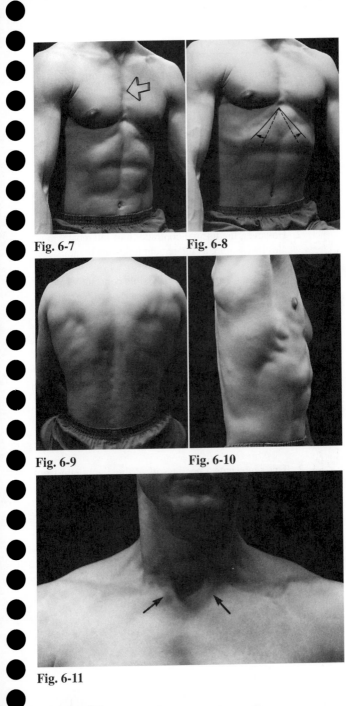

Fig. 6-7

Fig. 6-8

Fig. 6-9

Fig. 6-10

Fig. 6-11

E. Watch for Fleeting Inspiratory Retractions.

1. True retractions are transient, disappearing before end-inspiration.
   - They are visible as an indentation seen between the ribs, especially in the sixth through ninth interspaces between the sternum and anterior axillary line *(FIG. 6-12).*
   - Even if the patient holds his breath, true retractions vanish, since they last only as long as it takes air to enter.

2. However, the normal contraction of intercostal muscles last as long as the patient holds his breath.

3. Intercostal bulging may be visible constantly (pleural effusion or tension pneumothorax) or with expiration alone (airway narrowing).

F. Note Litten's Sign.

1. In thin individuals, motion of the diaphragm can be seen.
   - Have the patient lay supine. Adjust light, if possible to shadow the ribs. Observe on deep inspiration *(FIG. 6-13).*
   - A wave can be seen passing from the sixth interspace downward, then upward with expiration.

2. This represents a peeling-off of the diaphragm from the costal pleura.

3. When diaphragmatic motion is decreased, as by pleural fluid or air, so will be the wave on that side.

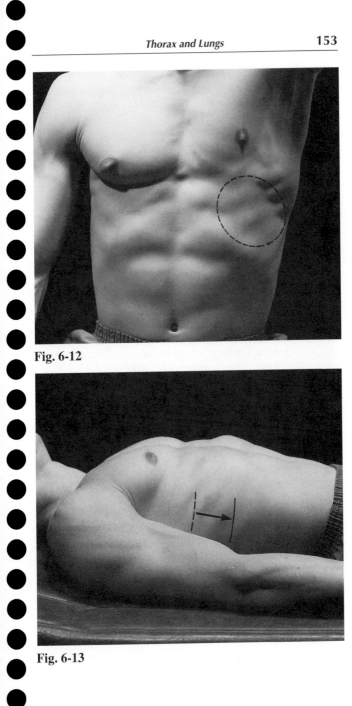

Fig. 6-12

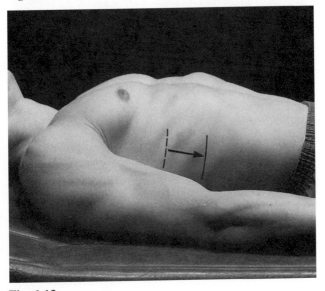

Fig. 6-13

G. Examine the Spine.

1. Inspect from the side, checking for thoracic kyphosis and lumbar lordosis *(FIG. 6-14).*

2. Check for scoliosis, first posteriorly:
   - With the patient standing, note the line formed by the posterior spinous processes *(FIG. 6-15).*
   - If the spines are not visible, have patient bend slightly forward *(FIG. 6-16).*
   - If they still cannot be seen, palpate and dot each spine with a washable marker, then view the dots from a distance.

3. Then anteriorly.
   - Note flank depth, the gap between the elbow and waist *(FIG. 6-17).*
     —Is it equal on each side?
     —The gap will be greater on the side of the major curve concavity.
   - Note the level of the shoulders. Does one droop lower than the other *(FIG. 6-18).*
   - Then, with the patient bending forward, check the level of the scapulas for symmetry *(FIG. 6-19).*
     —The scapula on the side of the major curve convexity is more prominent.

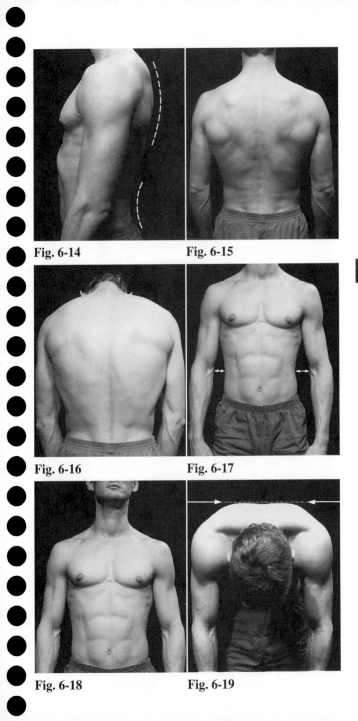

Fig. 6-14

Fig. 6-15

Fig. 6-16

Fig. 6-17

Fig. 6-18

Fig. 6-19

III. PALPATION.

A. Trachea.

1. See if one sternomastoid muscle insertion is more obvious than the other.

2. Bend the patient's head slightly forward, keeping the chin in the midline.

3. Then gently slip your finger between the trachea and sternomastoid insertion on each side *(FIG. 6-20)*.
   - If the finger slips in more easily on one side, the trachea is deviating away from that side.

4. Then check for deviation with inspiration.
   - Gently grasp the trachea with the thumb and fore-finger just under the cricoid cartilage *(FIG. 6-21)*.
   - Have the patient inspire deeply. The trachea should descend slightly in the midline. This is called *tracheal tug*.
     —A fixed trachea can indicate neoplasm or tuber-culosis restricting motion.
     —A trachea that deviates to one side during inspi-ration indicates unequal expansion of the lungs.

B. Tactile Fremitus.

1. The spoken voice vibrates lung tissue and, in turn, the chest wall.
   - A loud, low pitched voice produces the most vi-bration.
   - Fremitus is often softer when the adult voice is high pitched, as in many women.
   - In children, however, the thorax is smaller and vi-brates well even from a patient with higher pitched voice.
   - The most vibration is produced by the consonant "N" and prompts use of the words "ninety-nine" or "one-one."

2. Press firmly onto the skin with the base of the fin-gers or the ulnar side of the hand *(FIG. 6-22)*.
   - Have the patient say "ninety-nine" or "one-one" each time you touch *(FIG. 6-23)*.

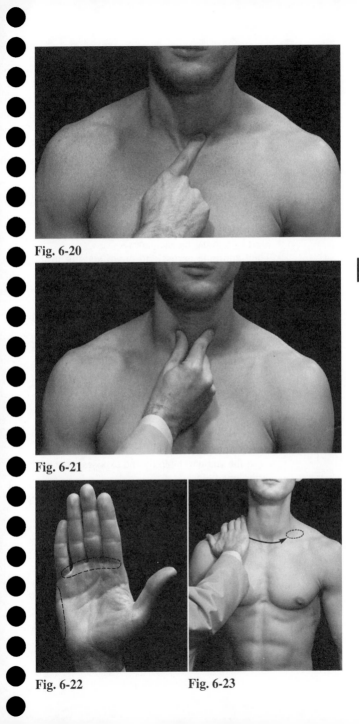

Fig. 6-20

Fig. 6-21

Fig. 6-22

Fig. 6-23

3. Use the *across-and-down pattern,* since each patient has a chest wall slightly different from another.
   - An acceptable guide for normalcy is to compare each side of the thorax for symmetry of findings.
   - This pattern allows the thorax to be examined side versus side, level by level, moving down stepwise.
     —A variation on this technique is to use both hands simultaneously, one on each side, stepping down about 2 inches at a time.

4. Begin anteriorly *(FIG. 6-24).*
   - Start by comparing each apex.
   - Then continue across-and-down staying in the midclavicular lines.
   - Use only one hand to palpate until you become accustomed to the sensation of fremitus.
   - In the female, gently displace the breast as needed to reach the chest wall.
   - Expect symmetric fremitus except where altered by normal anatomy:
     —Decreased fremitus over the region of the heart.
     —Increased fremitus over right upper lung field, due to straighter right mainstem bronchus.

5. Then check posteriorly *(FIG. 6-25).*
   - Have the patient fold his arms in front. This retracts the scapulas laterally and exposes more posterior lung field.
   - Always stay at the medial edge of the scapula, since scapular bone muffles vibration.
   - Follow the across-and-down pattern.
     —Once under the scapulas, descend in the midscapular line.
     —Expect more fremitus normally over the upper right lung fields and decreased fremitus when over increased thickness of fat or muscle.
     —Continue until the vibration ceases. This point, the approximate level of the diaphragm, is lower posteriorly than anteriorly.

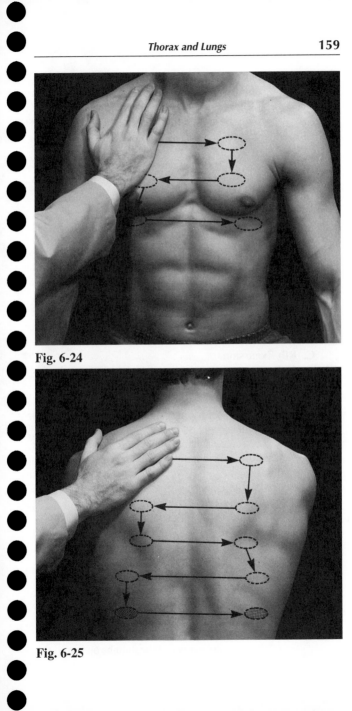

Fig. 6-24

Fig. 6-25

- Then estimate the diaphragmatic level more precisely by applying the ulnar hand downward in 2-inch steps until the vibration fades *(FIG. 6-26).*
  —The right hemidiaphragm level is slightly higher than the left.

6. Note any unexpected increase or decrease in the intensity of vibration against your hand. Record its location and symmetry.
   - Increased vibration implies:
     —An increase in lung density, such as with the consolidation of lobar pneumonia.
   - Decreased vibration implies:
     —A decrease in lung density, such as with obstructive lung disease, or by increasing the distance of the lung from the examining fingers as from pleural effusion, pneumothorax, or chest wall thickening by muscle or fat.

C. Rib Excursion.
1. Begin anteriorly near the upper lobes. Drape the fingers over the clavicle and medial shoulders.
   - Extend the thumbs.
   - Place the palms on the upper anterior chest wall near the clavicles.
   - Give some slack to the skin by moving the thumbs toward each other; they should nearly touch *(FIG. 6-27).*
   - Ask the patient to inspire deeply and allow the hands to move *(FIG. 6-28).*
   - Note divergence of the thumbs.

2. Then check near the right middle lobe and lingular segment.
   - Place the fingers high in the midaxillary line.
   - Rest the palms on the chest wall. Extend the thumbs at the level of the fifth interspace.
   - Move the thumbs medially again to raise some slack in the skin *(FIG. 6-29).*
   - Watch for divergence of the thumbs on inspiration *(FIG. 6-30).*

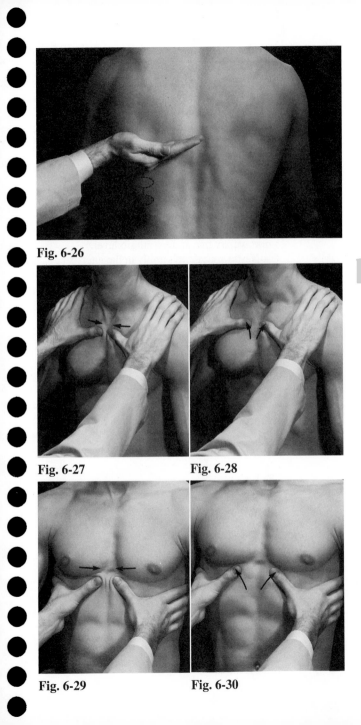

Fig. 6-26

Fig. 6-27

Fig. 6-28

Fig. 6-29

Fig. 6-30

3. Then at the costal margin:
   - Place a thumb in the midpoint of each costal margin and press firmly on the cartilage *(FIG. 6-31)*.
   - Watch for divergence with inspiration *(FIG. 6-32)*. Also observe for paradoxical motion (narrowing of the costal angle with inspiration).

4. Then examine posteriorly over the lower lobes.
   - Use the same method, placing the fingers at the tenth rib level *(FIGS. 6-33* and *6-34)*.
   - Another method is to place a thumb in the posterior axillary line at the tenth rib level.
     —Nestle your thumb firmly in the interspace.
     —With inspiration, it will be moved by the surrounding two ribs *(FIG. 6-35)*. Normal motion here is 1 to 3 cm.

5. Always note whether decreased excursion is symmetric or unilateral. Decreased excursion is commonly caused by:
   - Obstructive lung disease or pulmonary fibrosis, when symmetrically decreased.
   - Lobar pneumonia, pleural effusion, bronchial obstruction or pain, when unilaterally decreased.

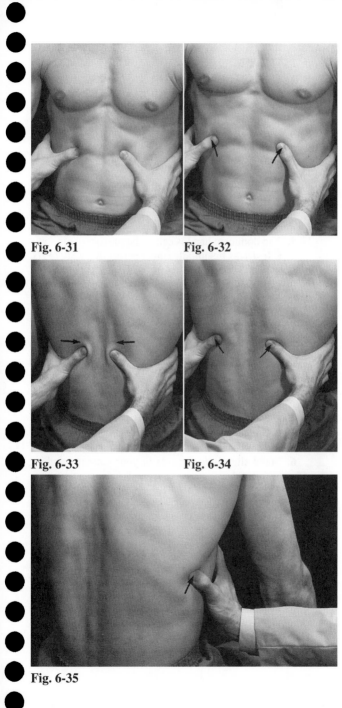

Fig. 6-31

Fig. 6-32

Fig. 6-33

Fig. 6-34

Fig. 6-35

IV. PERCUSSION.
A. Technique.
1. There is a separate technique for each hand.
2. The nondominant hand, which receives the strike, is called the pleximeter *(FIG. 6-36).*
   - The key point is to press the end of the middle finger firmly into the skin surface.
   - Firm contact produces a clear sound, whereas light contact muffles it.
   - The remaining fingers are slightly raised from the skin surface.
3. The dominant hand is called the plexor.
   - It strikes the middle finger perpendicularly *(FIG. 6-37).*
   - If it hits at any lesser angle, the volar pad is used and dampens the sound.
4. The two hands are held perpendicular to each other *(FIG. 6-38).*
   - This is the most comfortable position and prevents the fingernail from striking your finger.
5. The motion is a snapping one.
   - The wrist is thrown slightly forward by the forearm. As the wrist flexes, the middle finger extends.
   - After the strike, the finger bounces off.
   - Use the lightest strike that will produce a clear sound *(FIGS. 6-39* and *6-40).*
6. Stand slightly to the side of your patient, reaching your hands over.
   - In this way, your pleximeter hand can stay fairly horizontal while your plexor hand can hang vertically.
7. The percussion notes change with the density of tissues within 5 to 7 cm beneath the examining fingers.
   - As you percuss, it is useful to remember locations of the underlying viscera: heart, liver, gastric air bubble, and diaphragm.
   - In this way, you can roughly predict which areas should be resonant or tympanitic.

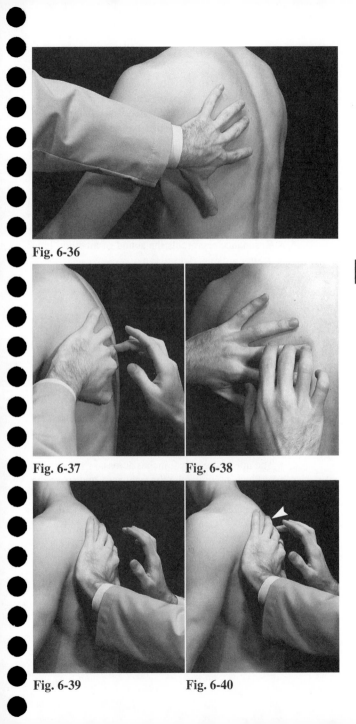

Fig. 6-36

Fig. 6-37

Fig. 6-38

Fig. 6-39

Fig. 6-40

8. You may wish to practice first in private, to gain a sense of the four normal percussion notes.
   - Flatness represents pure water, fat, or bone density.
     —It is brief and high pitched. Hear it by percussing your thigh.
   - Dullness represents the sound of a solid organ adjacent to tissues containing air, such as with the heart, liver, or spleen.
     —It has a soft "bass" note attached to it. Hear it by percussing 1 inch above your right costal margin, over your liver.
   - Resonance represents the sound of air-filled lung tissue.
     —It lasts longer and has a louder "bass" note attached to it. Hear it by percussing over your second right interspace.
   - Tympany represents the sound of an air-filled chamber, such as over loops of bowel.
     —It has a distinctly musical timbre. Hear it by percussing over your abdomen or puffed-out cheek.
   - Hyperresonance is an abnormal sound, a booming bass note, heard over hyperinflated lung tissue in obstructive pulmonary disease.

B. Examination Sequence.
   1. Begin anteriorly.
      - The apices are only 2 inches across.
        —Place a thumb over the right apex and strike the thumbnail *(FIG. 6-41)*.
        —Reach a middle finger behind the neck to the left apex *(FIG. 6-42)*.
      - Then continue across and down.
        —Stay in the midclavicular line and descend in 2-inch steps *(FIG. 6-43)*.
        —Continue until you reach dullness on each side.

   2. Then laterally.
      - Percuss high in the midaxillary line, moving downward in 2-inch steps.

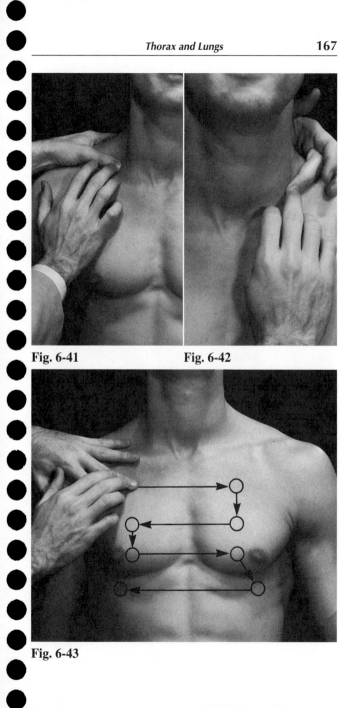

Fig. 6-41   Fig. 6-42

Fig. 6-43

3. Then check posteriorly.
   - Remember to have the patient fold his arms to retract the scapulas.
     —Check the apices above each medial scapular border.
   - Then follow the medial scapular border, using the across-and-down pattern *(FIG. 6-44).*
     —Under the scapulas, stay in the midscapular line.
     —Percuss downward until the resonance fades.
   - Determine the approximate level of the diaphragms with quiet breathing.
     —Percuss downward in 2-inch steps, noting the onset of dullness.
     —Percuss medial and lateral to the midscapular line *(FIG. 6-45).*
     —Remember that the right diaphragm will normally be a few centimeters higher than the left.
   - Determine diaphragmatic excursion.
     —On each side, percuss the onset of dullness inferiorly.
     —Compare the level found in full expiration versus full inspiration *(FIG. 6-46).* It is normally 4 to 6 cm.
       • A useful technique is to first percuss the middle finger of the pleximeter hand to locate the diaphragm position with full *expiration;* keep that finger in place.
       • Then, with the patient in full *inspiration,* locate the descended border with the index finger of the same hand. Your separated middle and index fingers now show the diaphragmatic excursion.
     —This motion is particularly reduced with obstructive pulmonary disease, since the diaphragms are already fully descended.

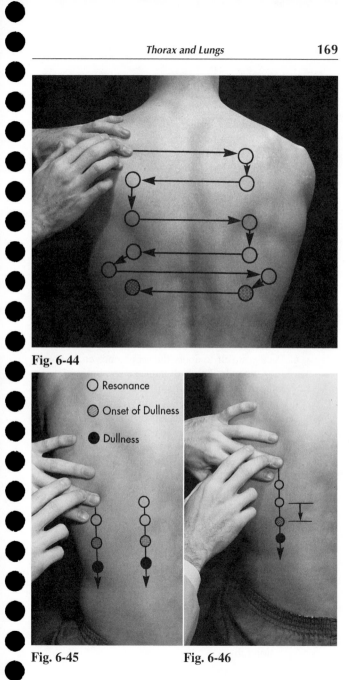

Fig. 6-44

○ Resonance
◉ Onset of Dullness
● Dullness

Fig. 6-45   Fig. 6-46

V. AUSCULTATION.

  A. Begin by Demonstrating Proper Breathing to the Patient:

    1. Say "Breathe through your mouth like this when I touch with my stethoscope."

    2. Breathe in deeply and exhale in a relaxed way, mouth open *(FIG. 6-47)*.

    3. Ask the patient to demonstrate back to you.

    4. This simple technique will amplify breath sounds and make any abnormalities easier to hear.

  B. Using the Diaphragm, follow the same across-and-down pattern as for percussion.

    1. Tap it lightly to make sure you are set to the diaphragm *(FIG. 6-48)*.

    2. Always apply the stethoscope to bare skin. Clothing can sometimes simulate crackling sounds.

    3. Try to make the room as quiet as possible. If in a patient's hospital room, turn down the television volume if on.

    4. Pace yourself to apply the scope once each three or four seconds. This will induce a respiratory rate between 15 and 20 breaths per minute, preventing symptoms of hyperventilation.

    5. In each case, the breath sounds will fade as you reach the level of the diaphragm.

  C. Start Anteriorly Over the Apices *(FIG. 6-49)*.

    1. Then down the midclavicular lines *(FIG. 6-50)*.

    2. Then laterally down the midaxillary line *(FIG. 6-51)*.

    3. Then posteriorly.

      ■ Have the patient fold his arms in front.

      ■ Listen first over the apices.

      ■ Then follow the medial scapular borders, moving further laterally once beneath them *(FIG. 6-52)*.

    4. Listen for changes in the quality of breath sounds (see pg. 177).

      ■ Vesicular versus bronchial breathing.

      ■ Amplitude of breath sounds.

      ■ The inspiration:expiration ratio.

      ■ Adventitious sounds: crackles, wheezes, and friction rubs.

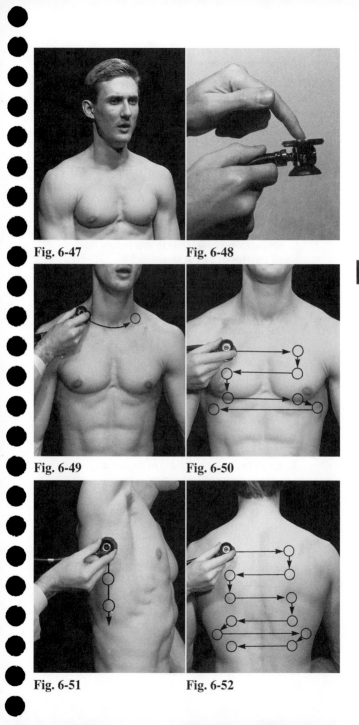

Fig. 6-47

Fig. 6-48

Fig. 6-49

Fig. 6-50

Fig. 6-51

Fig. 6-52

VI. OPTIONAL ADDITIONAL TESTS (Used if abnormalities are heard or suspected.)

A. Accentuate Wheezing Sounds by listening again during a forced expiration *(FIG. 6-53)*.

B. If Crackles Are Heard, see if they disappear after a few deep breaths.

    1. A few *transient* crackles can be heard normally if the portion of chest examined has been in the dependent position for a prolonged period of time. Crackles that persist are pathologic.

    2. They may also be caused by hair rubbing on the diaphragm; wetting the skin will reduce this.

C. Elicit Posttussive Crackles.

    1. Have patient inspire deeply, then exhale, then cough.

    2. Listen for crackles as patient inspires after cough.

D. Observe for Whispered Pectoriloquy.

    1. Listen over the suspected lung field as the patient whispers "one-two-three."

    2. With bronchial breathing (abnormal), the whispered voice will be heard more clearly.

    3. This typically occurs over consolidated lung tissue, as in lobar pneumonia, or over compressed lung tissue, as at the upper edge of a pleural effusion.

E. Listen for Bronchophony.

    1. Have the patient speak; note a change in intensity or clarity of the spoken voice.

    2. It will become louder and more distinct over an area of lung tissue consolidation or compression.

F. Listen for Egophony.

    1. Have patient vocalize the vowel "E."

    2. Over consolidated or compressed lung tissue, it will be heard through the stethoscope as "A." It often has a bleating, nasal quality.

G. If Patient Complains of Chest Pain with Breathing.

    1. Listen over the site of pain for a possible pleural friction rub *(FIG. 6-54)*.

VII. INTERPRETING FINDINGS.

    A. One Abnormal Finding Raises Suspicion of Disease, but the presence of many findings pointing to the same disorder are more confirmatory.

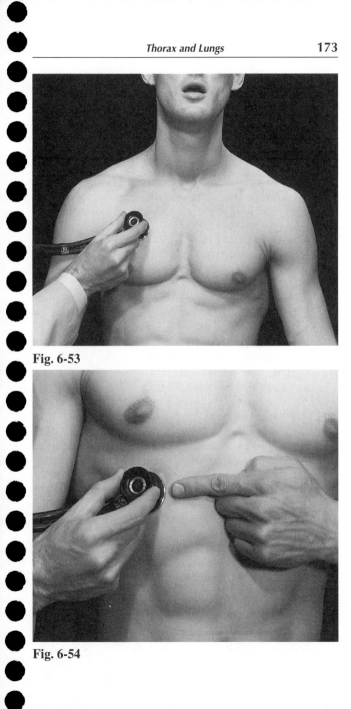

Fig. 6-53

Fig. 6-54

    B. Learn the Patterns of Abnormality, combining abnormal fremitus, percussion, and auscultation findings. For example:

      1. In lobar pneumonia, tactile fremitus is increased, percussion is dull, breath sounds are bronchial, and the adventitious sounds are crackles.

      2. In emphysema, tactile fremitus is decreased to absent, percussion tones are hyperresonant, breath sounds are faintly vesicular, and the adventitious sounds are wheezes.

VIII. NORMAL AND ABNORMAL BREATH SOUNDS.

    A. Normal Breath Sounds are heard over predictable regions of the chest *(FIG. 6-55).*

      1. *Bronchial* breath sounds are harsh, high pitched, and tubular. They are normally heard over the manubrium. When heard over the trachea in the neck, they are called *tracheal* breath sounds and are even louder and harsher.

      2. *Vesicular* breath sounds are soft, low pitched, and breezy, like wind blowing through the trees; heard normally over most of the lung fields.

      3. *Bronchovesicular* breath sounds are a mixture of bronchial and vesicular and are heard normally over the sternal angle or between the scapulas at about T-4 *(FIG. 6-56).*

    B. These Are of Diagnostic Value When Heard in Unexpected Locations.

      1. For example, bronchial breath sounds heard over peripheral lung indicate consolidation or compression of lung tissue.

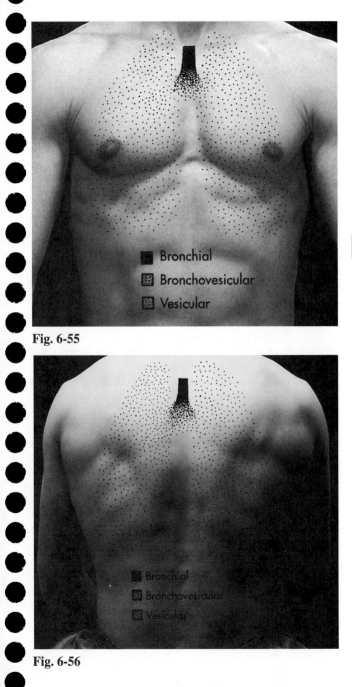

Fig. 6-55

Bronchial
Bronchovesicular
Vesicular

Bronchial
Bronchovesicular
Vesicular

Fig. 6-56

C. **The Inspiration:Expiration Ratio (I:E) Changes with the Type of Breath Sound.**
   1. Audible sound length is different when heard through stethoscope, compared with ear.

   2. Heard through the stethoscope: *(FIG. 6-57)*
      ▪ Vesicular sounds have an I:E ratio of 3:1
      ▪ Bronchovesicular sounds have an I:E ratio of 1:1
      ▪ Bronchial sounds have an I:E ratio of 1:3

   3. Airway narrowing, as with acute asthma or obstructive pulmonary disease, can also prolong the expiratory phase.

D. **Adventitious Sounds Occur in Disease States** *(FIG. 6-58).*
   1. *Crackles,* previously called rales, are discontinuous popping sounds, heard more during inspiration. They can be simulated by rubbing a lock of hair next to your ear.
      ▪ *Fine crackles* originate in smaller airways and are showers of brief high-pitched pops.
      ▪ *Coarse crackles* originate in larger airways and are lower in pitch and often longer in duration.

   2. *Wheezes,* previously called rhonchi, are continuous musical sounds from narrowed airways.
      ▪ Their pitch depends on the size of the airway
      ▪ Higher pitch equals smaller airway involvement.

   3. *Pleural rub* is a scratchy continuous sound, often very localized to one spot on the chest wall, which correlates with inflamed pleural surfaces. It is often quite transient.

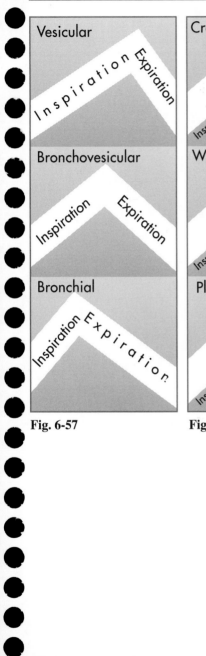

Fig. 6-57

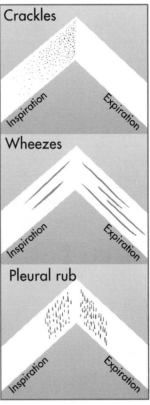

Fig. 6-58

7 *Breasts and Axillae*

I. TOPOGRAPHIC ANATOMY.

A. The Breast Lies Roughly Between the Second and Sixth Ribs, and Between the Anterior Axillary Line and Sternal Border.

B. It Is Composed of Lobes of Glandular Tissue Arranged in Circular, Spokelike Fashion.
1. Each lobule is drained by a duct leading to the surface of the nipple.
    - Intraductal papilloma typically causes bleeding from one or more ducts, which helps to signal its location.
2. The glandular tissue is supported by suspensory (Cooper's) ligaments that connect to both the skin and to muscle fascia.
    - A region of tumor or inflammation can exert traction on some of these ligaments, causing dimpling of the overlying skin.
3. Fat surrounds the breast and is the predominant tissue.

C. The Largest Portion of Glandular Breast Tissue Lies in the Upper Outer Quadrant.
1. A tail of breast tissue frequently extends from this quadrant into the axilla and is called the *tail of Spence*.
2. The majority of breast tumors are located in this quadrant and its extension.

D. For Purposes of Description, the breast can be divided into four quadrants by horizontal and vertical lines crossing at the nipple *(FIG. 7-1)*.
1. This divides the breast into upper outer and upper inner, lower outer and lower inner quadrants.
2. Lesions can also be described by viewing the breast as the face of a clock with the nipple at the center. Lesions can then be described as the "o'clock" and centimeters from the nipple.

E. Milk Lines: these exist as curving embryonic remnants that run from axilla to groin.
1. In some women, portions of the milk line persist, leaving a vestigial nipple with or without a small areola and glandular tissue. These are sometimes mistaken for nevi *(FIG. 7-2)*.

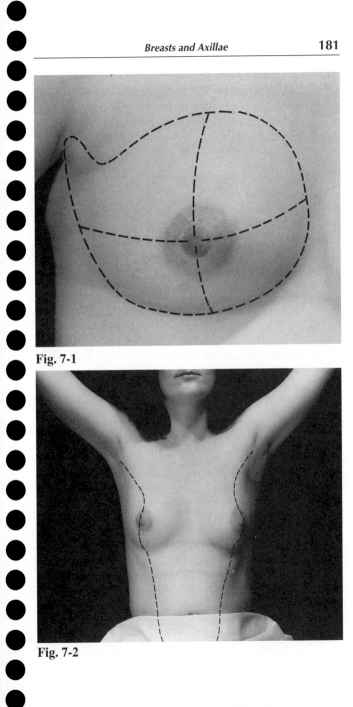

Fig. 7-1

Fig. 7-2

II. EXAMINER'S ATTITUDES.

A. It Is Normal for Beginning Students, Particularly Men, to Feel Awkward or Embarrassed About Performing the Breast Examination.

1. The learning of proper examination technique and repeated practice will build confidence.

III. PATIENT PREPARATION.

A. Emotional.

1. Some girls or women are embarrassed during the breast examination.
2. Take care to ensure privacy during the examination and to keep the breasts covered except during actual examination.
3. Explain the steps of the examination before you begin.
4. Assess her knowledge and practice of breast self-examination, since this examination can also serve as demonstration of the proper technique she can use herself.

B. Patient Positioning.

1. The patient should be seated, preferably on the side of the examination table, and disrobed to the waist *(FIG. 7-3)*.

IV. INSPECTION—OBSERVE:

A. Size and Symmetry (Mild asymmetry is normal.)

B. Contour: for masses, dimpling, or flattening.

1. Dimpling indicates retraction of the skin, often from underlying breast cancer and its associated fibrosis. It can also occur from breast surgery, such as a past biopsy.

C. Skin Characteristics: *(FIG. 7-4)*

1. The skin of the breast is of similar texture as that on the abdomen.
2. The areola are pigmented areas surrounding the nipples, with color varying from pink to brown and size varying greatly.
   - Sebaceous glands on the areola appear as small round elevations.
   - There may be scattered hair follicles around the areola.

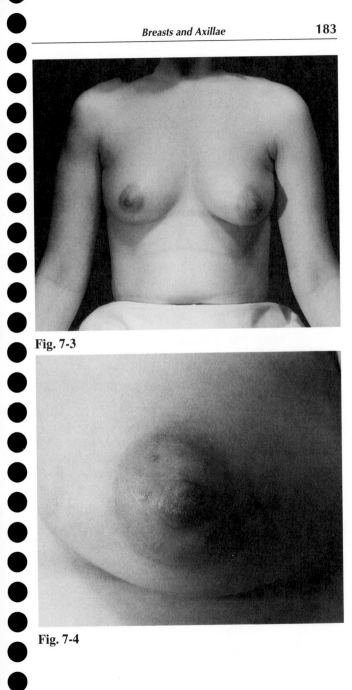

Fig. 7-3

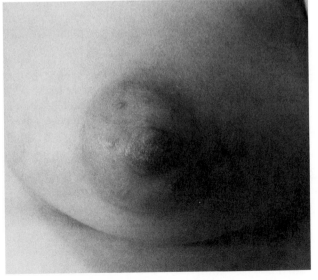

Fig. 7-4

3. The nipples are round, hairless, pigmented, and equal in size.
   - Their surface is convoluted, which gives them a wrinkled appearance. Their size varies among women.
   - If the breasts are symmetric, both nipples should point laterally and downward to the same degree.
   - Note any nipple inversion: is it congenital (benign) or of recent onset (consider tumor). Note any rashes, ulceration, or discharge.
     —Long-standing nipple inversion, although a normal variant, can cause problems with breast-feeding.

4. In light-skinned persons, a horizontal or vertical vascular pattern may be seen and is usually symmetric. Focal or unilateral patterns are abnormal.

5. Note any color changes (reddening or hyperpigmentation), edema, moles, or nevi.
   - *Peau d'orange* (orange peel) is a skin thickening with enlarged pores. It indicates lymphatic obstruction from underlying breast cancer.

D. **Perform Maneuvers That Pull on the Suspensory Ligaments** and may bring out early retraction. If these deviate the nipple, it will point toward the lesion.
   1. Have her raise both arms over her head. This usually results in an equal elevation of both breasts *(FIG. 7-5)*.

   2. Have her contract her pectoral muscles by:
      - Pressing her hands against her hips *(FIG. 7-6)*.
      - (Or) pressing her palms together *(FIG. 7-7)*.

   3. If the breasts are pendulous, have her lean forward (with your support in balancing her) *(FIG. 7-8)*. The traction caused by the breasts falling away from the thorax may bring out retraction.

   4. If you suspect a mass, gently move or compress the breast and watch for dimpling.

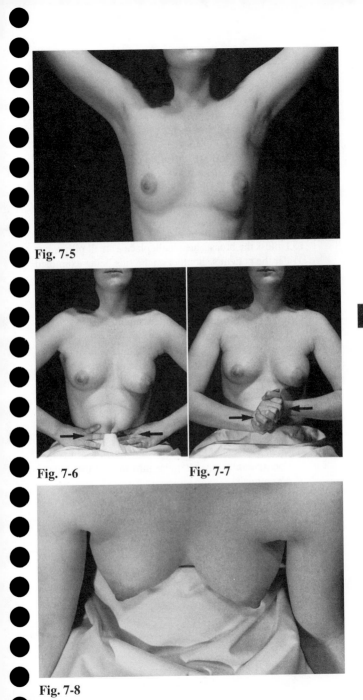

Fig. 7-5

Fig. 7-6

Fig. 7-7

Fig. 7-8

    E. In Adolescents, assess breast development according to
    Tanner's sexual maturity rating scale (see Appendix A).

V. PALPATION (The primary purpose is to discover masses.)
    A. Remember That the Breast Consistency Often Changes Cyclically.
        1. The breasts become engorged, lobular, and sensitive before menses. They decongest soon after.

    B. Position the Patient.
        1. Unless the breasts are small, place a small pillow under the patient's shoulder on the side being examined *(FIG. 7-9),* or she can place her ipsilateral arm behind her back, raising it slightly.
          ▪ This spreads the breast tissue more evenly across the chest and aids in finding nodules.

        2. The arm should be somewhat abducted to aid palpation of the tail of Spence. Expose only the breast being examined.

    C. Use the Pads of Three Fingers: *(FIG. 7-10)*
        1. Palpate in a rotary or to-and-fro motion.

        2. Movements should be gentle and even. Light palpation generally reveals more information than heavy pressure.
          ▪ In a large breast, palpate more firmly when trying to reach deeper structures.

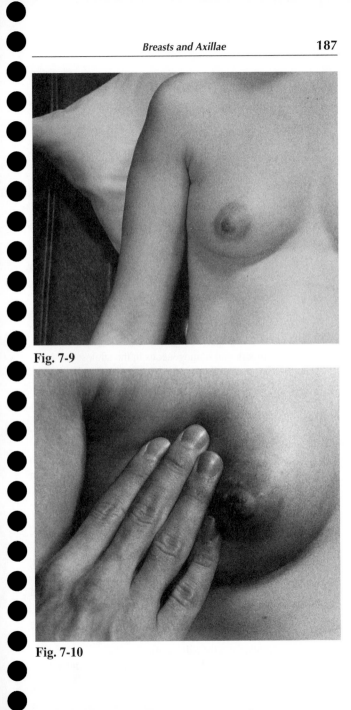

Fig. 7-9

Fig. 7-10

3. To ensure a thorough examination of the areola, periphery, and tail of Spence: *(FIG. 7-11)*
   ▪ Proceed systematically, such as:
     —Palpating in an outward spiral from the nipple.
     —Or in a series of concentric circles *(FIG. 7-12)*.
     —Or in a series of parallel lines running from midsternal or posterior axillary line toward the nipple line.
     —Or in wedge sections from breast periphery to center *(FIG. 7-13)*.
   ▪ Symmetry of the underlying disc of glandular tissue can be assessed:
     —Place the palm over the breast.
     —Tilt the hand from side to side to feel the disc of glandular tissue moving underneath *(FIG. 7-14)*.

D. **Note These Characteristics:**
   1. Consistency and elasticity: the normal breast feels granular and somewhat lumpy from the configuration of its lobes, and:
      ▪ Smooth and homogeneous in the adolescent.
      ▪ Somewhat stringy sensation in the elderly.
      ▪ Enlarged and more lobular in pregnancy.
   2. Any tenderness.
   3. Presence of nodules; if the patient mentions one, palpate the opposite breast first to use as a baseline. Define any mass by the following qualities:
      ▪ Location: by quadrant or clock method. You can also draw the mass within a simple circular diagram of the breast.
      ▪ The size in centimeters, describing its 3 dimensions.
      ▪ Its shape: round, discoid, regular, irregular, or matted (if several).
      ▪ Its consistency and elasticity: soft, firm, or hard; solid or cystic.
      ▪ Delimitation: whether its borders are well-defined or irregular.
        —Simple cysts have well-defined borders. Carcinoma often has poorly defined edges.
      ▪ Tenderness (to palpation).
        —Fibrocystic breast changes are often tender. Carcinomas are often painless.

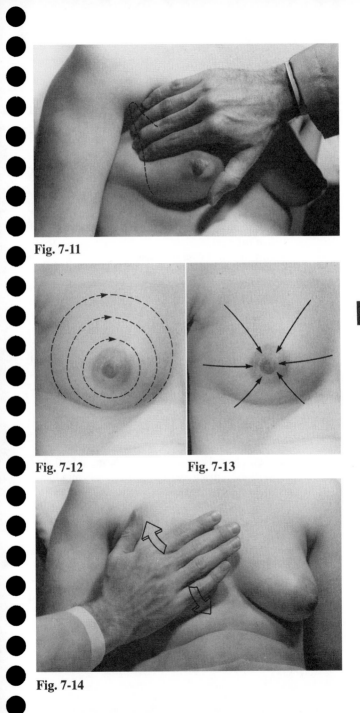

Fig. 7-11

Fig. 7-12   Fig. 7-13

Fig. 7-14

- Mobility: whether the mass is freely movable, movable only in certain directions, or fixed.
  —Try with and without her contracting her pectoral muscles (hands on hips).
  —Benign lesions and cysts are often freely movable. Carcinomas induce fibrosis and are adherent to overlying skin or underlying chest wall or muscle.
- Erythema or edema overlying the lesion.
  —Tender erythema often signals a breast infection. Edema raises concern of carcinoma *(peau d'orange).*
- Any dimpling over the mass.

E. **Palpate Each Nipple *(FIG. 7-15).***
 1. Gently compress the nipple and areola between thumb and index finger, attempting to elicit discharge.
 2. If discharge is seen or suspected:
  - Use your index finger to milk the lobes in radial sequence around the nipple.
  - Compression of the discharge-producing lobe will cause discharge to exude from the nipple *(FIG. 7-16).* Note which o'clock location induces the discharge.
  - Note its color: milky, watery, purulent or bloody.
    —Milky or watery discharge often relates to a hormonal influence.
    —Purulent discharge usually indicates infection.
    —Bloody discharge often indicates intraductal pathology, such as a papilloma or carcinoma.
 3. It is normal for the tactile stimulation of examination to cause transient erection of the nipple with wrinkling of the areola.

F. **Some Examiners also Palpate the Breast Through a Satin Cloth or with the Use of Baby Powder.**
 1. The slippery feeling that results sometimes aids in locating masses.

G. **Pendulous Breasts Can Be Palpated Bimanually by Compressing a Portion Between Both Hands *(FIG. 7-17).***
 1. In small breasts, this can falsely simulate a lump.

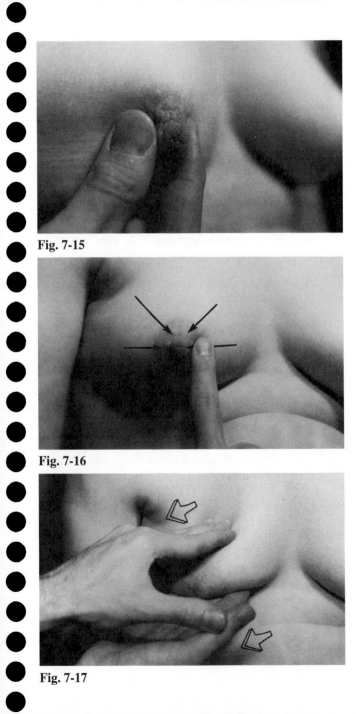

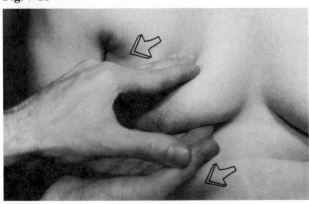

Fig. 7-15

Fig. 7-16

Fig. 7-17

VI. AXILLA.

A. Lymphatic Drainage: important because of the frequent spread of breast cancer through these channels *(FIG. 7-18)*.

1. Visualize the axilla as a four-sided pyramid:
   - Anterior (pectoral) nodes drain the anterior chest wall and most of the breast. They are located within the anterior axillary fold (1).
   - Posterior (subscapular) nodes drain the posterior chest wall and part of the arm. They are felt deep within the posterior axillary fold (2).
   - Lateral nodes drain most of the arm. They are felt against the upper humerus (3).
   - Medial (central) nodes drain all of the above. These are located high in the axilla and are the most frequently palpable (4).

2. From the central nodes, lymph drains into the infra- and supraclavicular nodes (5). Also, depending on the location of the lesion, spread may proceed directly to deeper channels or to the opposite breast.

B. Inspection *(FIG. 7-19)*.

1. Observe the skin for rashes, discoloration, edema, infection, bulging, or retraction.
   - The axilla is a common site for skin tags.
   - Erythema here is often an allergic response to underarm deodorants.

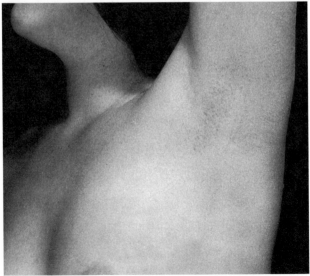

Fig. 7-18

Fig. 7-19

C. **Palpation (demonstrated for the left axilla).**
   1. Support her left wrist or hand with your left arm *(FIG. 7-20)*.
      - This relaxes the muscles, as well as abducting the arm. Your right fingers should lie directly behind the pectoral muscles, pointing toward the mid-clavicle.
   2. Lift your fingers high into the axilla, then press inward *(FIG. 7-21)*.
   3. Maintaining pressure against the ribs, slide your fingers downward over the central nodes *(FIG. 7-22)*. (The maneuver is actually performed with the arm lowered.)
   4. Then feel inside the anterior axillary fold behind the lower edge of the pectoral muscle, feeling for pectoral nodes.
   5. Feel inside the posterior axillary fold for the subscapular nodes *(FIG. 7-23)*. This is more easily done from behind.
   6. From the same posterior position, feel against the humerus for the lateral nodes.
   7. Finally, feel above and below the clavicle for supra- and infraclavicular nodes *(FIG. 7-24)*.
   8. Small (0.5 cm) soft, movable nodes are often present normally.
   9. Repeat on the right axilla, palpating with your left hand.

VII. **MALE BREAST EXAMINATION.**
   A. **Inspect the Nipple and Areola for Nodules, Ulcerations, or Edema.** The four positions (arms over head, etc.) are unnecessary.
   B. **Palpate for Masses** in the nipple, areola, or small rim of breast tissue.
      1. Male breasts are often enlarged with obesity.
      2. Adolescent boys will sometimes have normal and transient gynecomastia, where the disc of glandular breast tissue is enlarged. It is often unilateral.
   C. **Inspect and Palpate the Axilla** as above.

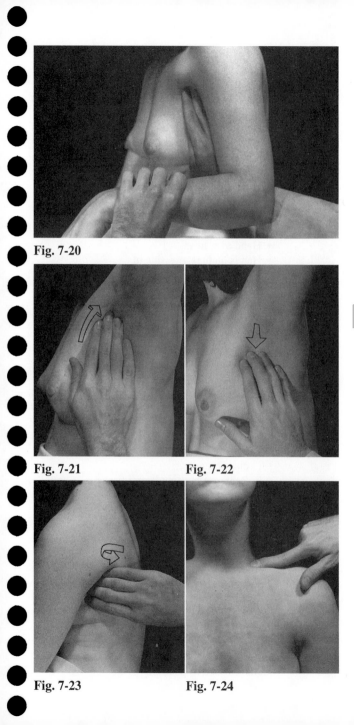

Fig. 7-20

Fig. 7-21

Fig. 7-22

Fig. 7-23

Fig. 7-24

VIII. BREAST SELF-EXAMINATION.

A. During the History-Taking, assess the patient's knowledge and practice of breast self-examination.

B. After Your Examination, which can serve as a demonstration, emphasize the following:

    1. Breasts should be examined each month between the fourth and seventh days of menses, when the breasts are least congested.

    2. Have her inspect the breasts using the four positions:

- Hands at sides.
- Hand over head.
- Hands on hips, pressing in.
- Leaning forward, braced against a chair.
  - —A mirror is necessary for adequate inspection. Watch for skin changes, discharge, and dimpling, as described previously.

    3. Show her how to palpate the breast, including the areola, and milking the nipple for discharge.

- Use a systematic approach. The *concentric circle* approach is the easiest to teach.
  - —Remind her to use the opposite hand for each breast. Show her how to press with the pads of two or three fingers.
  - —Have her touch the nipple, as a landmark, then palpate in two or three "larger and larger" circles around it.
  - —Reassure her that breast tissue is "normally lumpy," and that the goal of breast exam is to notice any *new* lumps.
- Some patients prefer to self-examine in the shower, using soap and water to facilitate the sliding motion of palpation.

    4. Show her how to palpate her axilla in the supine position. In patients with large breasts, the entire palpation portion of breast self-examination should be done in the supine position.

    5. Have her demonstrate self-examination for you to reinforce her memory of it.

    6. She should report any change to a health professional as soon as possible.

8 The Abdomen

I. **TOPOGRAPHIC ANATOMY: These lines and landmarks assist the caregiver in locating areas for examination and in documenting the location of findings.**
  A. **Reference Lines.**
     1. Anteriorly: *(FIG. 8-1)*
       ■ The midsternal line, from xyphoid process to pubic ramus.
       ■ The midclavicular line, from midclavicle to inguinal ligament.
     2. Laterally: *(FIG. 8-2)*
       ■ The anterior axillary line, extending downward from the anterior axillary fold
       ■ The midaxillary line, descending from the midaxilla.
  B. **Surface Landmarks of the Abdomen.**
     1. Posteriorly, the costovertebral angle is formed by the junction of ribs and vertebral column *(FIG. 8-3)*.
     2. The abdominal wall is bounded above by the *inferior costal margin (FIG. 8-4)*.

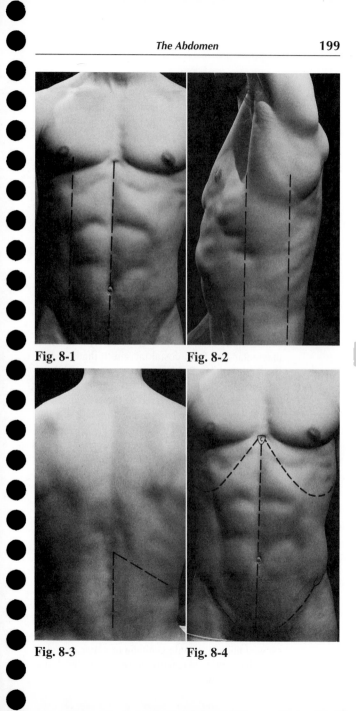

Fig. 8-1

Fig. 8-2

Fig. 8-3

Fig. 8-4

- But its contents extend upward to the dome of the diaphragm.
3. The *midline* runs from the xiphoid process through the umbilicus to the superior edge of the pubic bone.
4. The *inguinal ligament* extends upward from the pubic ramus to the anterior superior iliac spine.
   - This marks the inferior boundary of the abdominal wall, but its contents extend below to fill the pelvic basin.

C. **Anatomic Mapping.** There are two commonly used methods of subdivision.
   1. Four quadrants *(FIG. 8-5)*.
      - Formed by two lines, the first line runs vertically from sternum to pubis. The second line runs perpendicular to the first, intersecting at the umbilicus.
      - This divides the abdomen into right and left upper and lower quadrants.
   2. Nine zones *(FIG. 8-6)*.
      - In this method, two lines drop vertically in the mid-clavicular line from costal margin to inguinal ligament (near the lateral borders of the rectus abdominus muscles)
      - Two horizontal lines intersect at the level of the inferior costal margins and the anterior superior iliac spines.
      - The central third, with its three divisions, is referred to most often. From top to bottom, they are named:
        —Superior third: epigastric
        —Middle third: umbilical
        —Inferior third: suprapubic

D. **The Order of Examination Techniques Is:**
   1. Inspection.
   2. Auscultation.
   3. Percussion.
   4. Palpation.
      - Auscultation precedes percussion and palpation, as any contact with the bowel can increase its motility.
      - The rectal examination is an important component of the abdominal examination. In this text, it is reviewed under the male genitalia or pelvic examination chapters. It is usually performed at the end of the examination.

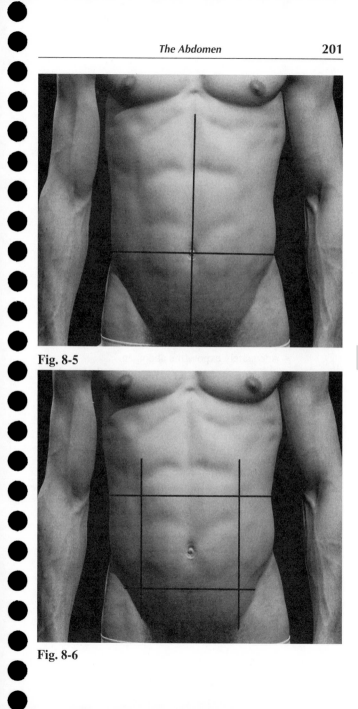

Fig. 8-5

Fig. 8-6

II. INSPECTION.

  A. Position the Patient *(FIG. 8-7)* in order to relax the abdominal muscles.

    1. The patient should:
- Lay supine.
- Have arms at sides or folded over the chest, not over or behind the head, since this tenses the abdominal muscles.
- Have an empty bladder before the examination begins.
- Breathe quietly and slowly.

    2. The examiner should:
- Ensure that the patient and the examination room are comfortably warm.
- Support the patient's head with a small pillow. The patient will often try to watch the examination by lifting up his head, thus tightening the abdominal muscles.
- Adequately expose the abdomen.
  —Keep the chest covered to the level of the lower sternum.
  —The abdominal skin should be exposed from the sternum to pubis.
  —The inguinal area should be visible, but the genitals covered.
- Explain the examination before you start, and continue reassurance during the examination. This gentle, ongoing narrative can be very comforting for the patient and promotes relaxation.
- Use adequate lighting.
  —A single light source is best.
  —Position it tangentially to highlight surface detail, either aiming across from left to right, or downward from over the patient's head.

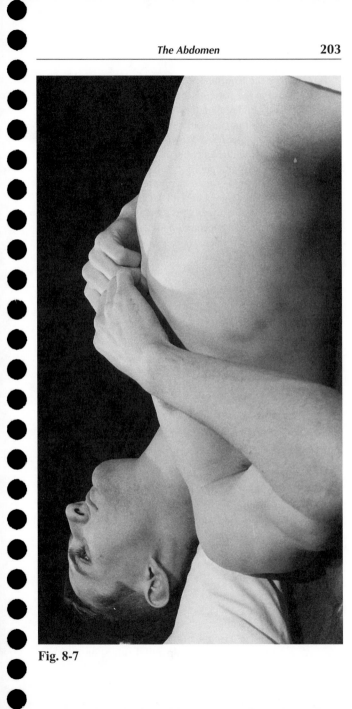

Fig. 8-7

B. Observe the Contour of the Abdomen.

1. Stand to the patient's right side, with your head only slightly higher than the abdomen *(FIG. 8-8)*.
   - The abdomen should swell and recede easily with breathing *(FIG. 8-9)*.
   - Seen from the side, the abdomen is usually:
     —Flat from xiphoid to pubis.
     —Or symmetrically depressed (scaphoid).
       • This can occur with cachexia.
     —Or symmetrically protuberant.
       • This can occur with ascites, pregnancy, gaseous distension, and other causes.
   - A rounded contour is normal in infants and small children.
     —In adults, this indicates poor abdominal muscle tone and/or obesity.

2. Note any fullness above or below the umbilicus, since this may represent enlargement of a specific organ.
   - Note whether the umbilicus is inverted, flat, or everted.
     —The umbilicus can be deeply inverted with obesity and everted with pregnancy, ascites, and large abdominal masses.
     —An umbilical hernia can also evert the umbilicus.

3. Watch for motion on the abdominal surface *(FIG. 8-10)*.
   - You can normally see the aortic pulsation in the epigastric area.
   - Visible peristalsis can be seen occasionally in thin individuals, but not normally in an abdominal wall of average thickness.
   - Peristaltic waves, when visible:
     —Usually result from motion in the stomach or small intestine.
     —Are seen as elevated oblique bands that begin near the left upper quadrant and move slowly downward and rightward.
     —Occasionally cause parallel ridges on the skin, forming a ladder pattern.

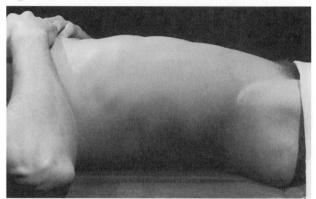

Fig. 8-8

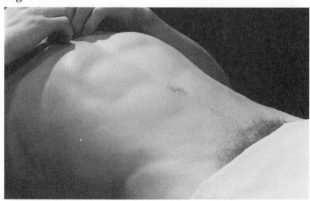

Fig. 8-9

Fig. 8-10

C. **Observe for Symmetry of Contour.**
   1. Stand near the foot of the bed or examination table *(FIG. 8-11)*.
   2. Have the patient breath deeply; enlargement of the liver or spleen may show as a bulging in the right or left upper quadrants.
   3. Note any bulging of the flanks (as in ascites).
   4. Check for abdominal wall herniations.
      ▪ Look in particular: *(FIG. 8-12)* (1) down the midline, (2) near the umbilicus, and (3) near the inguinal ligaments.
      ▪ Ask the patient to lift his head and shoulders off the pillow. This increases intraabdominal pressure, causing most hernias to visibly bulge.

D. **Inspect the Skin.** The abdominal region is very useful for inspection since it contains a large single expanse of skin.
   1. Is the skin soft and velvety (its normal texture) or tense and shiny (indicating intraabdominal mass or fluid).
      ▪ Marked flaccidity can indicate recent wasting and weight loss.
   2. Note any:
      ▪ Surgical scars (location and length). Some common scars are:
         —Cholecystectomy: diagonal right upper quadrant (or three healed pencil-width holes if by laparoscopic approach).
         —Appendectomy: diagonal right lower quadrant
         —Herniorrhaphy: diagonal scar parallel to and near the inguinal ligament.
         —Cesarean section: curved suprapubic incision, or vertical below umbilicus if classical Cesarean.
         —Laparotomy: vertical midline scar, above and/or below umbilicus.
      ▪ Disorders of pigmentation, such as jaundice.
         —The abdominal skin often renders jaundice or hyperpigmentation more visible, since it is usually protected from the sun and is therefore less tan.
         —When looking for jaundice, use daylight illumination. The yellowish color of flourescent lights can mask the jaundice.

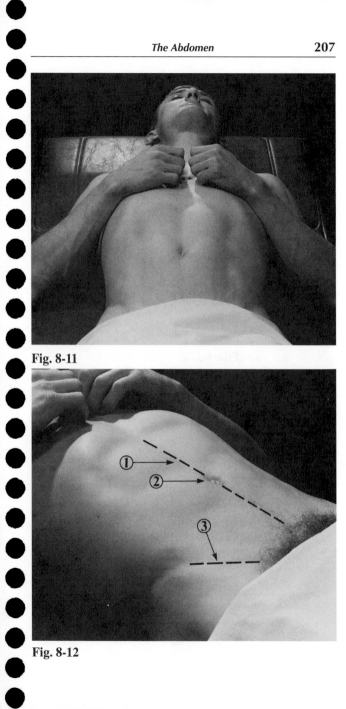

Fig. 8-11

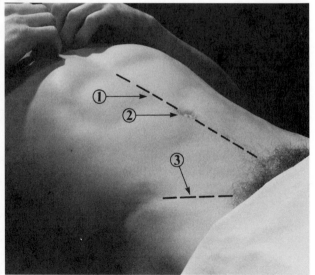

Fig. 8-12

- Skin lesions, such as spider angiomas or nevi.
- Hair distribution.
  —Patients with advanced cirrhosis often have decreased body hair.
- Striae (stretch marks).
  —These appear as irregular lines or streaks, usually in the lower quadrants.
  —Recently formed striae are pink or violet. Older ones fade to a silvery white color.

3. Inspect for visible veins.
   - Check the epigastric and suprapubic areas.
   - Superficial veins are not normally visible unless the patient is emaciated.
   - Engorged abdominal veins indicate obstruction of venous return, usually through the portal vein or vena cava.
   - Determine the direction of venous return.
     —Place two index fingers on a segment of engorged vein *(FIG. 8-13)*.
     —Empty it by spreading your fingers a few inches *(FIG. 8-14)*.
     —Lift one finger and watch the speed of refilling *(FIG. 8-15)*.
     —Repeat and lift the other finger *(FIG. 8-16)*. The rate of refilling is usually faster in one direction, indicating the direction of flow in that venous collateral.
   - Normal venous return is directed away from the umbilicus.
     —With obstruction of the portal vein, the superficial veins are often visibly engorged but their direction of refilling is normal. This radiating spoke-like pattern is termed *caput medusae.*
     —With obstruction of the inferior vena cava, venous collaterals in the lower abdomen will show *upward* flow toward the umbilicus. Obstruction of the superior vena cava causes *downward* flow from the upper abdomen toward the umbilicus.

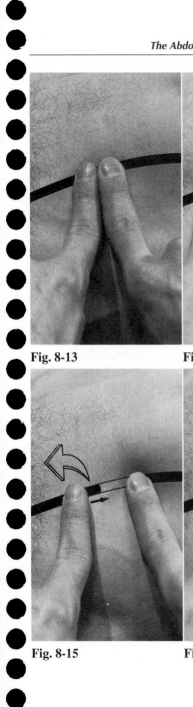

Fig. 8-13

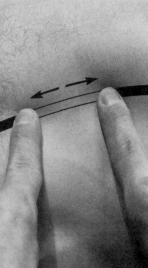

Fig. 8-14

Fig. 8-15

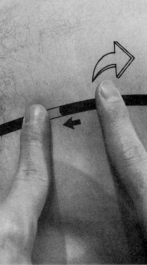

Fig. 8-16

III. AUSCULTATION. Listen for three kinds of sounds:

A. Peristaltic Sounds.

    1. Warm the stethoscope in your hand for a few seconds *(FIG. 8-17).*

        ■ Cold will induce muscle contraction or shivering.

    2. Place the diaphragm lightly on the skin *(FIG. 8-18).*

        ■ If possible, let it rest by its own weight.

        ■ Deep pressure from the stethoscope can induce vascular bruits or can raise the pitch of bowel sounds, simulating pathology.

    3. Note the frequency and pitch of the sounds.

        ■ This is the sound of air and fluid moving through the gut, indicating its motility.

        ■ There is a wide range of normal sounds.

          —Generally, the sounds are soft, medium-pitched clicks or gurgles that occur every five to fifteen seconds.

          —There may also be long pauses or bursts of continuous sound.

        ■ Bowel sounds are widely transmitted throughout the abdomen.

          —It is only necessary to listen in one quadrant, usually the right lower, since the ileocecal valve produces active sounds.

          —Listen in all four quadrants if abnormalities are suspected.

        ■ Always try to relate the peristaltic sounds to the patient's clinical condition.

          —For example: loud, rushing bowel sounds are more clinically significant in a patient with diarrhea than in one who recently drank a carbonated beverage.

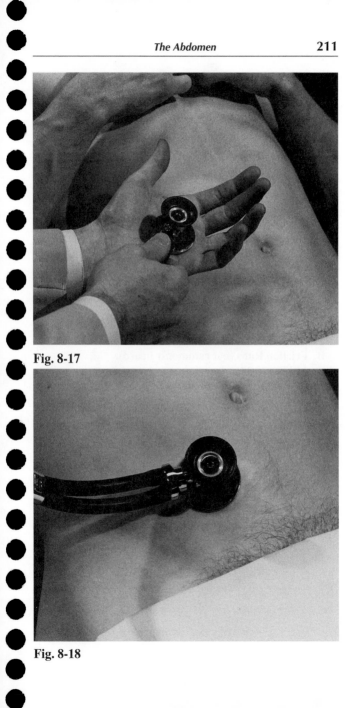

Fig. 8-17

Fig. 8-18

4. Listen in particular for two abnormalities:
    ▪ Hypoactive or absent bowel sounds.
        —If peristaltic sounds are not immediately audible, listen for a full five minutes, measured by your watch, before concluding they are absent *(FIG. 8-19)*.
        —Try to stimulate peristalsis by flicking the abdominal wall with your finger.
        —Silence suggests the immobile bowel in peritonitis or paralytic ileus.
    ▪ High-pitched tinkling bowel sounds.
        —These sound like faint wind chimes and indicate tightly distended loops of bowel in intestinal obstruction.
        —Ask if there is cramping when the sounds peak in frequency and intensity. This indicates that waves of increased peristalsis are trying to push fluid through a stenotic bowel.

B. **Friction Rubs (not commonly heard).**
    1. Place the diaphragm over each costal margin, over the region of the liver *(FIG. 8-20),* or spleen *(FIG. 8-21).*

    2. Have the patient breathe slowly and deeply.
        ▪ The friction rub is a creaking or grating sound like two pieces of leather rubbing together. It is heard only during the motion of breathing.
        ▪ The rub is rare, even in the presence of disease.
            —It is useful to listen, though, if a patient has localized pain over these areas.
            —It may occur with hepatic inflammation or tumors, or with splenic infarction.

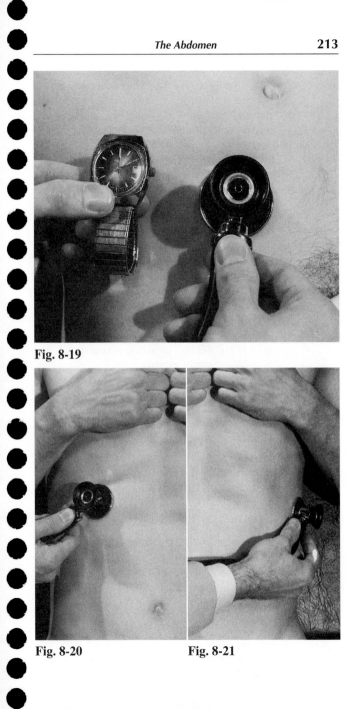

Fig. 8-19

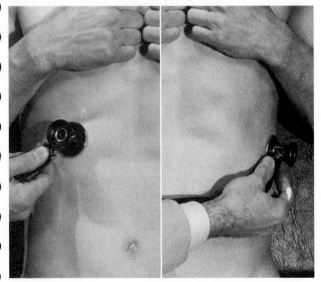

Fig. 8-20   Fig. 8-21

C. **Vascular Sounds.**

    1. *Bruits* are particularly present in patients with hypertension or lower extremity vascular disease; they are soft and high-pitched.

- Using the bell of the stethoscope, press just enough to maintain an air seal with the skin.
- Listen over:
  - —The *abdominal aorta;* in the upper midline *(FIG. 8-22).* A benign bruit is sometimes heard, particularly in young adults.
  - —The *renal arteries,* below each costal margin *(FIG. 8-23)* or on the back over each costovertebral angle.
  - —The *iliac arteries;* in the center of each lower quadrant *(FIG. 8-24).* Or estimate their course with a line drawn from 1 inch below the umbilicus to each femoral pulsation.
  - —The *femoral arteries:* listen below the midpoint of each inguinal ligament. Apply only light pressure *(FIG. 8-25).* The artery is superficial, and firm pressure may induce a bruit.
  - —Whenever you hear a bruit, listen again to the heart *(FIG. 8-26).* Some murmurs will radiate to the abdomen, especially those of aortic valve origin.

    2. Venous hum *(FIG. 8-27).*

- Listen on or below the right costal margin.
  - —This may occur over venous collaterals formed secondary to liver disease, such as with portal venous hypertension.
  - —It is softer than a bruit and continuous rather than systolic in timing.

D. **Succussion Splash** (optional).

    1. This is performed when there is suspicion of gastric outlet obstruction.

    2. Place both hands on the abdomen. Under one of your hands, in the right upper quadrant, press the stethoscope diaphragm onto the skin.

    3. While listening though the stethoscope, vigorously shake the abdomen from side to side. Listen for a sloshing sound, as if from a partially filled water balloon. The test is positive if the splash is audible more than six hours after a meal.

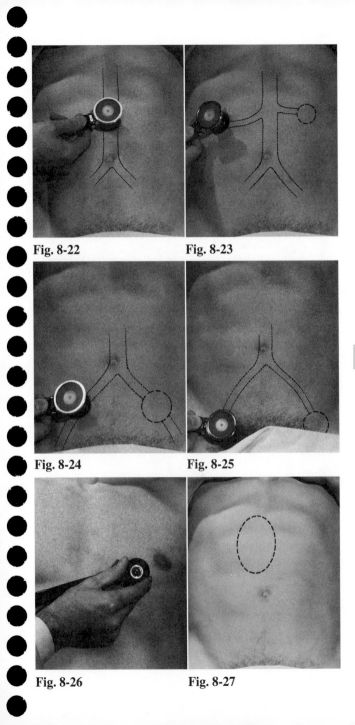

Fig. 8-22

Fig. 8-23

Fig. 8-24

Fig. 8-25

Fig. 8-26

Fig. 8-27

IV. PERCUSSION.
A. See Chapter 6, Thorax and Lungs, for Technique.

B. General Survey.
1. Percuss lightly in each quadrant *(FIG. 8-28)*.

2. This produces a general picture of the areas of tympany or dullness.
   - Tympany usually predominates, depending on the amount of gas in the colon.
   - Solid masses will percuss as unexpected areas of dullness.
     —Percuss over any area of unexpected bulging.
     —For example: a distended bladder will produce lower midline dullness.

C. Percuss the Gastric Air Bubble *(FIG. 8-29)*.
1. Percuss horizontally and vertically in the area of the lower anterior left ribcage.
2. The air bubble has a lower and louder percussion note than the nearby intestine.
3. Its size is variable and depends on the time elapsed since the last meal eaten.
4. A significant rightward shift of the gastric air bubble may occur with massive splenomegaly.

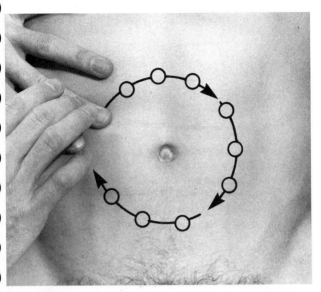

Fig. 8-28

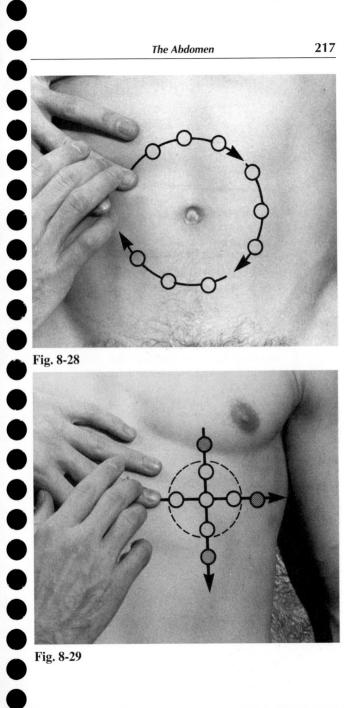

Fig. 8-29

D. Estimate Liver Size.

   1. Percuss first in the right midclavicular line.

   ▪ To locate the upper border:

      —Begin percussing from an area of resonance, usu-
      ally the fourth interspace *(FIG. 8-30).*

      —Percuss downward in 1-inch steps until the note
      first changes to dullness. Mark this point as the
      upper border. It is usually in the fifth to seventh
      interspace *(FIG. 8-31).*

   ▪ To locate the lower border:

      —Begin percussion from an area of tympany, as
      near the umbilicus. Always begin low in case the
      liver is enlarged *(FIG. 8-32).*

      —Percuss upward in 1-inch steps until the percus-
      sion note changes to dullness. Again, mark this
      point. In healthy patients, it is usually at or slighly
      above the costal margin.

   ▪ It is useful to have the patient hold his breath in mid-
   expiration as you percuss, since moving borders will
   give a falsely increased or decreased size.

   ▪ Measure the vertical distance between these points
   (FIG. 8-33).

      —It is normally 6 to 12 cm in the midclavicular line

      —Size will vary with sex and body build. The liver
      is generally larger in males than females. It is also
      larger with a larger bone structure.

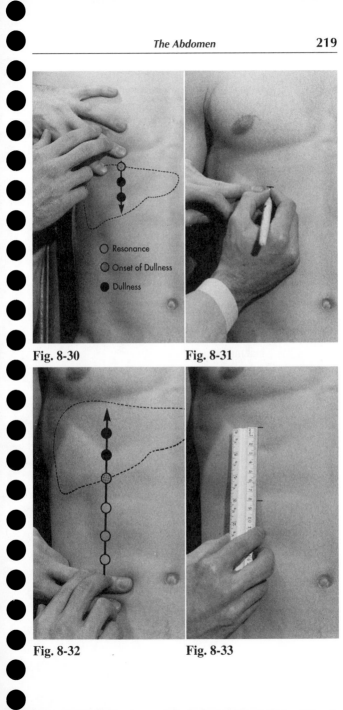

Fig. 8-30

○ Resonance
◉ Onset of Dullness
● Dullness

Fig. 8-31

Fig. 8-32

Fig. 8-33

- If you have trouble locating a border:
  —Repeat your measurement during a deep inspiration.
  —Both borders will shift downward 2 or 3 cm *(FIG. 8-34)*. An exception to this is in patients with chronic obstructive pulmonary disease, such as emphysema, where the diaphragms are already fully depressed.

2. If the liver seems enlarged, percuss again:
  - In the midsternal line *(FIG. 8-35)*.
  - In the anterior axillary line.
  - By percussing in multiple locations, you can better confirm your suspicion of hepatomegaly.

3. Variations in size and location.
  - Both upper and lower borders may be shifted:
    —Downward by emphysema or pectus excavatum.
    —Upward by ascites, pregnancy, or a large abdominal tumor.
  - The upper border of dullness may be:
    —Falsely elevated by pleural effusion or pulmonary consolidation adjacent to the upper border.
    —Falsely lowered by free air under the diaphragm, as in a perforated viscus (e.g., peptic ulcer).
  - The lower border of dullness can be falsely elevated by gas in the hepatic flexure of the colon.

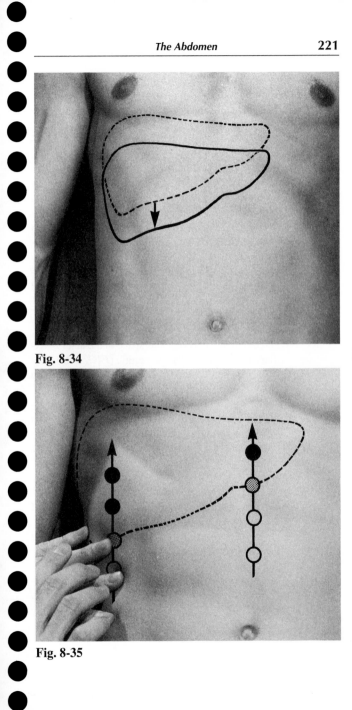

Fig. 8-34

Fig. 8-35

E. Percuss the Spleen (two methods).
   1. Region of dullness.
   - The spleen lies near the tenth interspace just poste-
     rior to the midaxillary line.
   - Percuss from the midline in several directions to-
     ward the anticipated area of splenic dullness *(FIG.
     8-36)*.
   - Try to outline its border.
     —The spleen is usually less than 7 cm wide by per-
       cussion.
     —Dullness detected below the ninth interspace in
       the midaxillary line may indicate splenic enlarge-
       ment.
     —False positives can occur with left lower lung con-
       solidation, pleural effusion, or with an enlarged
       left lobe of the liver.

   2. Shifting inferior border.
   - Percuss over the lowest interspace in the anterior ax-
     illary line; it is usually tympanitic *(FIG. 8-37)*.
   - Continue percussion as the patient takes a deep
     breath.
     —During inspiration, the spleen moves down, me-
       dially, and slightly forward.
     —With a normal spleen, the note will remain tym-
       panitic; with enlargement, the note may shift to
       dullness.

   3. In either case, the spleen can appear:
   - Falsely enlarged by feces in the splenic flexure of
     the colon.
   - Falsely normal in size (when truly enlarged) by the
     presence of gastric or colonic air.

   4. When an enlarged area of splenic dullness is found, al-
     ways palpate more thoroughly for splenic enlargement.

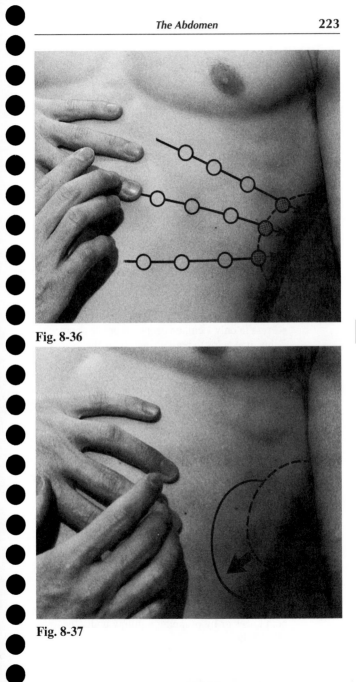

Fig. 8-36

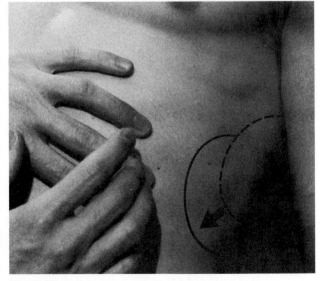

Fig. 8-37

V. PALPATION.

A. Patient Preparation.

1. Warm your hands.
   - Beginners usually have cold hands because of anxiety, which passes with practice. Until then, wash your hands in warm water before you begin.

2. Approach the patient slowly. Avoid quick motions onto the skin surface.

3. If you suspect any tender areas, palpate them last.

B. Light Palpation: This is very useful for detecting slight tenderness, large masses, and muscle guarding.

1. Position your hand with fingers together, hand and arm parallel to the abdominal skin. Press with the pads of the fingertips *(FIG. 8-38).*

2. Move slowly and feel with light, pressing motions.
   - Press in only 1 cm, no deeper. A gentle approach at this time helps to reassure and relax the patient.
   - Feel in each quadrant for:
     —Muscle tone; normally rubbery resistant.
     —Tenderness; if present, use caution later with deeper palpation.
     —Obvious masses.
   - Watch the patient's face for any signs of discomfort, since he may not say anything.

3. If the abdominal wall remains tense, it is most likely secondary to:
   - Voluntary guarding (tightening of abdominal muscles), from patient ticklishness or anxiety, cold examiner's hands, or too vigorous pressure during palpation.
   - The involuntary guarding (abdominal wall muscle spasm) of peritoneal irritation.

4. Try to increase relaxation by having the patient flex both knees or by propping a pillow under the knees *(FIG 8-39).*

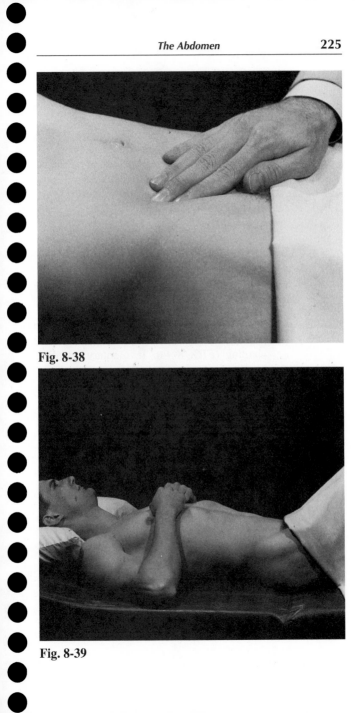

Fig. 8-38

Fig. 8-39

- Attempt to reduce ticklishness, if present.
  —Place the patient's hand under yours. Palpate a few times. The patient cannot be tickled by his own hand *(FIG. 8-40).*
  —Then reverse hands, with yours on the bottom, and palpate again *(FIG. 8-41).*
  —As the patient's abdomen relaxes, place the patient's hands back by his chest or sides.
- See if the wall relaxes somewhat during slow expiration *(FIGS. 8-42* and *8-43).*
  —When it does, it is called voluntary guarding. This is typical in ticklishness or anxiety.
  —Involuntary guarding or rigidity will not relax with expiration. It is a protective spasm of the abdominal muscles caused by peritoneal irritation. When present, see if it is unilateral or bilateral.
- Try palpating with the stethoscope.
  —The patient generally does not associate this with pain, and he may not react as much with muscle guarding *(FIG. 8-44).* Involuntary guarding, though, will persist.

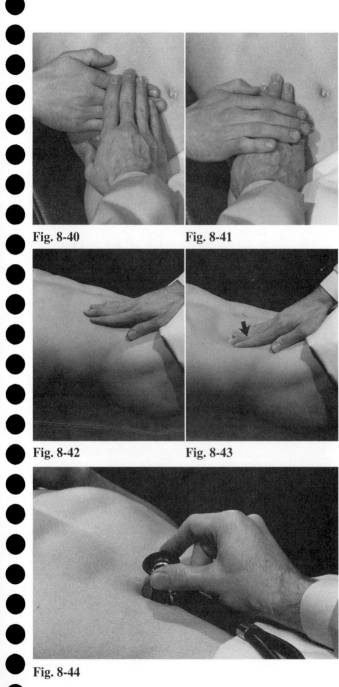

Fig. 8-40

Fig. 8-41

Fig. 8-42

Fig. 8-43

Fig. 8-44

C. Palpate for Internal Organs.

1. Liver (two methods). Remember the location of the lower liver border by percussion; this will indicate the likelihood of a palpable edge.

    ▪ Bimanual method.

      —Stand to the patient's right side.

      —Place your left hand under the ribcage at the posterior inferior costal margin *(FIG. 8-45).*

      —Place your right hand by the umbilicus, lateral to the rectus abdominus muscle *(FIG. 8-46).* (The rectus muscles are firm and can prevent deep palpation.)

        • Always begin this low in case the liver is enlarged. You can aim your fingers vertically or obliquely to his upper left.

      —Now lift up with the left hand and press slightly in with the right; this raises the liver toward the examining hand *(FIG. 8-47).*

      —Then have the patient take a deep breath. Feel for the liver edge as it descends *(FIG. 8-48).*

      —If you don't feel an edge, raise your right hand 1 inch upward and try again.

        • Continue until your fingers reach the costal margin, and slightly under it *(FIG. 8-49).*

        • You can release right hand pressure at the peak of inspiration. This allows the right hand to ride up over the liver edge as it descends.

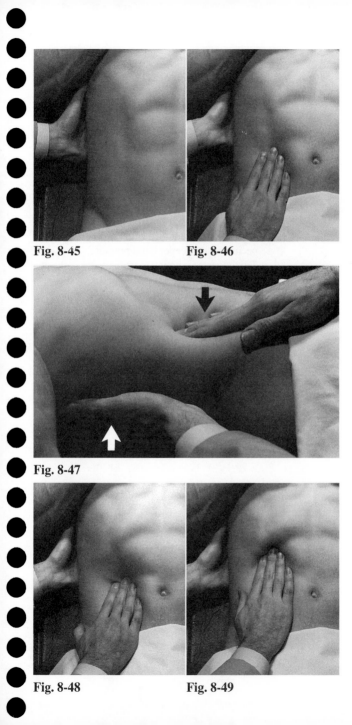

Fig. 8-45

Fig. 8-46

Fig. 8-47

Fig. 8-48

Fig. 8-49

—The liver edge is often not palpable.
- When it is, you can feel it touch and slide under your fingers. Or it may feel like an increase sense of resistance. It is often more palpable in thin, slender individuals.

—If you feel the edge, check for tenderness, texture, and nodularity *(FIG. 8-50)*.
- The normal liver is firm and rubbery. Its edge is sharp and regular with a smooth surface. It is usually located at or slightly below the right costal margin, and it may be mildly tender, especially with deeper hand pressure.
- Try to locate its boundaries: medially in the epigastrium *(FIG. 8-51)* and laterally, at the anterior axillary line *(FIG. 8-52)*.
- Percuss its size again. The liver may be positioned lower than normal without being enlarged.

—Whenever the liver is enlarged:
- Feel carefully for enlargement of the spleen.
- For both liver and spleen, when extreme enlargement is suspected, search for the liver or spleen edge low in the abdomen.

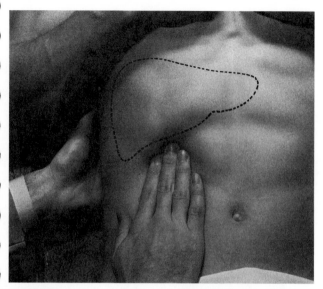

Fig. 8-50

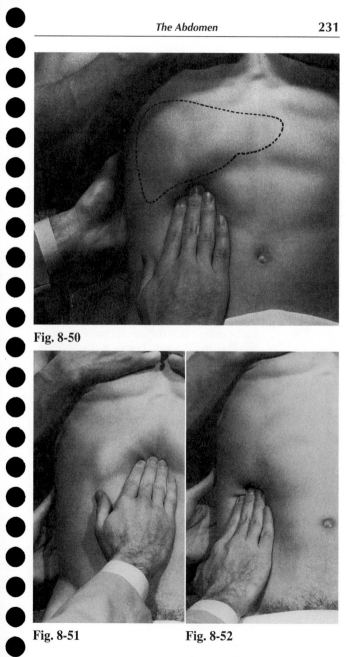

Fig. 8-51   Fig. 8-52

- Hooking maneuver.
  —Stand above the patient, facing toward his feet.
  —Place both hands side by side below the level of liver dullness, usually near the right costal margin *(FIG. 8-53)*.
  —Ask the patient to breathe deeply. As he does, curl your fingertips inward and upward; this allows you to feel for the edge with all fingers at once.
- Additional liver palpation techniques.
  —Fist percussion *(FIG. 8-54)*.
    • Place the palm of the left hand on the lateral inferior costal margin. Strike it lightly with the right fist.
    • Compare the sensation to percussion at the left costal margin.
    • Right-sided tenderness often indicates inflammation or congestion of the liver.
  —Gallbladder (not normally palpable).
    • If enlarged, it will be felt at the right inferior costal margin near the lateral border of the rectus muscle. The gallbladder is a soft, cystic mass 6 to 8 cm wide that moves with respiration. Tenderness limited to this site suggests gallbladder inflammation.
    • Always feel for a gallbladder if the patient is jaundiced.
  —Murphy's sign *(FIG. 8-55)*.
    • The gallbladder is palpated during a deep breath; as it descends, it touches the examining hand.
    • When inflamed, this causes pain, and the patient will catch his breath during midinspiration.
  —Scratch test: a combination of palpation and auscultation. This maneuver is particularly useful when the liver is believed to be enlarged but the edge is difficult to palpate.
    • Using the left hand, place the stethoscope diaphragm below the right costal margin in the midclavicular line. Place your index finger in the left lower quadrant.
    • While listening through the stethoscope, lightly scratch the patient's skin as you move your fin-

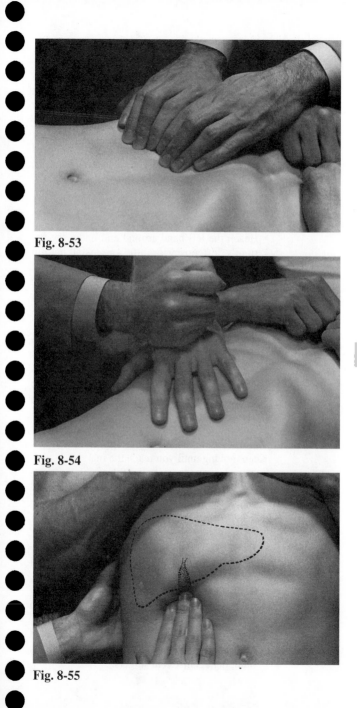

Fig. 8-53

Fig. 8-54

Fig. 8-55

ger toward the stethoscope. Repeat this in several distant locations in the left upper and right
lower quadrants, always moving toward the
stethoscope.
- As the finger scratches over the liver edge, the
  intensity of the scratching sound, as heard
  through the stethoscope, will suddenly increase.

2. Spleen.
   - Bimanual method.
     —Stand to the patient's right side.
       - Reach the left hand around and under the pa-
         tient's left posterior inferior costal margin
         (FIG. 8-56).
       - Place the right hand near the umbilicus with the
         fingers aimed upward toward the spleen. Again,
         always begin low so as to not miss a grossly en-
         larged spleen.
     —Lift up with the left hand to displace the spleen
       anteriorly.
     —Press gently in with the right hand.
     —Feel as the patient breathes deeply. If present, you
       will feel a firm edge with the peak of inspiration
       (FIG. 8-57).
     —If you don't feel an edge, move toward the left
       costal margin an inch and try again *(FIG. 8-58)*.
       Keep moving until you reach the margin.
       - It is easiest to reach under the margin by start-
         ing an inch away so the skin has some slack and
         can stretch underneath.
     —The edge is seldom palpable.
       - Occasionally a spleen tip can be felt normally
         in a thin and relaxed patient. If palpable, de-
         scribe the edge in centimeters below the left
         costal margin.
       - The splenic edge is more firm and blunt than
         the liver edge. When grossly enlarged, it often
         has a notch on its medial border.
       - When massively increased, you will feel a firm
         mass that slides out from under the margin,
         bumping against your fingers.

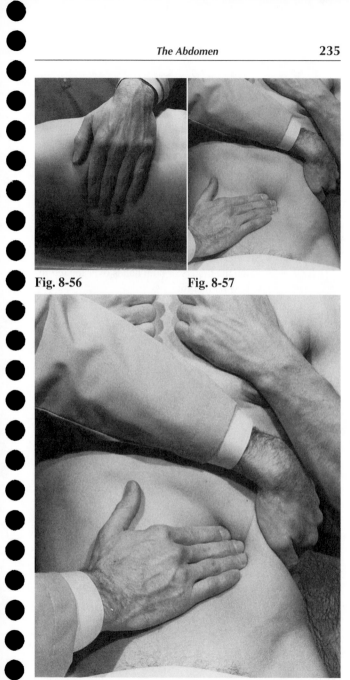

Fig. 8-56   Fig. 8-57

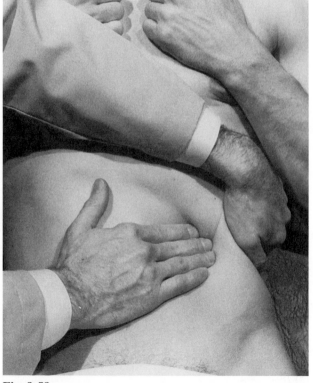

Fig. 8-58

—If you suspect enlargement but don't feel an edge
- Roll the patient onto his right side with his knees and hips slightly flexed *(FIG. 8-59).* In this position, gravity brings the spleen forward and medial.
- Attempt palpation again.
- Alternate method.
  —Have the patient lay supine.
  - Place his left fist and forearm under the small of his back. This will displace the spleen more anteriorly.
  —Use the hooking maneuver described earlier.
  - Stand at the patient's left side.
  - Hook the fingers of both hands over the left inner costal margin.
  - Press the fingers in and upward as the patient breathes deeply *(FIG. 8-60).*

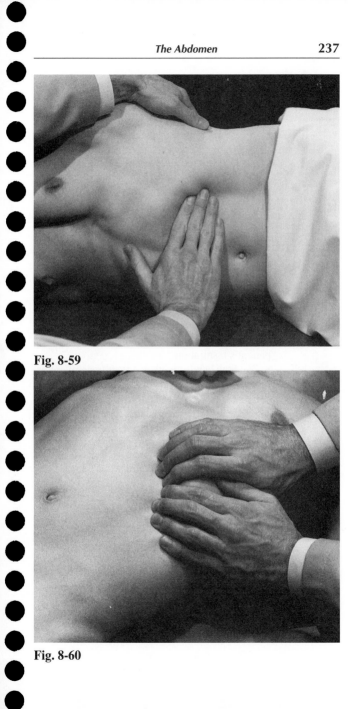

Fig. 8-59

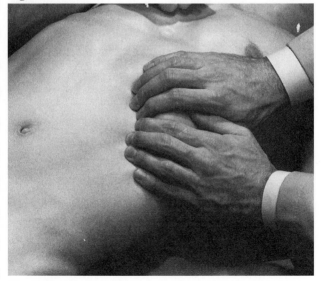

Fig. 8-60

3. Kidneys.
- Right kidney.
  —Support the flank with your left hand *(FIG. 8-61)*. Place the hand behind and below the right costal margin; this helps to displace the right kidney anteriorly.
  —Place your right hand below the right costal margin with the fingertips positioned to the left *(FIG. 8-62)*.
  —Press the two hands together and feel during a deep breath *(FIG. 8-63)*.
    - In a thin individual, you can feel the rounded lower pole as it descends during inspiration.
    - If palpable, describe its size, contour, and any tenderness.
    - The kidney is felt as a smaller, rounded, more localized mass compared to the longer, sharp, rubbery liver edge.
  —Attempt to capture the kidney at the peak of the patient's inspiration:
    - Cup both hands together at their upper margins; exert more pressure with the upper hand *(FIG. 8-64)*.
    - Ask the patient to exhale and hold it.
    - Slowly release the pressure of your fingers *(FIG. 8-65)*.
    - If the kidney is captured: you will feel it slip upward and out from your fingers.
- Left kidney: The left kidney is higher than the right and is seldom palpable normally.
  —Remain at the patient's right side. Palpate in the same manner as for the spleen, but aim the right hand more toward the left flank.
  —Attempt to capture the left kidney by moving to the patient's left side and using the same two-handed technique, this time with your *right* hand underneath the patient's flank.

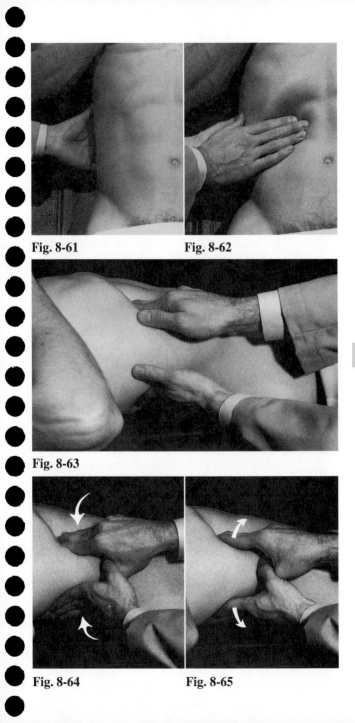

Fig. 8-61

Fig. 8-62

Fig. 8-63

Fig. 8-64

Fig. 8-65

4. Aorta.
   - Press the fingertips of the right hand deeply into the epigastric area slightly left of the midline *(FIG. 8-66)*.
     —It is common to feel the aortic pulsation, especially in thin individuals, and this may normally produce mild tenderness.
   - If the pulsation is prominent, suggesting an abdominal aortic aneurysm, try to gauge the width of the pulsation.
     —In thin individuals: *(FIG. 8-67)*
       - Encircle the pulsation with your thumb and fingers, and press inward.
       - The normal aorta is 2.5 to 4 cm wide. An aortic aneurysm is much wider; most are present at or slightly above the umbilicus.
     —In obese individuals:
       - Press the fingertips of both hands deeply in on either side of the aortic pulsation *(FIG. 8-68)*.
       - Sense the size of the aorta, as your fingers are pushed apart with each pulsation.
       - Estimate the width according to the abdominal wall thickness. An increased wall thickness will make the aortic pulsation seem wider.
   - When a prominent pulsation is felt:
     - Listen again for a possible aortic bruit.
     - Then palpate for iliac artery aneurysms in each lower quadrant *(FIG. 8-69)*.
     - Finally, see if the femoral pulses are present or absent *(FIG. 8-70)*.

5. Urinary bladder: felt as a tense suprapubic mass if distended by urine. It may be more readily outlined by percussion.

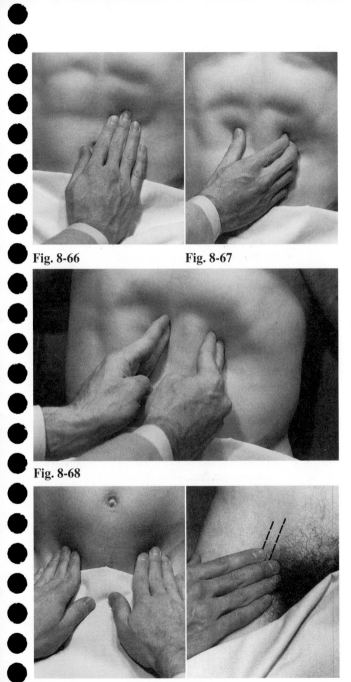

Fig. 8-66

Fig. 8-67

Fig. 8-68

Fig. 8-69

Fig. 8-70

D. Survey the Abdomen for Masses.

    1. Palpate with a two-handed technique; this is useful when additional pressure is needed to palpate the deeper abdominal structures.

- Place your nondominant hand on the abdomen.
- Rest your dominant hand on top with the distal pads of the fingers touching the nails of the lower hand.
- In this method, the upper hand applies pressure while the lower hand feels the structures beneath. This increases sensitivity of the palpating hand, since it loses sensitivity if it must exert pressure at the same time.
- The motion has three components.
   —First, push the hands forward. This gives some slack to the skin *(FIG. 8-71).*
   —Then push down with the fingertips of the upper hand. Your fingertips will curl as you press inward *(FIG. 8-72).*
   —Then press and pull back, rolling the deeper structures under your fingers *(FIG. 8-73).*

    2. Palpate thoroughly in each quadrant; always begin at the same location so you don't skip any areas.

- If the patient is apprehensive:
   —Distract him with idle conversation or review the abdominal history.
   —Begin palpating over a nontender area. Palpate tender areas last.
   —Continue watching the patient's face as you palpate. Note wincing or changes in facial expression.
- Remember that you can palpate more deeply when the patient exhales.

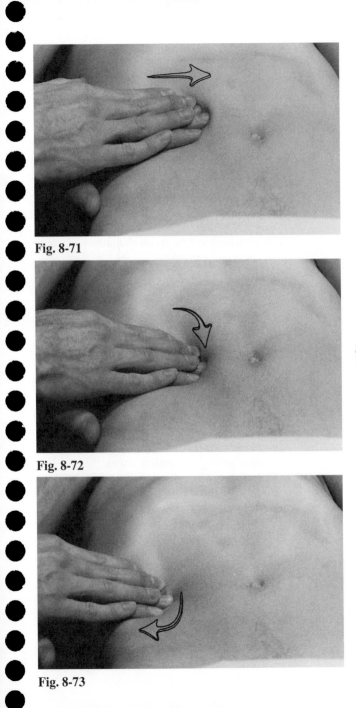

Fig. 8-71

Fig. 8-72

Fig. 8-73

3. If a mass is palpated:
   - Note its size, shape, location, consistency or texture, mobility, and whether it moves with respiration.
     —The knee-chest position may help in palpating a tumor of the omentum, stomach, lower, or transverse colon.
   - Be aware of the many "normal" masses palpable in the abdomen *(FIG. 8-74).*
     —Xiphoid process, protruding downward from the junction of the right and left inferior costal margins.
     —Lateral border of the rectus abdominus muscle or its rectangular segments.
     —Stool-filled ascending or descending colon.
       • Or sigmoid colon low in the left lower quadrant, felt as a tender, tubular structure.
     —Distended bladder or pregnant uterus.
     —Sacral promontory; felt usually in thin individuals.
       • It presents as a fixed, stony hard mass deep in the abdomen below the umbilicus.
       • Its location and consistency resembles a tumor mass to the unaware.
     —Aorta or iliac arteries.
   - If you can't tell if a mass or tender area is deep or in the muscle wall: *(FIG. 8-75)*
     —Palpate again as the patient strains.
       • Have him lift his head off the pillow. In young patients, ask them to raise their feet a few inches above the examination table.
     —As the muscles tighten *(FIG. 8-76).*
       • Masses or tenderness in the wall itself will remain prominent.
       • Deeper masses will become less palpable and visceral tenderness will be less prominent, since the tensed abdominal wall now acts as a barrier to deep palpation.

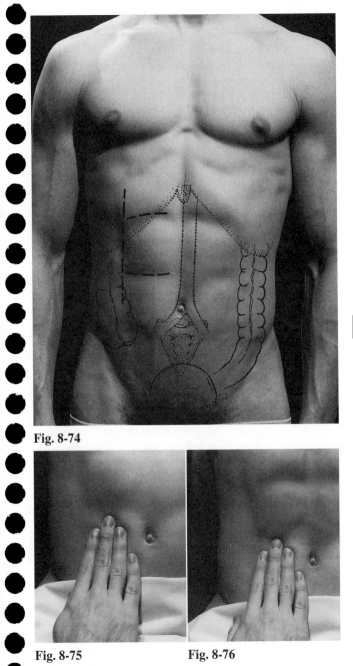

Fig. 8-74

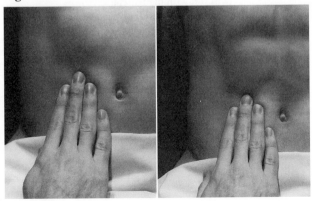

Fig. 8-75   **Fig. 8-76**

VI. ADDITIONAL TESTS.

A. **Ascites** (free intraabdominal fluid) often presents as an enlarged abdomen with bulging flanks. It can be confirmed by percussion or palpation.

1. Percussion: check for shifting dullness.
   - This test relies on the fact that, in ascites, air-filled loops of bowel always rise to the most superior portion of the abdomen, floating on the ascites fluid.
   - With the patient supine, percuss from the umbilical area outward in several directions *(FIG. 8-77)*. Map the lateral border between tympany and dullness.

     —In normal subjects, there will be patchy distribution of tympany and dullness across the superior abdomen.

     —In patients with ascites, the central abdomen will be prominently tympanitic, representing air-filled loops of bowel, with a more well-defined circular border of dullness, representing the settling out of ascites fluid.
   - Then roll the patient onto one side. Percuss and mark the border again between tympany and dullness.

     —In normal subjects, the borders usually remain constant through the change in position. In other words, the areas of tympany and dullness will roll with the patient.

     —With ascites: *(FIG. 8-78)*, as the patient rolls to one side, the area of tympany will rise to the uppermost flank, now the most superior portion of the abdomen. The air-filled loops of bowel are "floating to the top." The level of dullness will also rise nearer to the umbilicus, as the air-filled loops of bowel are displaced upward by fluid.

2. Palpate for a fluid wave *(FIG. 8-79)*. This sign is most positive with gross ascites.
   - Place your hand on either flank.
   - Have an assistant press the ulnar edge of his hands down into the midline of the abdomen. Or, have the patient place his/her hand in the same location.

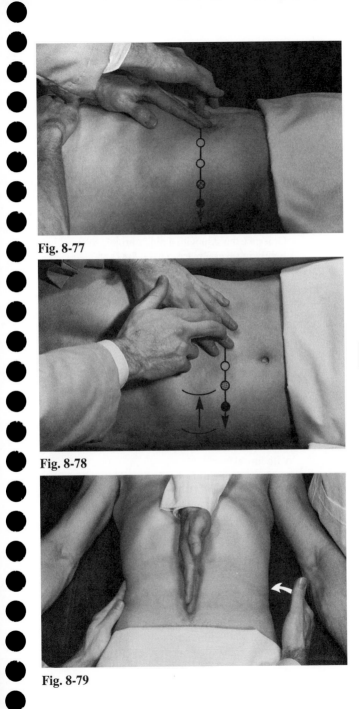

Fig. 8-77

Fig. 8-78

Fig. 8-79

—This prevents transmission of a wave through the abdominal wall.
- Tap sharply with one hand.
- With ascites, you will feel an impulse (fluid wave) strike the other hand.

B. Tests for Peritoneal Inflammation: use caution, since even localized peritonitis can be painful.

  1. Check for cutaneous hyperesthesia.
- Gently pull at the skin; lift a fold away from the underlying muscle; do not pinch *(FIG. 8-80)*.
- Or stroke the skin with a pin or broken tongue blade lightly in several places *(FIG. 8-81)*.
- Ask if this feels sharper or painful in a particular location: an indication of peritonitis.

  2. Rebound tenderness: This is usually assessed when greater than normal tenderness is present.
- CAUTION! Perform this test near the end of the examination, since the pain and subsequent muscle spasm that may occur can interfere with further probing.
- Press the fingertips firmly but slowly into the abdomen near the suspicious area *(FIG. 8-82)*.
- Then quickly remove them *(FIG. 8-83)*.
- Rebound tenderness is present if pain occurs during withdrawal.
    —The patient will feel a sharp stab of pain; this indicates the parietal peritoneum is inflamed. Having the patient cough may produce the same result.
- Have him point to the site of pain. It is often quite removed from your palpating fingers.
    —In acute appendicitis, test for rebound by pressing in the left lower quadrant. Sudden release may cause pain in the *right* lower quadrant. This is known as *Rovsing's sign.*
- An alternate method is to lightly percuss the abdominal wall with one finger. The patient will feel irritation at the site of peritoneal inflammation.

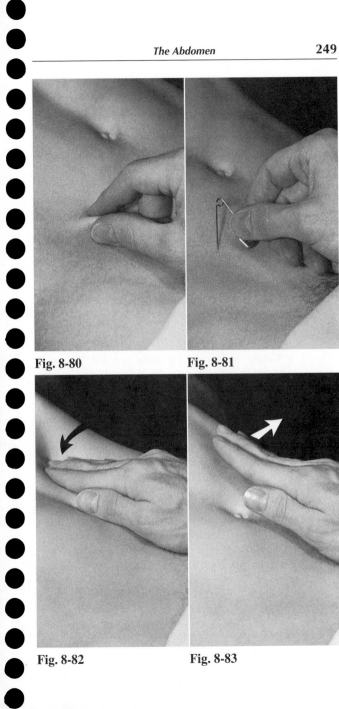

Fig. 8-80

Fig. 8-81

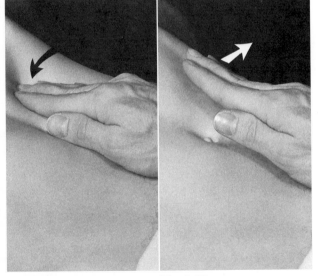

Fig. 8-82

Fig. 8-83

3. Psoas muscle test.
   ▪ There are two methods.
     —With the patient supine, ask him to flex his thigh. Resist this motion with your hand above his knee *(FIG. 8-84).*
     —With the patient on his left side (or vice versa), passively extend the right leg at the hip *(FIG 8-85).*
   ▪ Inflammation near the psoas muscle, as with an extrapelvic appendicitis, causes lower quadrant pain on the side tested.
4. Obturator muscle test.
   ▪ With the patient supine, flex the knee and hip 90 degrees.
   ▪ Grasp the ankle and rotate the hip internally and externally *(FIG. 8-86).*
   ▪ Intrapelvic inflammation, often from appendicitis, will cause lower quadrant pain on the affected side.
5. In children, a very useful screening test for peritonitis is the *jump* test.
   ▪ Simply ask the child to jump in place. With peritoneal irritation, the child will complain of abdominal pain.
   ▪ In adults, this phenomenon is demonstrated during the patient's ride to the hospital or doctor's office. Simply ask "How was the ride here?" With peritoneal irritation, the patient will complain they felt pain with each bump in the road.
6. Finally, whenever peritonitis is uncertain by the previous tests, perform a rectal or pelvic examination. These are described further in Chapters 9 and 10.
C. **Renal Percussion Tenderness.**
   1. If you suspect costovertebral angle tenderness, begin very gently! In acute pyelonephritis, this can be very painful.
   2. First, place your fingers over the costovertebral angle and lightly "jiggle" the skin. If no pain results, proceed further.
   3. Place your left palm over one costovertebral angle.
   4. Percuss lightly, then firmly with your right fist *(FIG. 8-87).* Check each side.

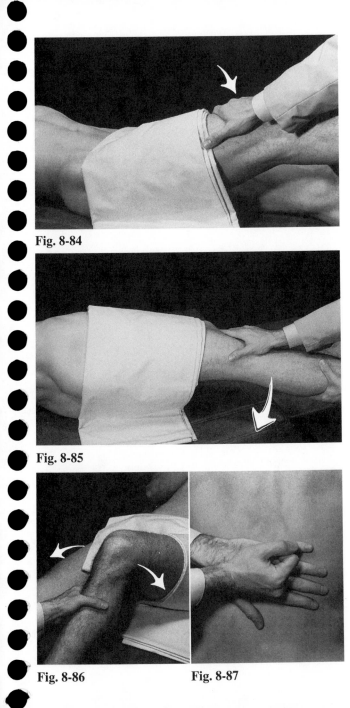

Fig. 8-84

Fig. 8-85

Fig. 8-86

Fig. 8-87

5. The patient should normally feel the impact, but not pain.
   - Pain in this location can signal either pyelonephritis or paraspinal muscle tenderness. The tenderness in pyelonephritis tends to be more localized, whereas paraspinal muscle tenderness tends to run the length of the lumbar paraspinal muscle.

9 Male Genitalia

I. ITEMS NEEDED FOR EXAMINATION:

A. Disposable Examination Gloves, Lubricant, Gauze Squares, Tissues.

B. Strong Light Source (flashlight, otoscope, or transilluminator).

C. Materials for Bacteriologic Evaluation.

1. Thayer-Martin or similar media.
2. Chlamydia test media or DNA probe.
3. Sterile calcium alginate swabs.
4. Glass slides and cover slips.

D. Occult-Blood Test Paper and Developer.

II. EXAMINER'S ATTITUDE

A. It Is Normal for the Beginning Student to Feel Anxious or Awkward About Examining the Male Genitalia.

1. The learning of proper examination technique and repeated practice will build confidence.
2. Let your own feelings of awkwardness be a reminder of the vulnerability the patient feels in receiving this examination.

III. PATIENT PREPARATION.

A. Emotional.

1. Because of past experiences in sports-related activities and the normal trials of growing up, most males are aware of the extreme sensitivity of their genitals to touch and, in particular, to pressure.
   - The examiner should be aware of this and should approach this portion of the examination slowly and gently.

2. Some patients, out of modesty, will be reluctant to have their genitals examined by a female practitioner. In most cases, after the initial reluctance, the patient will allow the examination to continue.
   - Just as with the pelvic examination, a few patients have a strong and declared preference for a same-sex examiner, and their wishes should be respected, if possible.

3. The patient will occasionally have an erection during the examination, regardless of the sex of the examiner. This is a normal and autonomic response.
   - When this does occur, reassure him that an erection sometimes occurs and is normal.

B. Patient Comfort.

1. The room should be comfortably warm.

2. If your hands are cold, warm them in running water before you begin.

3. The patient may remain gowned and may also wear additional clothing on the upper torso.
   - If the patient is uncomfortably cool, the scrotum may contract, making palpation of its contents more difficult.

C. Patient Positioning.

1. He may be supine or standing, depending on his ability.

2. If the patient is standing, seat yourself.

3. Although the pictures that follow show ungloved hands, using disposable gloves is a recommended technique.
   - If the patient has a latex allergy, use vinyl gloves.

IV. GENITAL EXAMINATION.

A. Assessment of Sexual Maturity (in adolescents).

1. Using Tanner's stages according to three criteria (see Appendix B).

2. In general, if a boy's testes have increased in size to 2.5 centimeters or more, or if his pubic hair has reached stage 2, he can be reassured that sexual development has begun. The time of onset of adult sexual characteristics is extremely variable.

3. In the adult male, the pubic hair rises in the midline toward the umbilicus.

B. Penis.
   1. Inspection *(FIG. 9-1)*.
      - Patients are sometimes concerned whether their penis is too small or too large. It is important to be aware of his overt or covert concerns.
      - Grasp the shaft gently with thumb and forefinger and inspect all sides of the glans.
         —Note its color, which varies from pink to light brown in Caucasians and from light to dark brown in African-Americans.
         —Note any scars, ulcerations, nodules, or signs of inflammation.
            • If an ulceration is seen, palpate it with a gloved finger for tenderness and consistency.
            • Painless penile ulcerations commonly occur in primary syphilis. Painful clusters of ulcerations are more often herpes simplex.
      - If the patient is uncircumcised, retract the foreskin or ask the patient to do it.
         —The foreskin should be easily retractable from the glans, and easy to return to its original position *(FIG. 9-2)*.
            • Phimosis exists when the foreskin cannot be retracted.
            • If the foreskin has been left retracted for too long, or in other causes of inflammation, it swells, termed *paraphimosis,* and cannot be returned to its original position.
            • Note any fissuring in the edge of the foreskin, which may represent infection. When inflammation is present, culture any discharge for causative agents (which can be aerobic, anaerobic, or fungal).
         —Some whitish material, termed smegma, may be found under the glans.

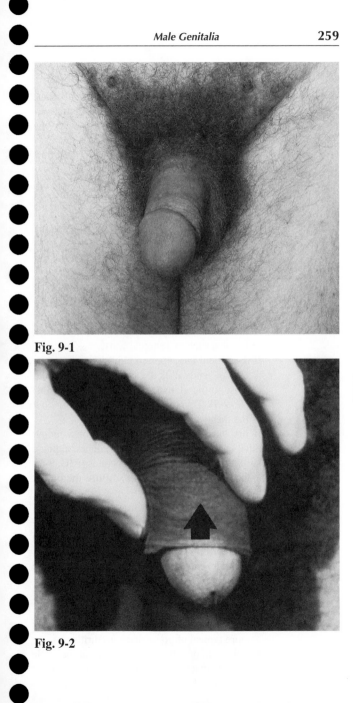

Fig. 9-1

Fig. 9-2

- Note the size and position of the urethral meatus *(FIG. 9-3)*.
  —Should be positioned rather centrally on the glans.
  - When the urethra is located on the ventral surface, anywhere along the shaft down to the perineum, it is termed *hypospadias*.
  - When the urethra is similarly displaced dorsally, it is termed *epispadias*.
  —When hypospadias or epispadias is seen, describe the location of the urethral meatus as precisely as possible:
  - For hypospadias, the locations are glandular, penile, penoscrotal, or perineal.
  - For epispadias, describe it as glandular, penile, or complete.
- Then gently compress the glans and inspect the meatus. This opens the distal end of the urethra for inspection *(FIG. 9-4)*.
  —Observe for patency, inflammation, discharge, or lesions, such as venereal warts.
  —If the patient has reported a discharge but none is visible, gently milk the shaft of the penis from its base to the glans (or have the patient do it) *(FIG. 9-5)*. This may bring some discharge out of the meatus.
  —If discharge is present, note its consistency: thick or watery. Gently insert a calcium alginate swab and let it absorb for 15 seconds *(FIG. 9-6)*.
  - Inoculate an appropriate culture media for gonorrhea.
  - Swab a glass slide for Gram stain *(FIG. 9-7)*.
  - Swab the appropriate receptacle for *Chlamydia* testing, or use a DNA probe, which often tests for both *Chlamydia* and gonorrhea.
  —Discharge can help determine the causative agent. Although not absolute:
  - Scant watery discharge is more typical of chlamydial urethritis.
  - Thick, copious yellow-green discharge is more typical of gonorrheae urethritis.
  - If present, note the color and size of the circle of dried discharge on the patient's underwear as a clue.

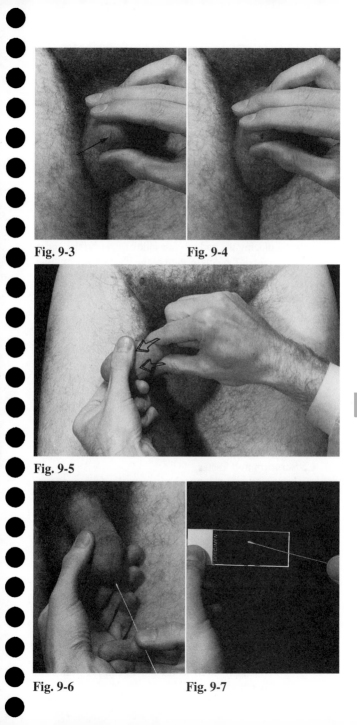

Fig. 9-3

Fig. 9-4

Fig. 9-5

Fig. 9-6

Fig. 9-7

2. Palpation.
   ▪ While still gently holding the glans in one hand,
     inspect and palpate the shaft between the thumb
     and fingers of the other hand *(FIG. 9-8)*.
       —It should feel smooth and semifirm in consis-
         tency.
       —The overlying skin appears slightly wrinkled
         and feels slightly movable over the underlying
         structures.
       —Note swellings, nodules, and induration.
   ▪ The urethral area can be palpated more directly by
     placing the pad of your index finger on the under-
     side of the penile shaft at the base (in the midline)
     and pressing gently upward. Continue palpating in
     steps upward to the glans.
       —Feel for local tenderness or thickening.
   ▪ If you retracted the foreskin, return it to its usual
     position before you continue *(FIG. 9-9)*.
   ▪ Examine the base of the penis for rashes or signs of
     pubic lice *(FIG. 9-10)*.
       —If you suspect pubic lice, look closely at the pu-
         bic hair shafts for attached lice (brown-black) or
         nits (white). An ophthalmoscope serves nicely
         as an illuminated and highly powered magnifier
         to identify lice.

C. **Scrotum and Testes.**
   1. Functional anatomy.
      ▪ The scrotum is a musculocutaneous pouch that
        contains the testes, epididymides, and spermatic
        cords.
      ▪ It functions as a thermal regulator, keeping the
        testes 1° or 2° cooler than normal body tempera-
        ture.
      ▪ Its external appearance varies with different con-
        ditions.
          —In children, or when cold, it is wrinkled and
            short and is contracted firmly around the testes.
          —In the elderly, or when warm, the scrotum hangs
            loosely with the testes within.
      ▪ Normally, both testes are in the scrotum at or
        shortly after birth.

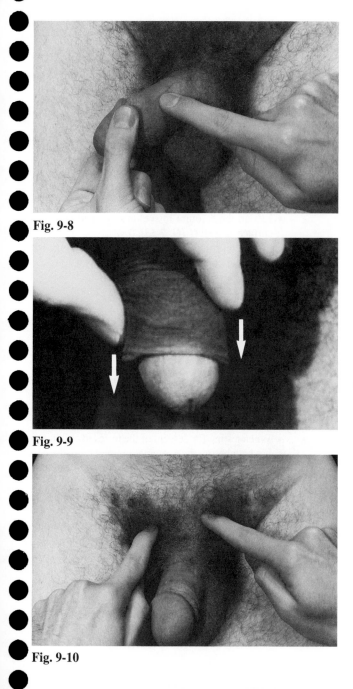

Fig. 9-8

Fig. 9-9

Fig. 9-10

2. Inspection.
  ▪ Either you or the patient should lift the penis out of
    the way to facilitate observation of the scrotal skin.
    If possible, the patient should be standing *(FIG.
    9-11).* Note:
    —Its general size, shape, symmetry, and any
      swelling. The left scrotal sac usually hangs
      slightly lower than the right.
    —Its skin for nodules, inflammation, ulcerations,
      or other lesions *(FIG. 9-12).* The skin is nor-
      mally wrinkled.
  ▪ Lift up the scrotum to see its sides and posterior
    surface as well *(FIG. 9-13).*
    —The scrotum and inner thighs (especially the
      area in contact with the scrotum) is a common
      site for fungal infections.

3. Palpation.
  ▪ This should be performed very gently for several
    reasons.
    —Pressure on the testicles causes a very unpleas-
      ant deep aching sensation.
    —Stimulation of the scrotum activates the cremas-
      teric reflex, which causes the scrotal muscula-
      ture to contract. This renders palpation more dif-
      ficult.
  ▪ When testing for descent of the testes in children, a
    hot bath before the examination may relax the cre-
    masteric muscle and allow the testis to descend
    into its normal scrotal position.
    —If a testis is in the inguinal canal, attempt to
      draw it into the scrotum as follows:
      • Stand on the same side as you wish to examine.
      • Form your index and middle finger into an in-
        verted "V." Place it over the midpoint of the
        inguinal ligament and gently push toward the
        scrotum.
      • The testicle, felt as a soft, marblelike mass,
        will be felt by the examining fingers of the
        other hand.
    —A truly undescended testicle cannot be moved.

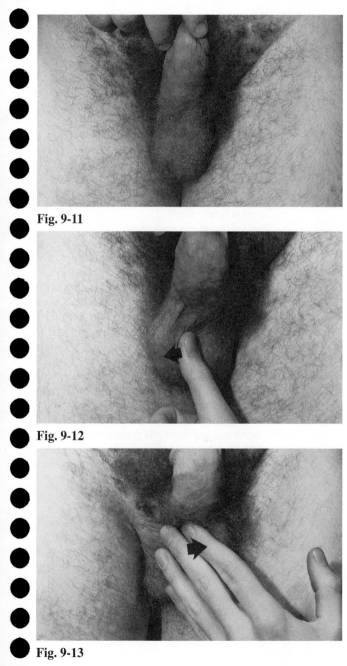

Fig. 9-11

Fig. 9-12

Fig. 9-13

- Gently grasp each testicle between thumb and first two fingers *(FIG. 9-14)*.
  —Note their size, shape, consistency, and any tenderness. After puberty, the normal testes are:
    - About 4 cm in length and ovoid in shape.
    - Smooth and rubbery (softer texture in the elderly).
    - Freely movable and equal in size.
    - They usually lie in the scrotum with their long axis in the vertical position.
  —Palpate carefully for nodules or other masses. If a mass is felt, note:
    - Its size and any tenderness.
    - Whether the mass is attached to the testicle (such as a tumor or spermatocele) or if it comes from above (such as a hernia).
    - If attached, note its position in relation to the testis; anterior, above, or behind.
    - Whether it transilluminates (see p. 268).
  —If one or both of the testes are not palpable in adults, try to find it within the inguinal canal (see technique on p. 264).
- Palpate the epididymis overlying each testicle.
  —This is a soft ridge of tissue adherent to the back, top, and lateral side of each testicle.
  —Gently brace one testicle in front with your thumb and forefinger and palpate the epididymis with the other hand *(FIG. 9-15)*.
    - Use a gentle pinching motion, probing each part of the epididymis; it is more irregular and granular in texture than the testes.
    - Palpate for masses or tenderness.
    - In some cases of inflammation, termed *epididymitis,* the testes and epididymis are indistinguishable, and usually *very* tender.

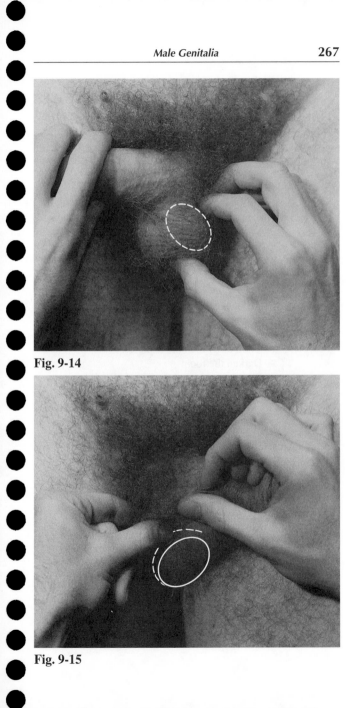

Fig. 9-14

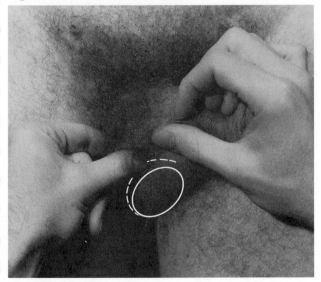

Fig. 9-15

- Palpate the spermatic cord.
  —Grasp the soft, tubular structure as it emerges from the base of the epididymis, using the thumb and forefinger *(FIG. 9-16).*
  —The vas deferens is felt as a distinct but movable cord within. The accompanying vessels and nerves are felt as thin fibers near the vas.
    • Palpate for tenderness or beading.
    • A varicocele is a collection of dilated veins surrounding the vas, usually in the left scrotum. It will feel warm and spongy to the touch, often with a "bag of worms" sensation. If you feel this, repeat the examination with the patient supine. The veins will collapse.
  —Follow the cord upward to its entrance into the inguinal canal.
- Further test any scrotal masses with transillumination. This is used to evaluate any swelling in the scrotum other than the testicles.
  —Darken the room.
  —Place a strong light source behind the scrotum and shine it through the mass *(FIG. 9-17).* You can use a flashlight, transilluminator attachment, or an otoscope without its plastic speculum.
  —Look for transmission of the light as a red glow.
    • This occurs normally or with clear cystic masses, such as a hydrocele.
    • Light will not transmit through a solid tumor or a blood-filled cyst.

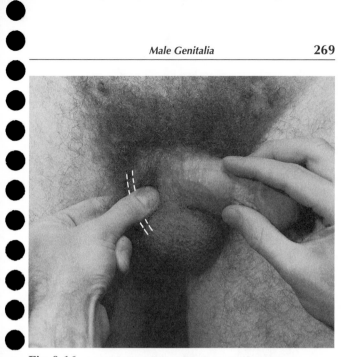

Fig. 9-16

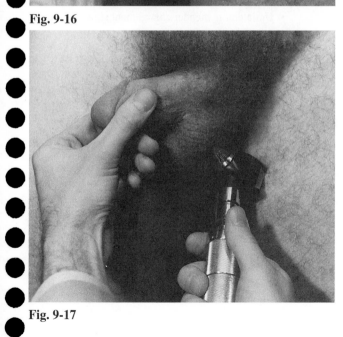

Fig. 9-17

V. PALPATION OF INGUINAL LYMPH NODES.
A. Lymph Nodes.
1. Anatomy *(FIG. 9-18)*.
   - The superficial inguinal nodes are formed in two clusters.
     —The horizontal group (1), which are located just under the midpoint of the inguinal ligament. These drain the region of the penis, scrotal skin, anal canal, and gluteal region.
     —The vertical (or subinguinal) group (2), located a few centimeters more inferior and medially. These drain the lower leg, excluding the heel.
     —Drainage from the urethra and testes passes to the iliac and periaortic nodes, which are not normally palpable.
   - Unilateral tender enlargement of these palpable nodes should prompt a search for signs of infection on the penis (such as herpes simplex), scrotum, or ipsilateral leg (such as a cellulitis).
   - Unilateral nontender enlargement signals a similar search for malignancy.

2. Method
   - Palpate each side with a rolling motion *(FIG. 9-19)*. Small (0.5 cm.), soft, nontender, movable nodes are palpable normally.

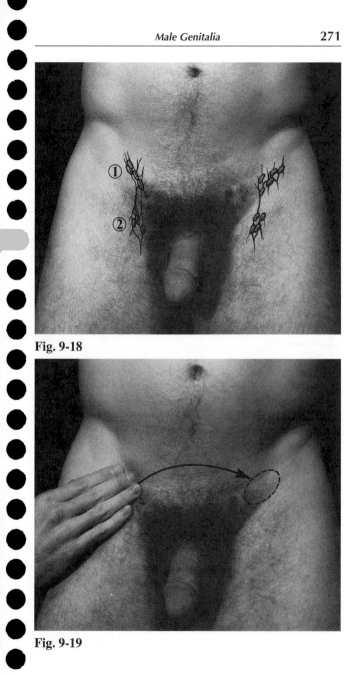

Fig. 9-18

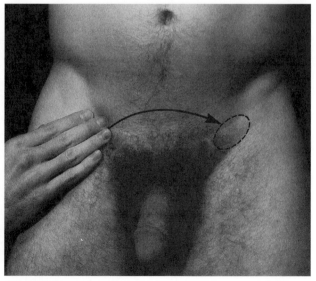

Fig. 9-19

VI. HERNIAS: Screening is advised for all patients.

A. Patient Position: Best done with the patient standing, but can also be done supine if the patient is debilitated.

B. Anatomy: The inguinal canal is a narrow tunnel through the abdominal wall *(FIG. 9-20)*.
1. Its internal opening (internal inguinal ring), lies about 1 cm above the midpoint of the inguinal ligament, and its external inguinal ring opens near the pubic ramus.

2. The inguinal canal allows the structures within the spermatic cord, especially the vas deferens, to pass into the abdomen.

3. Weakening of the inguinal canal produces inguinal hernias.
   - Either *direct,* through the canal wall.
   - Or *indirect,* traveling through the internal inguinal ring and sometimes into the scrotum.
   - These are usually seen as a bulging near the pubic ramus but above the inguinal ligament, which is marked by a groin crease.

4. Weakening of the femoral canal produces femoral hernias, seen as a bulging near the pubic ramus but below the inguinal ligament. They are not common in men.

C. Inspection *(FIG. 9-21).*
1. Locate the inguinal ligament by drawing an imaginary line from the anterior superior iliac spine to the edge of the pubic ramus.

2. Ask the patient to bear down. Straining is preferred to coughing because a more sustained pressure occurs. Also, the impulse of a cough sometimes mimics the impulse of a hernia.

3. Watch for bulging above (inguinal hernia) or below the inguinal ligament (femoral hernia).

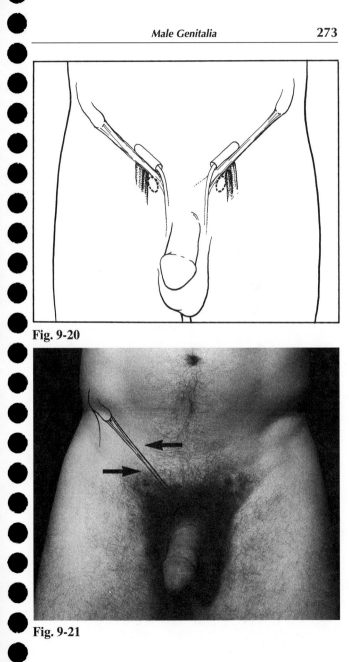

Fig. 9-20

Fig. 9-21

D. Palpation: Inguinal Hernias. Use your right hand for the patient's right side and your left hand for his left side.

1. Place your right index finger low on the anterior-lateral surface of the right scrotum. This will give the skin some slack needed to probe further *(FIG. 9-22).*

2. Infold the skin as you guide your finger upward, following the spermatic cord *(FIG. 9-23).*

3. When you reach the external inguinal ring, it will feel like a triangular slitlike opening through which the spermatic cord passes.
   - Invaginate the skin with your index finger and enter the external ring *(FIG. 9-24).*
   - Then turn your finger slightly outward, so the pad of your fingertip is aiming both posteriorly and inferiorly.
   - Gently enter the inguinal canal and attempt to reach the internal inguinal ring. Your finger is now parallel to the inguinal ligament and is aimed toward the anterior superior iliac spine.
   - Stop at any point if you feel resistance or the patient voices discomfort.

4. If no mass is felt, ask him to cough or bear down *(FIG. 9-25).*
   - A direct inguinal hernia, if present, will be felt as a soft mass pressing against the ventral pad of your fingertip.
   - An indirect inguinal hernia will be similarly felt, but descending onto the tip of your finger.

5. Remove your finger and use your other hand for the left side. Inform him that he may experience a transient aching sensation in this area (from slight stretching of the inguinal canal).

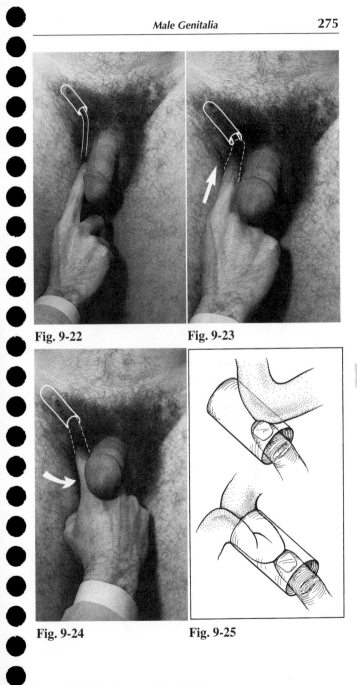

Fig. 9-22

Fig. 9-23

Fig. 9-24

Fig. 9-25

E. Palpation: Femoral Hernias.
  1. Estimate its location:
  - Place your right index finger on the right femoral pulse *(FIG. 9-26)*.
  - Your middle finger then lies over the femoral vein and your ring finger on the femoral canal.

  2. Ask the patient to strain, and feel for bulging.
  - If present, the hernia presents as a reducible bulge below the inguinal ligament.
  - It is usually firm, small, and may resemble an enlarged lymph node.

  3. Repeat on the left side.

F. If You Find a Large Mass, either inguinal, scrotal, or femoral and suspect it may be a herniation:
  1. Ask the patient to lie down on the examination table. The mass may return to the abdomen by itself.

  2. If it does not, try to gently reduce it back into the abdominal cavity using sustained pressure with your fingers *(FIG. 9-27)*.
  - Do not attempt this if the mass is tender, or if the patient feels nausea.
  - Do not persist if this pressure causes pain.

  3. You can also ask the patient if he has been able to reduce it himself, and ask him to demonstrate.

  4. Listen to the mass with a stethoscope to see if bowel sounds are present *(FIG. 9-28)*.

  5. A tender or nonreducible mass may be an incarcerated hernia, and requires surgical evaluation.

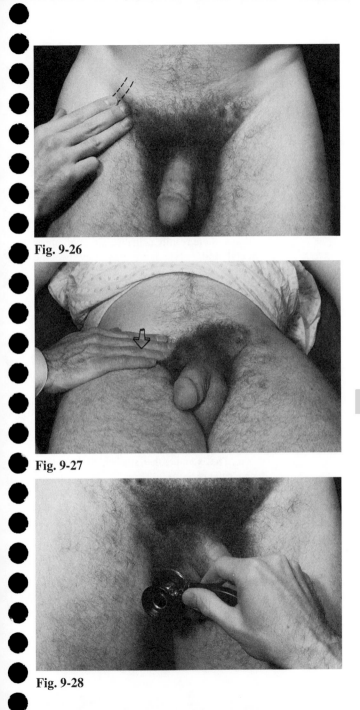

Fig. 9-26

Fig. 9-27

Fig. 9-28

VII. RECTAL AND PROSTATE EXAMINATION.
A. Preparation.
  1. Patient positioning: three positions can be used:
   - The left-lateral (Sims) position.
     —The patient is positioned on his left side near the edge of the examination table *(FIG. 9-29)*. A pillow is placed under his head.
     —The superior thigh and knee are flexed, bringing the knee close to the chest.
     —This moves the rectal ampulla into a more inferior and posterior position, making any rectal masses more readily palpable, although upper rectal and pelvic structures may become slightly less palpable.
     —This position is usually the most comfortable for the patient.
   - The knee-chest position *(FIG. 9-30)*.
     —The patient kneels on the examination table, then flexes forward to rest his head and shoulders on the table's surface. His knees are positioned more widely apart than the hips.
   - The standing position *(FIG. 9-31)*.
     —The patient bends forward over the examination table, supporting himself on his elbows.
     —This position and the knee-chest position are widely used for prostatic evaluation and massage. The examiner then sits behind the patient on a stool.
   - In debilitated patients, the lithotomy position can be used, with the patient supine and hips and knees flexed and drawn up on either side.
     —This hinders prostate palpation but does allow bimanual bladder palpation.

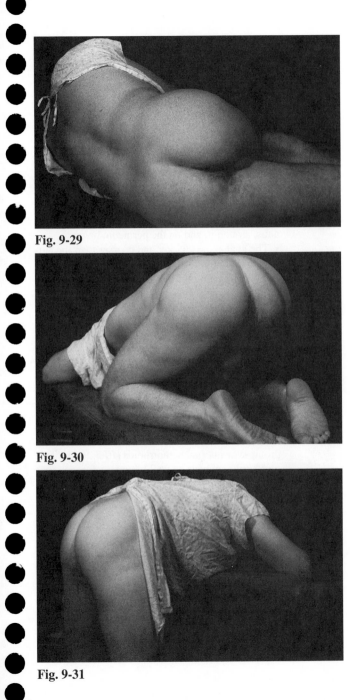

Fig. 9-29

Fig. 9-30

Fig. 9-31

2. Urine samples.
    ■ It is best to collect a routine specimen before rectal examination.
    ■ Prostatic manipulation can force secretions into the posterior urethra. If this secretion contains pus, a voided specimen collected after palpation will be contaminated by it.

B. Anal Inspection: wear disposable gloves on both hands.

1. Spread the buttocks and inspect the skin on the anus, around it, and on the perineum below.
    ■ The anal skin is darker and coarser than the surrounding area *(FIG. 9-32).*
    ■ Note any skin tags, external hemorrhoids or fistula openings, signs of inflammation, and condyloma acuminata (genital warts).

2. Gently stretch the anal skin with thumb and forefinger and look for an anal fissure.
    ■ This is a painful triangular split of the skin, usually posteriorly, just at or within the anal margin.
    ■ There may be a small "sentinel" skin tag at the anus, just distal to the fissure.

3. Ask the patient to bear down and inspect for rectal prolapse or internal hemorrhoids *(FIG. 9-33).* This may further expose an anal fissure.

4. Also inspect the sacrococcygeal area for pilonidal cysts or sinus openings.

5. Describe any lesions by locating them on the face of a clock, with the 12 o'clock position directly superior *(see Fig. 10-75).*

6. If an anal fissure is found, digital rectal examination should be either performed very cautiously or postponed.

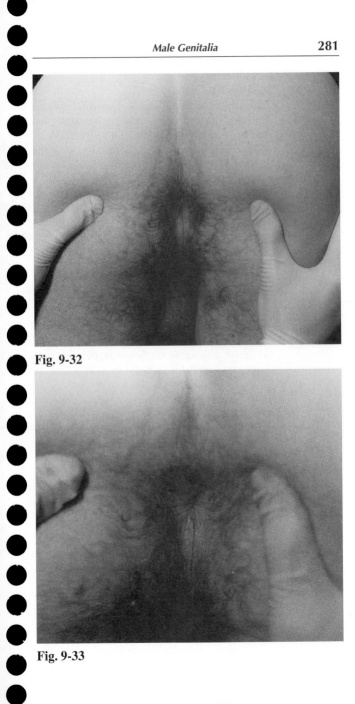

Fig. 9-32

Fig. 9-33

C. Rectal Palpation.

  1. Anatomy *(FIG. 9-34).*
     - The anal canal goes directly inward for about 3 cm then angles sharply upward, becoming the rectum, and follows the curve of the sacrum.
     - The anal canal is wrapped distally with the sphincter muscles and proximally with the levator ani muscle.
     - The prostate gland indents the rectum and is palpable through its anterior wall.

  2. Apply lubricant *(FIG. 9-35).*
     - Either allow the gel to drop onto your gloved fingers,
     - Or place some gel onto a square of sterile gauze (see *Fig. 10-47*). Swab your fingers through it.
     - *Never* allow your examining fingers to touch the tube's opening. This may cause contamination of the tube. If this happens, discard the tube.
       —Small, disposable single-use tubes or packets are also available to avoid the contamination potential of multi-use tubes.

  3. Inform the patient.
     - By its nature, the examination causes some discomfort.
     - Explain what you are going to do, and that it will be briefly uncomfortable but not painful. Also mention this may produce a sensation of having to move his bowels; the sensation will stop as soon as you remove your finger.
     - Tell the patient you will now apply some lubricant to the anus.

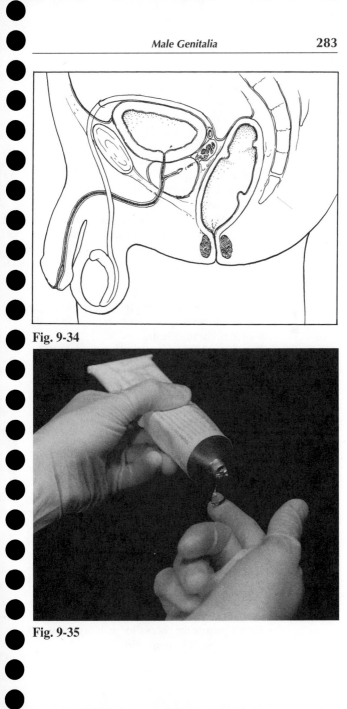

Fig. 9-34

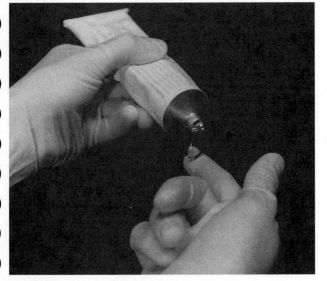

Fig. 9-35

4. Make initial contact. This description assumes a right-handed examiner. Reverse sides if you are left-handed.
   - Spread the patient's left buttocks with your left hand *(FIG. 9-36).* Apply some of the lubricant from your finger onto the anus.
   - Place the pad of your right index finger on the anus and apply gentle pressure.
     —Wait a few seconds. This relaxes the anal sphincter.
       • Attempting to enter too quickly can result in sphincter spasm and a painful examination.
     —Ask the patient to bear down, as if having a bowel movement.

5. Insert the finger *(FIG. 9-37).*
   - Gently increasing finger pressure, let the finger slip into the anal canal. Aim your finger in the direction of the umbilicus.
   - The anal sphincter should admit the finger with some resistance but without pain.
     —If the sphincter tightens, wait a few seconds before continuing. Do not persist if it causes pain.

6. Palpate the anal canal.
   - As you enter, note the tone of the anal sphincter.
   - Rotate your finger to examine the entire muscular ring.
   - Then ask him to tighten his muscles around your finger; this is a useful measure of sphincter strength. Sphincter laxity may indicate neurogenic disease.
   - Palpate for the levator ani muscle over its posterior and lateral attachments to the rectal wall. This is done by feeling the proximal portion of the anal canal just before it widens into the rectum.
   - Gently palpate the coccyx for mobility and sensitivity; it should be nontender.

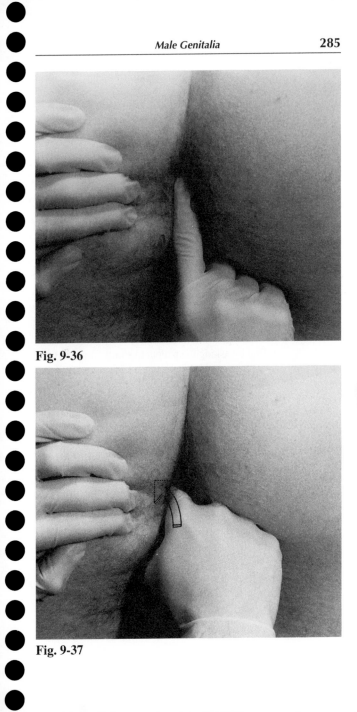

Fig. 9-36

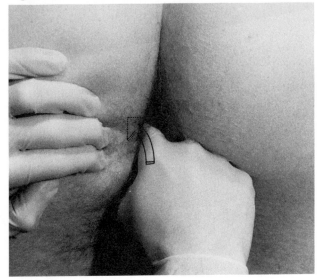

Fig. 9-37

7. Palpate the rectum, turning your finger to face each side in turn *(FIG. 9-38)*.
   ▪ Feel the anterior, left lateral, posterior, and right lateral rectal walls *(FIG. 9-39)*. Note how the rectum curves backwards, following the curve of the sacrum. Make sure to rotate your finger through the entire 360 degrees at different levels.
     —Be aware that the rectum between the 12:00 and 3:00 o'clock positions is hard to reach. You may need to turn slightly away from the patient to rotate your right index finger counter-clockwise enough.
   ▪ The walls should normally feel smooth to the examining finger. Note the presence of tumors or polyps.
     —Feces simulate carcinoma but can be squashed and moved around.
     —True carcinoma is quite firm and, if not in a polyp, is often immobile.
   ▪ End by asking the patient to strain. This can bring masses another 7 to 10 cm higher within reach. Palpate deeply for rectal lesions that are barely out of reach *(FIG. 9-40)*.
     —Rectosigmoid carcinomas, felt as an induration in the rectal wall, are often located at this upper border of reach.

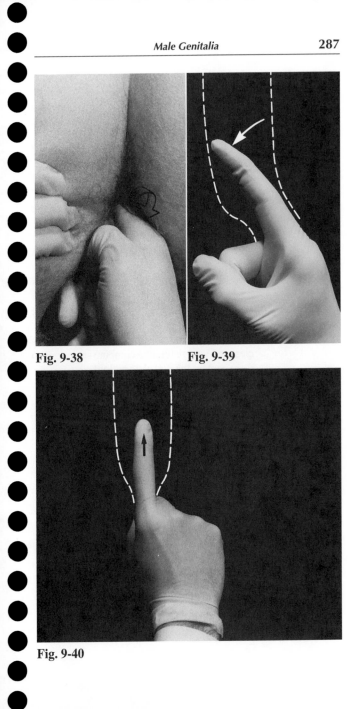

Fig. 9-38   Fig. 9-39

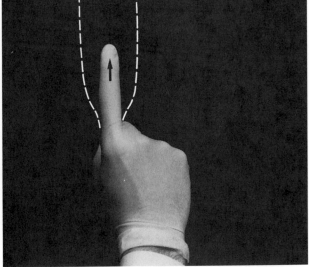

Fig. 9-40

D. Prostate Palpation.
  1. Anatomy *(FIG. 9-41)*.
   - Posteriorly, the prostate is 2 to 3 cm long and roughly triangular in shape, being wider at the top where it joins the bladder neck.
   - Its two lateral lobes are separated by a central groove (1).
   - The seminal vesicles are two soft, corrugated structures (2).
     —They extend upward and laterally from the junction of the prostate gland and bladder.
     —At their attachment to the prostate, they join with the internal portion of the vasa deferentia (3).
       • Neither seminal vesicles or vasa deferentia are normally palpable.
       • With infection, they may become firm and tender.
     —These three structures; prostate, seminal vesicles, and vasa deferentia combine secretions to form semen, the ejaculatory fluid.
   - The gland is located just anterior to the rectum and is palpable through the anterior rectal wall.

  2. Palpation. (The patient may feel the urge to urinate during prostate palpation and should be told this beforehand.)
   - Direct your finger anteriorly and outline its surface *(FIG. 9-42)*.

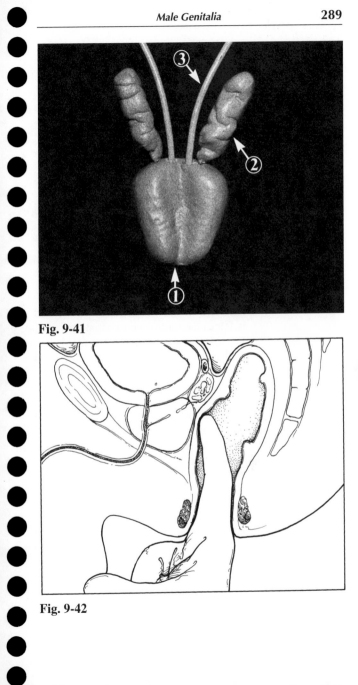

Fig. 9-41

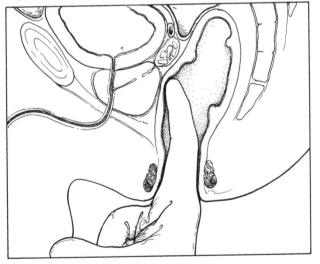

Fig. 9-42

- Note:
  - —Its width *(FIG. 9-43)*, normally about 2 to 3 cm.
  - —Length *(FIG. 9-44)*, normally about 3 cm.
  - —Central groove *(FIG. 9-45)*, which is more prominent closer to the junction with the bladder above.
    - The sulcus is often absent with prostatic hypertrophy or carcinoma.
  - —Consistency *(FIG. 9-46)*, which is normally firm and rubbery, similar to the thenar eminence when the thumb is pressed tightly to the little finger.
    - Softening (bogginess) can occur with infection.
    - Stony hardness can occur with carcinoma, chronic fibrosis, or prostatic calculi.
  - —Mobility *(FIG. 9-47)*.
    - Moderate mobility is normally present and is felt as the fingertip presses into the midline sulcus and moves from side to side.
    - With advanced carcinoma, the gland is fixed because of local extension through the gland's capsule.
  - —Tenderness.
    - The gland is normally nontender, although there is a vague visceral discomfort felt with finger pressure.
- Also note:
  - —Any enlargement of the gland.
    - Graded 1 to 4, for bulging from 1 to 3 cm into the rectal lumen.
  - —The presence of nodules.
    - Early prostate carcinoma is often found on the posterior lobe as a stony-hard area with a distinct border within the gland.
    - An infected area more likely has a diffuse border and may be tender.

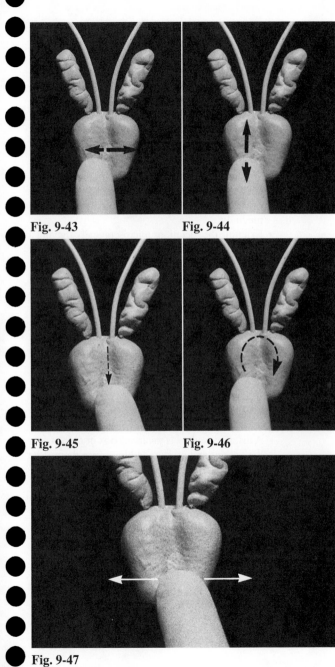

Fig. 9-43

Fig. 9-44

Fig. 9-45

Fig. 9-46

Fig. 9-47

3. Prostatic massage (optional): used most often as a
   diagnostic procedure when prostatitis is suspected.
   - Do not perform in cases of severe prostatitis or
     purulent urethritis (to prevent obstruction), or
     prostate carcinoma (to prevent further spread).
   - With a rolling motion, use the pad of the index
     finger to express secretions into the prostatic ure-
     thra.
   - Start laterally and superiorly and massage toward
     the midline *(FIG. 9-48).*
   - Finally, milk the seminal vesicles downward and
     medially.
   - Examine the secretions microscopically (having a
     glass slide ready to place at the urethra) and by
     culture *(FIG. 9-49).*
     —If no secretion is obtained, have the patient
       void only a few drops of urine. This will usu-
       ally contain adequate secretion for examina-
       tion.

**E. Finally, Examine the Nature of Any Feces Clinging
   to the Glove.**
   1. Test a sample for occult blood *(see Fig. 10-80).*

   2. Also, gently wipe the anal area with a tissue, or of-
      fer the patient a tissue to do it himself.
      - A discrete method is to place a box of tissues near
        the patient and encourage him to use them if he
        wishes. Then leave the room for him to redress.

F. Let the Patient Dress before discussing your findings
   with him.
   1. This gives you an opportunity to check the prosta-
      tic secretions, if taken.

   2. It also gives the patient a moment to relax from the
      stress of examination. In this way, he can benefit
      more from subsequent discussion with the examiner.

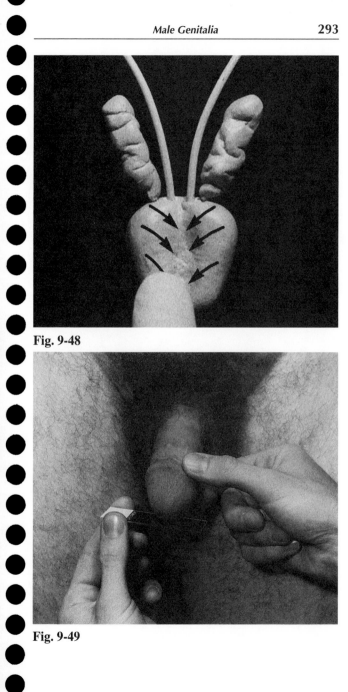

Fig. 9-48

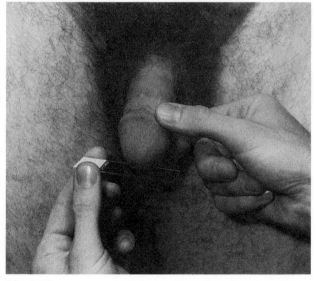

Fig. 9-49

10 Female Genitalia

I. ITEMS NEEDED FOR EXAMINATION.
A. Disposable Gown and Drape.

B. Adjustable (Flexible-Neck) Light Source.

C. Vaginal Specula of Appropriate Sizes.

D. Materials for Papanicolaou Studies:
1. Sterile cotton applicators.
2. Cervical (Ayre) spatulae and cytobrush.
3. Rectal swabs, or cotton balls, and a long forceps.
4. Three glass slides, marked "E," "C," and "V," or a single slide with three marked divisions.
   - Some slides simply have two marked sections for cytobrush and spatula. These are often prepackaged by the laboratory used by each office.
5. Fixative spray or solution.
6. (Optional) Thin-prep kit, consisting of cytobrush, spatula, and a vial of fixative.

E. Materials for Bacteriologic Evaluation.
1. Plain glass slides and cover slips.
2. 10% potassium hydroxide solution.
3. 0.9% saline solution.
4. Optional Thayer-Martin media or DNA probe.

F. Disposable Examination Gloves, Lubricant, Tissues, Hand Mirror, Gauze Squares, Basin Filled with Warm Water (for metal speculae).

II. EXAMINER'S ATTITUDE
A. It Is Normal for the Beginning Student to Feel Anxious or Awkward About Performing the Pelvic Examination.
1. The learning of proper examination technique and repeated practice will build confidence.
2. Let your own feelings of awkwardness be a reminder of the vulnerability the patient feels in receiving this examination.

III. PATIENT PREPARATION.
A. Emotional.
1. By its very nature, the pelvic examination is uncomfortable. Most women view it with at least some apprehension, often from:
   - The discomfort of prior examinations, since the pelvic viscera respond with an aching sensation even with acceptable examination technique.
   - Painful or embarrassing experiences during prior examinations.
   - The fear of first examination, such as with an adolescent patient.
   - The fear of discovery of disease.

2. Behavior that seems an obstacle to examination may actually help in understanding the patient's underlying problem.
   - One example is "protective" body language: adduction of the thighs, pelvic floor muscle contraction, and pulling away.
     —It is helpful to bring this reaction to the patient's attention. Ask if anything is worrying her.
     —Find out if this also occurs during normal sexual relations, as this posture may reflect underlying anxieties.

3. Adequate time for history taking and discussion greatly helps in reducing your patient's apprehension.
   - Understand that the examination causes the patient to feel extremely vulnerable.
   - This feeling can be offset by treating the patient with kindness and respect and, by your manner, maintaining the patient's dignity.

4. Properly inform the patient:
    - On what procedures you will perform.
      —This typically consists of a speculum examination with Pap test, bimanual examination, rectovaginal examination and, in older patients, a rectal examination.
    - On her own genital anatomy (if she wishes it.) A plastic model of the pelvic organs is useful for demonstration, particularly on the patient's first examination.
    - On when physical contact is made.
      —Always make first contact on the upper inner thigh, not on the genitals.
      —Avoid any unexpected moves.
    - (Very important) on any questions she may have concerning the examination.
      —Medical history-taking is best done while the patient is dressed and seated, not when she is in the lithotomy position.

B. **Patient Comfort.**
    1. The room should be comfortably warm. If your hands are cold, warm them in running water before you begin.

    2. The patient should not douche for at least 24 hours before the examination, since it interferes with the evaluation of cytologic and bacteriologic studies.

    3. Ask the patient to empty her bladder before you begin.
        - The patient will be more comfortable during the bimanual examination with an empty bladder.
        - Since a urinalysis may be performed during the same visit, this is a convenient time for specimen collection.

    4. When the practitioner is male, patients often prefer to have a female nurse or assistant in the room.

C. Patient Positioning.

1. Extend the lower end of the examination table.

2. The patient should change into an examining gown *(FIG. 10-1).*
   - Help her move to the supine position.
   - Place a pillow to support her head.
   - Her arms should be at her sides or comfortably folded across her chest.

3. Place a drape over her legs and lower abdomen, according to her preference.
   - Some patients wish to watch the examination, whereas others prefer the drape for reasons of modesty.

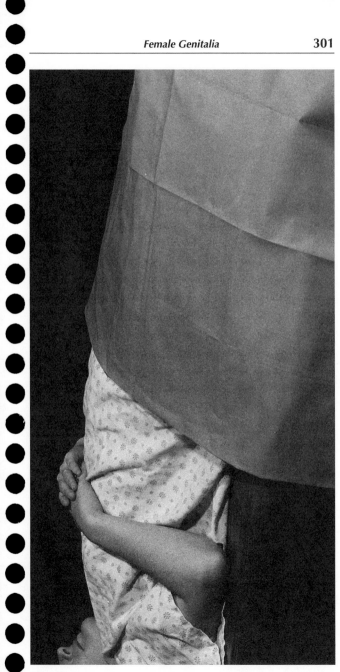

Fig. 10-1

4. Extend the stirrups and angle them outward to 45 degrees; they should be spread far enough out so the patient's knees can flex to about 70 degrees *(FIG. 10-2)*.
   ▪ Help her place one heel, then the other into the stirrups. Shoes may be more comfortable than bare feet.
   ▪ This is the "lithotomy" position: with the patient supine, knees flexed, and hips flexed and abducted *(FIG. 10-3)*.

5. Have her move toward the end of the examining table until her buttocks extend just over the table's edge. Assist her by:
   ▪ Aiding her movement with your hands on her hips *(FIG. 10-4)*.
   ▪ Or, alternatively, placing your hand at the table's edge, off center, to signal an endpoint for her motion. Say "come towards the edge until you feel my hand."

6. Last, seat yourself.
   ▪ Depress the drape so you can maintain eye contact with the patient. Glove both hands.
     —If the patient has a latex allergy, use vinyl gloves.

7. In debilitated patients, the left lateral (Sims) position may be used *(see FIG. 9-29):*
   ▪ The patient lies on her left side, as close to the edge of the examination table as safety allows.
   ▪ Her left thigh is slightly flexed, and her right thigh is flexed to about 90 degrees.
   ▪ The examiner stands behind and to the side, to allow inspection and palpation as detailed in the following.

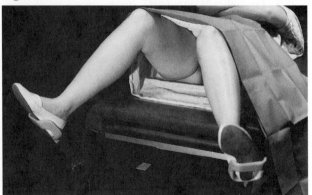

Fig. 10-2

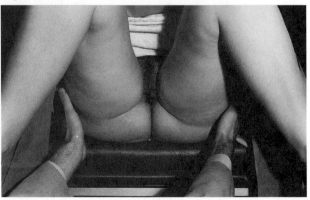

Fig. 10-3

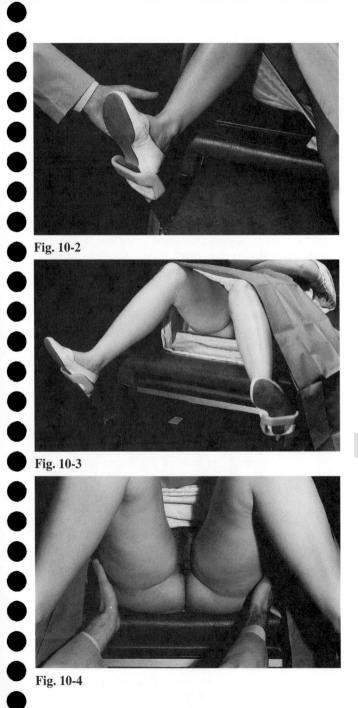

Fig. 10-4

IV. EXTERNAL GENITALIA: INSPECTION.

A. Assessment of Sexual Maturity (in adolescents).

1. Note pubic hair and breast changes.
   - In adolescents, rate according to Tanner's stages (see Appendix A).
   - In the adult, the pubic hair appears roughly as an inverted triangle with the base near the mons pubis and the apex extending downward to the labia.
     —In some women with familial hirsuitism, the hair may extend up the abdomen to the umbilicus, resembling the more diamond-shaped male hair distribution.

B. The Labia Majora *(FIG. 10-5)*.

1. This is the outermost region of the external genitalia. (The external genitalia are collectively called the vulva.)
2. They are seen as two folds of adipose tissue that surround the inner lips (which are termed the labia minora). The skin of the vulvar area is slightly more pigmented.
   - In the nulliparous patient, the lips nearly touch, whereas in the parous patient, the lips are separated.
3. Note any ulcerations, signs of infection, changes in pigmentation, or other lesions.
   - If you suspect pubic lice, look closely at the pubic hair shafts for attached lice (brown-black) or nits (white). An ophthalmoscope serves nicely as an illuminated and highly powered magnifier to identify lice.
4. To inspect further, inform the patient you will make contact, then touch her inner thigh with the *back* of your gloved hand *(FIG. 10-6)*.
   - This avoids startling the patient and prevents protective adduction.
   - Begin by touching the inner thigh near the knee, then move down in six inch steps.
     —If her legs adduct, say "let your legs fall to the sides," as you continue moving down in steps.
   - Before you touch the touch the genitalia, say "you'll feel my fingers."
   - Separate the labia so all skin surfaces can be visualized *(FIG. 10-7)*.

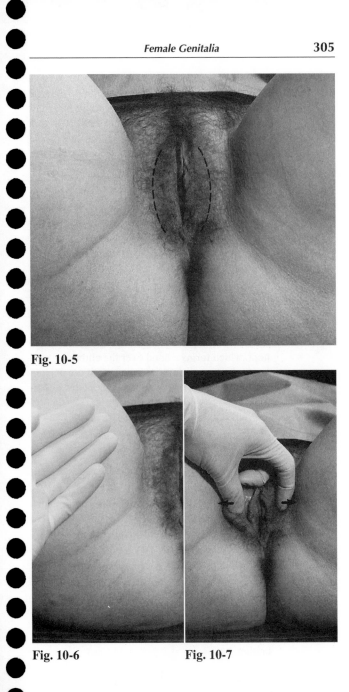

Fig. 10-5

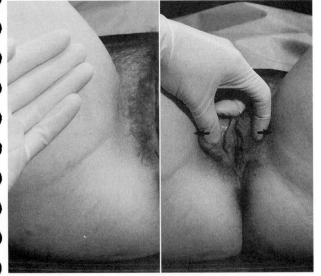

Fig. 10-6   Fig. 10-7

C. **The Labia Minora** (1) *(FIG. 10-8).*

   1. Seen as two thin folds of skin extending from the midline just over the clitoris and ending on either side of the vaginal opening. Note their dark pink color.

   2. The vestibule is a boat-shaped area between the inner surfaces of the labia minora.

     ▪ The skin is much more delicate than that of the labia majora.

     ▪ It is the most common site of the granulomatous and ulcerative lesions in younger women and of malignant changes in the elderly.

      —Inspect for discharge, redness, masses, and atrophic changes.

D. **The Clitoris** (2).

   1. It is normally 1 to 1.5 cm long and pink-gray in color.

     ▪ It is covered in part by the junction of the labia minora, which forms a hood over the clitoris.

     ▪ Inflammatory conditions of the clitoris are uncommon. Enlargement may relate to endocrine abnormalities.

E. **The Urethral Meatus** (3).

   1. It is visible between the clitoris and vaginal opening.

     ▪ It normally appears slitlike or stellate in shape and is the same color as the surrounding mucous membranes.

     ▪ In the young, nulliparous patient, the opening may be concealed by surrounding tissues. It may appear adjacent to the anterior vaginal border.

   2. Inspect for discharge, erythema, or polyps visible at the urethral opening.

   3. In older women, the urethra often prolapses, becoming inflamed and tender.

     ▪ In cases of chronic urethritis, especially in postmenopausal women, a small polyp (urethral caruncle) may be seen on the posterior surface of the urethra.

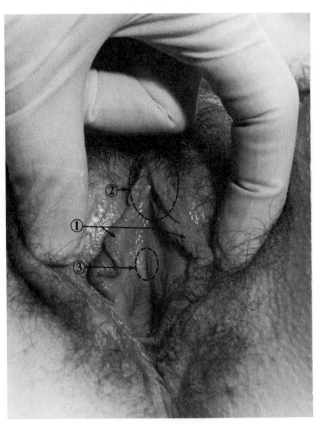

Fig. 10-8

F. The Vaginal Opening (introitus).
    1. The hymen, or hymenal remnant, appears just inside the introitus *(FIG. 10-9)*.
- In the virgin, its size and thickness varies considerably.
- It will normally admit one finger, and occasionally two or more.

    2. Observe any uterine prolapse. In such cases, the cervix would appear at or external to the introitus.

    3. Note any inflammation, ulceration, or vaginal discharge. If swellings or nodules are present, palpate them.

G. The Fourchette *(FIG. 10-10)*.
    1. Seen as a midline seam of skin that terminates at the anus. This overlies the muscular perineal body.

    2. Note any scars of an episiotomy, the healed incision often performed during childbirth.

    3. At this time, also briefly inspect the anus, particularly for hemorrhoids. This will be examined in more detail during the rectal examination.

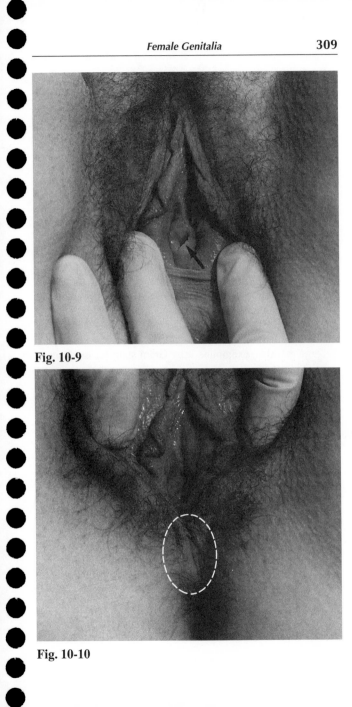

Fig. 10-9

Fig. 10-10

V. EXTERNAL GENITALIA: PALPATION.

A. First, Palpate Any Visible Abnormality. Note size, texture, mobility, and tenderness.

B. Then Palpate the Labia; they should feel soft and their texture should be homogenous.

C. If Urethritis Is Present or Suspected, Palpate Skene's Glands *(FIG. 10-11)*.

1. These are a series of small paraurethral glands along either side of the urethra. They are often involved in gonorrheal or chlamydial infections.

2. Gently insert your index finger, pad upward, about 4 cm into the vagina *(FIG. 10-12)*.
   - Gently milk the urethra by pressing upward as you withdraw your finger.
   - If discharge appears from or around the urethral orifice, culture it for gonorrhea and/or chlamydia. Also, examinine it by Gram stain for evidence of gonorrhea.

D. If There Is Labial Swelling or a History of It, Check for Enlargement of Bartholin's Glands *(FIG. 10-13)*.

1. These are located at the inner edge of the labia at about the 4:00 and 8:00 o'clock positions.

2. Palpate each side of the labia between thumb and forefinger *(FIG. 10-14)*.
   - Place one finger outside and one inside the introitus, sweeping them along the length of the labia majora.
   - Feel for tenderness or cystic swelling. The glands are not normally palpable.
     —Swelling may be inflamed (infection) or noninflamed (simple glandular obstruction). Both types of swelling are palpable beneath the labia majora and may involve the labia minora.

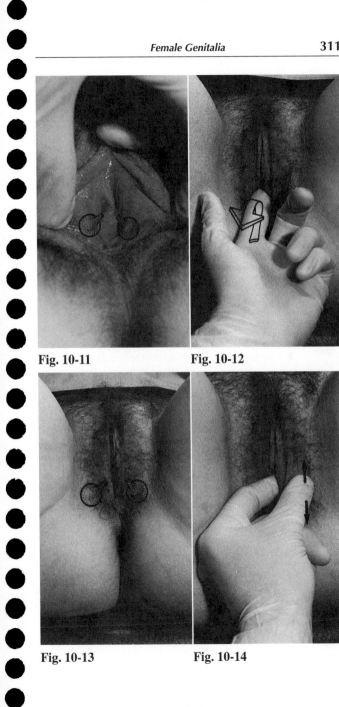

Fig. 10-11

Fig. 10-12

Fig. 10-13

Fig. 10-14

E. Assess Muscle Tone.
   1. Insert your index and middle fingers into the vagina.
      - Ask the patient to constrict her vaginal muscles *(FIG. 10-15)*.
      - A nulliparous patient will demonstrate a high degree of tone; in the multiparous patient, less so.

   2. Separate your fingers and ask the patient to bear down; watch for: *(FIG. 10-16)*
      - Bulging of the vaginal walls anteriorly (cystocoele) or posteriorly (rectocoele).
      - Protrusion of the urethra (urethrocoele) and any associated urinary incontinence.
         —If incontinence is suspected, ask the patient to cough. Shield the urethra and watch for a spurt of urine.
         —Always ask "any leaking of urine?" Patients seldom reveal this information unless directly asked.
      - Any uterine prolapse, where the cervix drops down and becomes visible at or protrudes from the introitus.

   3. With the fingers still in place, feel the thickness of the perineal body.
      - This is a muscular layer in the posterior and more external portion of the vagina. After an episiotomy, the perineum often feels thinner and more rigid because of the healed incision.

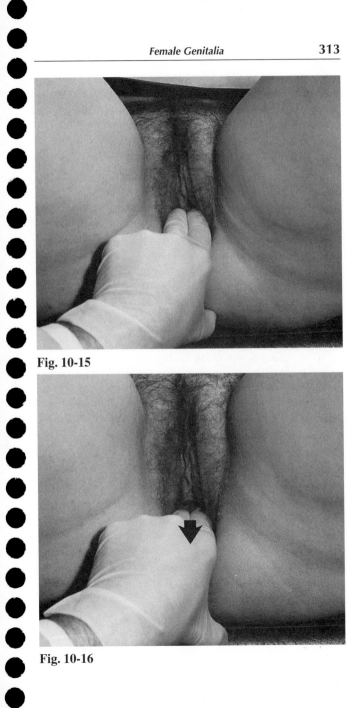

Fig. 10-15

Fig. 10-16

VI. **SPECULUM EXAMINATION:** Some clinicians prefer
to precede speculum insertion with a brief digital
examination to assess the size of the introitus and
vaginal canal, any obstructing anomalies and the
position of the cervix. Use 1 or 2 gloved fingers
lubricated only with water.

   A. **Information on Vaginal Specula:** Two basic shapes
   are generally used.

      1. The Graves model *(FIG. 10-17).*
         ▪ These have wider blades and are used more com-
           monly in the sexually active adult.
         ▪ Their lengths vary from 8 to 13 cm, ranged small,
           medium, and large.

      2. The Pederson type, which has narrower blades for
      use with a smaller introitus *(FIG. 10-18).*
         ▪ It is used for the adolescent, virginal, or elderly pa-
           tient, or when it is prefered by the patient for com-
           fort.

      3. The plastic, disposable models are usually the
      Graves type *(FIG. 10-19).*
         ▪ Being plastic, they are not cold on contact with the
           perineum.
         ▪ This model typically makes a loud click when
           opened or released, and the patient should be in-
           formed of this before it is used.

      4. Two parts of the specula are adjustable.
         ▪ The thumb rest, used for levering the blades open,
           has a set screw just above it.
         ▪ The center sliding section, used for vertically
           widening the blades, has its set screw in the front
           of the speculum handle. The plastic models have
           similar adjustments, which click into place.
         ▪ Become familiar with these two adjustments and
           practice widening, locking, and releasing the
           blades.

      5. Use a strong light source, such as a flexible-neck
      lamp aimed through the speculum.
         ▪ Some plastic speculae have a built-in light guide, de-
           signed for a light source that plugs into the handle.

      6. Place the appropriately sized speculum in warm wa-
      ter (if a metal one: *[FIG. 10-20]*). Use no lubricant
      yet, since it is bacteriostatic and will also distort cells
      for cytologic studies.

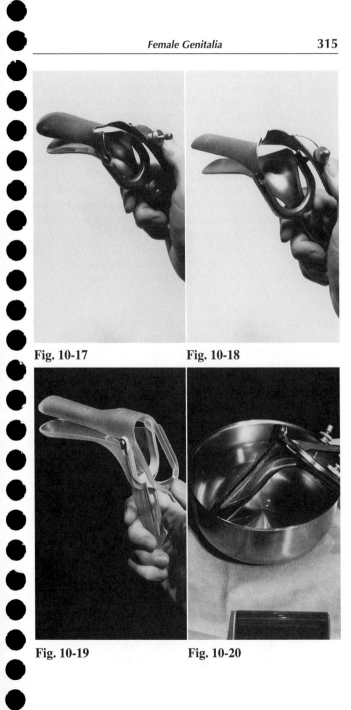

Fig. 10-17

Fig. 10-18

Fig. 10-19

Fig. 10-20

B. Insert the Speculum.

1. Initiate contact by touching the patient's inner thigh.

2. Place two gloved fingers just inside the introitus *(FIG. 10-21).* Inform the patient she will feel some pressure, then spread the fingers slightly and press gently down.

3. Use your thumb to retract the left labia. This prevents the labial lip and any pubic hair from being pulled on during speculum insertion *(FIG. 10-22).*

4. Hold the speculum blades at an angle, tilted 45 degrees from horizontal.

   ▪ This takes advantage of the 'H' configuration of the relaxed vagina. It also prevents contact with the more sensitive clitoris and urethra.

   ▪ As you hold the speculum, press your thumb upward under the thumbrest to keep the blades closed during insertion.

5. Ask the patient to bear down, as if with a bowel movement. This helps to open the vaginal orifice and relax the perineal muscles.

6. Insert the speculum blades at an angle over your fingers *(FIG. 10-23).*

   ▪ Aim 45 degrees downward as you enter, again to avoid the urethra.

   ▪ Once in, rotate the blades back to the horizontal position *(FIG 10-24).*

7. Keeping gentle posterior pressure, look through the blades and guide them further in to the end of the vagina *(FIG. 10-25).*

   ▪ Then open the blades by bracing the handle and pressing on the thumb rest *(FIG. 10-26).*

   ▪ If the skin of the vagina appears to stretch or blanch, stop and withdraw the blades until tension is released. You may be aiming at the wrong angle. Use similar caution if the patient expresses pain.

     —If so, check again to see if the speculum is pinching mucosal tissues or pulling on nearby pubic hairs.

   ▪ If the patient is especially tense, stop insertion but leave the blades in place. Ask her to take a few slow deep breaths to aid relaxation before you continue.

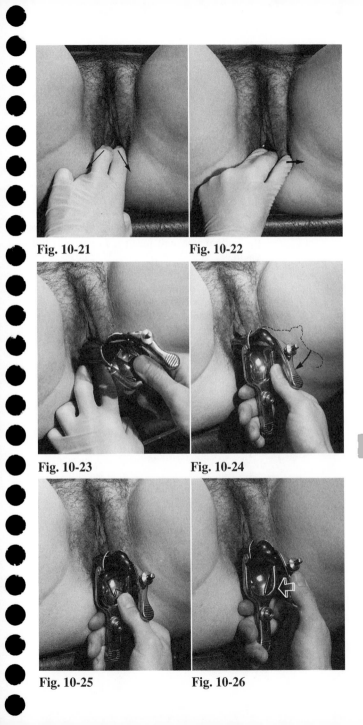

Fig. 10-21

Fig. 10-22

Fig. 10-23

Fig. 10-24

Fig. 10-25

Fig. 10-26

8. If the cervix is not visible:
   - Withdraw the speculum halfway and reinsert it in a different plane.
   - Since the most common uterine position is anteversion, the cervix usually enters the anterior vaginal wall and points posterior and downward.
   - It is then most useful to reinsert the blades aiming more posteriorly until the cervix becomes visible.
   - If after several attempts, you still cannot find the cervix:
     —Remove the speculum completely and inform the patient you will insert a finger into the vagina.
     —Wet your gloved index finger with water and insert. The cervix is usually easily found, often deeper and more posterior than you expected.
     —Make a mental note of cervix position and reinsert the speculum.

9. When the cervix is seen:
   - Open the blades until they slip into the anterior and posterior fornices *(FIG. 10-27).*
   - Widen them to fully expose the cervix (without causing patient discomfort) and lock them in place *(FIG. 10-28).*

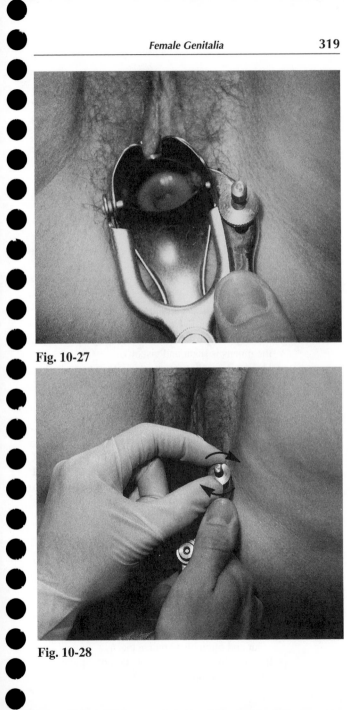

Fig. 10-27

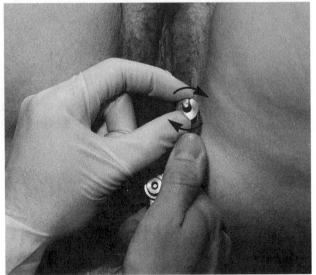

Fig. 10-28

C. **Inspect the Cervix** *(FIG. 10-29).*
   1. Anatomy.
      - The normal cervix is about 2 to 3 cm in diameter and also in length. A diameter larger than 4 cm is considered hypertrophy.
      - It is round or conical in shape and is the same color as the vaginal walls.
      - The uterus is anteverted in about 80% of patients, with the cervix protruding from the anterior wall and pointing posteriorly.
      - Its opening, or os, is round and small in the nulliparous patient.
        —The external os normally measures 3 to 5 mm in diameter.
        —After childbirth the os typically appears slit-like.
   2. Note any secretions, which vary in quality with the menstrual cycle.
      - During premenstrual and postmenstrual periods, the mucus is scant and viscous.
      - During preovulatory and ovulatory periods (because of high estrogenic activity), secretions are thin and copious.
      - After menopause, there is little or no cervical secretion.
   3. Look for nodules, ulcerations, or masses.
      - One common benign condition is the presence of nabothian cysts. These are smooth, round, small (under1 cm) yellow lesions caused by obstruction of the cervical gland ducts.
      - Another is eversion of the squamocolumnar junction.
        —The columnar epithelium, which lines the endocervical canal, sometimes extends outward to the ecto- (external) cervix.
        —It produces an area of beefy redness forming a relatively symmetric circle around the os.
        —The margins of an eversion are usually uniform, whereas in carcinoma they are raggedly irregular and often bleed on contact.
      - If any lesions are in question, colposcopic examination is recommended.

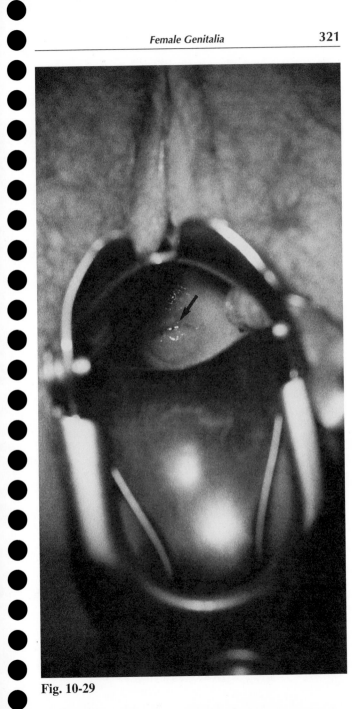

Fig. 10-29

4. If the patient wishes, help her to see her own cervix with a hand mirror.

- Raise the head of the exam table to 45 degrees and arrange the drape so it does not obstruct her vision.
- Assist her in holding the mirror to reflect her vision through the speculum.

D. Obtain Specimens: Generally, this includes a Pap test, a culture for gonorrhea, and a wet smear, in cases of vaginal infection.

1. Pap test (Papanicolaou study of cervical cytology)

- There are three methods: endocervical swab, cervical scrape, and vaginal pool specimen.
  —Most clinicians and pathologists use the cervical scrape and one or both of the other two methods. Consult the cytopathologist at your laboratory for locally recommended procedures.
- Have the appropriate items organized on a tray within reach (see Materials Needed) *(FIG. 10-30)*.

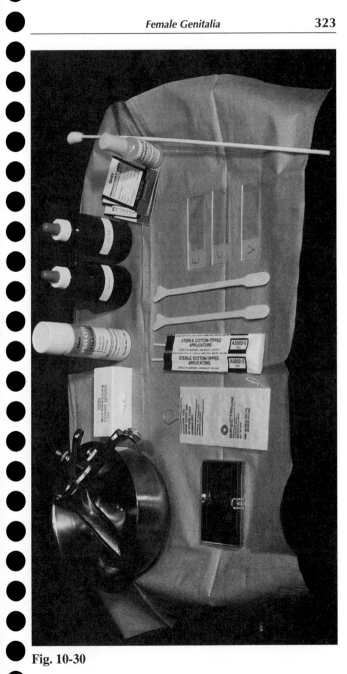

Fig. 10-30

- Endocervical sample:
  —If cervical mucus is present, remove it with the rectal swab or equivalent *(FIG. 10-31).*
  —Gently insert a cytobrush fully into the os and rotate 360 degrees several times *(FIG. 10-32).* (As of this writing, a plain cotton applicator is recommended only during pregnancy, since it collects a lower yield of cells.)
  —Remove it and gently *unroll* the secretions onto the slide marked E (or portion of slide marked for cytobrush) *(FIG. 10-33).*
    - These are fragile columnar epithelial cells. Rolling the swab too vigorously against the slide will distort the cells.
    - Position the swab so all surfaces are transferred to the slide.
    - The smear should be thin and evenly spread, avoiding thick areas that are difficult to examine.
  —Spray immediately with fixative or place in a standard ether-alcohol solution *(FIG. 10-34).*
- Cervical scrape:
  —Place the longer end of a cervical spatula into the os. When the longer, curved portion of the spatula is placed in the os, the rim of the cervix fits between the two wooden humps.
  —Apply moderate pressure and rotate 360 degrees *(FIG. 10-35).* This scrapes the entire circumference of the squamocolumnar junction.
  —Smear on the "C" slide (or portion of slide marked for spatula) and spray or fix as before *(FIG. 10-36).*
  —When using the Thin-Prep method, the cytobrush and spatula samples are stirred into a vial of fixative liquid and the vial is submitted as the specimen.

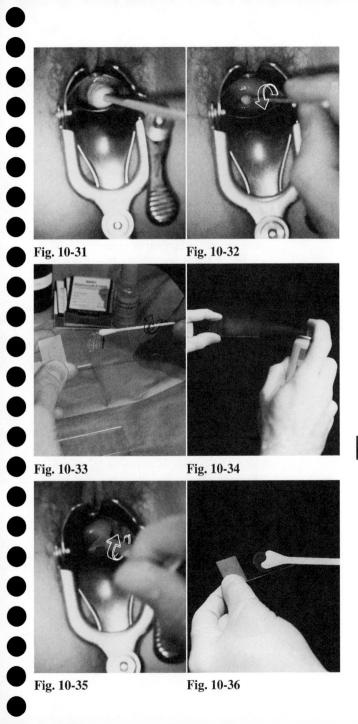

Fig. 10-31

Fig. 10-32

Fig. 10-33

Fig. 10-34

Fig. 10-35

Fig. 10-36

- Vaginal pool (optional):
  —Use the opposite, paddle-shaped end of the spatula *(FIG. 10-37)*. (Some clinicians prefer the cotton-tipped applicator.)
  —Collect material from the floor of the vagina under the cervix. If the cervix has been removed, collect material from the cuff of remaining vagina.
  —Smear on the slide marked V and fix as before.
- The specimen is usually submitted with selected information about the patient:
  —Her age and last menstrual period.
  —Whether she is pregnant or taking hormonal supplements or contraceptives.
  —Prior history of abnormal Pap tests.
- Remember that this is primarily a test of *cervical* cytology. A negative study does not rule out the presence of neoplasia in the endometrium, fallopian tubes, or ovaries.

2. Gonorrheal culture. This is an optional measure during pelvic examination of the sexually active patient. There are two methods.
   - Direct culture:
     —Swab the endocervix with a sterile calcium alginate applicator *(FIG. 10-38)*. Cotton-tipped swabs contain traces of fatty acids that can be bacteriostatic.

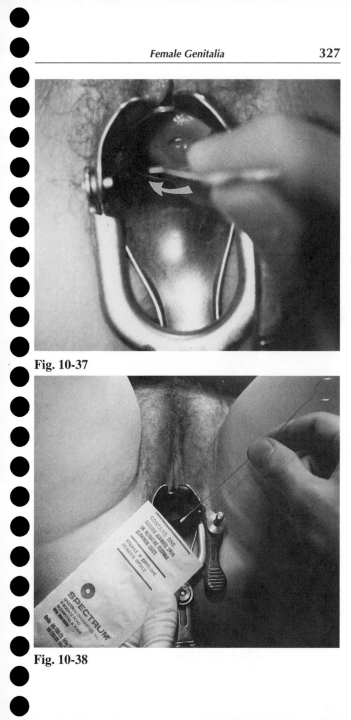

Fig. 10-37

Fig. 10-38

—Inoculate a Thayer-Martin (or other compatible media) at room temperature.
- Streak the swab across the plate in a continuous 'Z' pattern, exposing all surfaces of the swab *(FIG. 10-39)*.
- Return the culture plate to a warm, anaerobic environment.

■ DNA probe (usually a prepackaged kit.)
—Clean the endocervix with a cotton-tipped applicator, then insert a second swab and leave it for 30 seconds.
—Drop the swab into the included vial of transport medium and break off the stick to fit the vial.
—This test often includes detection of *Chlamydia trachomatis* as well.

■ Anal swab (optional).
—Gently insert the sterile swab into the anal canal.
—Rotate 360 degrees and leave it in for about 20 seconds to ensure saturation. If the swab contains feces, discard it and try again with a fresh swab.
—Culture as before.

3. Wet (hanging drop) specimen: Used in cases of suspected vaginal and cervical infection.
■ Mark a glass slide on one edge with the letter S; have dropper bottles of 0.9% saline and 10% potassium hydroxide and cover slips ready.
■ With a cervical spatula or cotton-tipped applicator, obtain material from the floor of the vagina. Material can also be taken from the inferior blade of the speculum, where secretions often pool.
■ Smear two small (0.5 to 1 cm) circles on the slide *(FIG. 10-40).* Add a drop of saline to the circle nearest the 'S' and a drop of potassium hydroxide (KOH) solution to the other.
■ Add cover slips and examine microscopically. This is usually done while the patient is redressing.
—Check the saline preparation for motile trichomonads, white cells, bacteria, or "clue" cells and the KOH preparation for the buds or hyphae of *Candida albicans*.

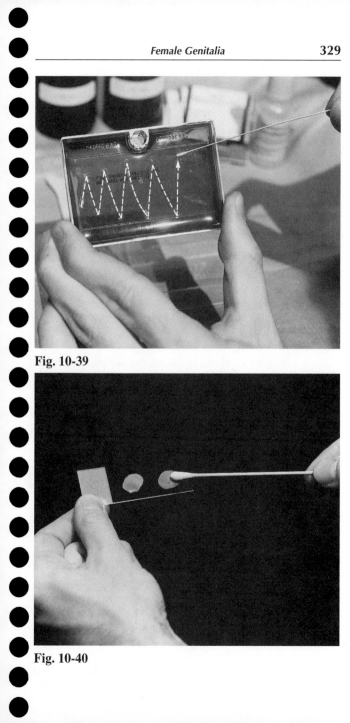

Fig. 10-39

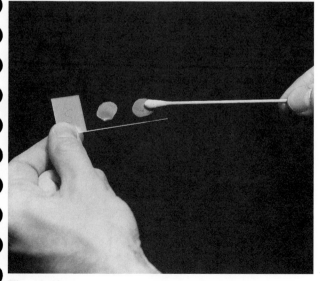

Fig. 10-40

- The motile trichomonads stop their motion within minutes, so try to view the "saline" slide as quickly as possible.

E. Inspect the Vaginal Walls. Note their color and texture during speculum insertion, while in, and during removal.

1. Withdraw the speculum blades until the blades clear the cervix *(FIG. 10-41).* Place your thumb on the thumbrest to keep the blades open, then release the set screw *(FIG. 10-42).*

2. Slowly withdraw the blades and carefully inspect the vaginal mucosa *(FIG. 10-43).*
   - Note its color and any inflammation, ulcerations, discharge, or masses.
     —The color is normally pink and uniform.
     —With inflammation, the walls are reddened and often coated with discharge.
   - Turn the blades so the anterior and posterior walls are visible.
   - Note the normal transverse folds, or rugae. These folds give the vagina its distensibility. After menopause, the folds greatly diminish.
   - Then return to the horizontal position and inspect the lateral vaginal walls.

3. When the speculum is half out, have the patient bear down. Check for vaginal wall relaxation (cystocoele or rectocoele) and uterine prolapse.

4. Slowly close the blades as they are removed.
   - Use care not to pinch mucosal tissues or catch hairs between the blades.
   - Continue inspecting throughout speculum removal *(FIG. 10-44).*
   - Again, as the ends of the blades near the urethra, angle their tips downward as you lift the speculum out of the introitus.

5. Inspect the speculum for odor, then either discard it if disposable or, if metal, place in a soaking solution.

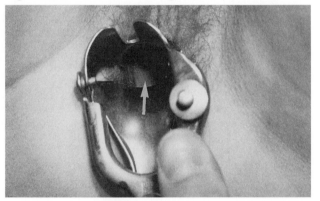

Fig. 10-41   Fig. 10-42

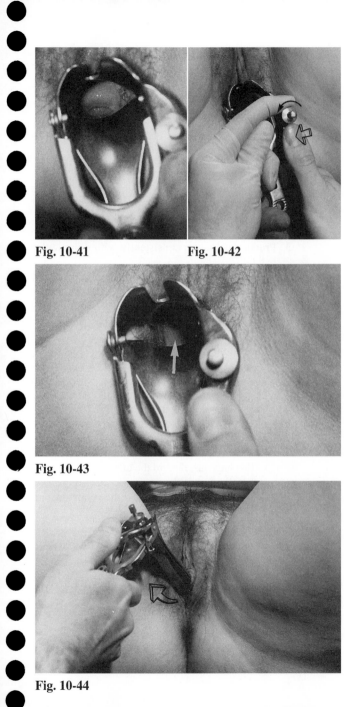

Fig. 10-43

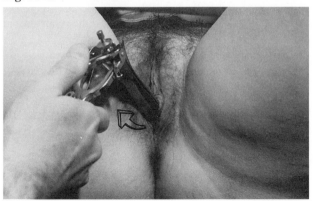

Fig. 10-44

VII. Internal palpation. This consists of the bimanual and rectovaginal examination. It allows the examiner to outline the pelvic organs between the two hands.

   A. Preparation.
   1. Move to the standing position.

   2. Have a small stool ready to support your foot, or pull out the built-in step in the exam table, if present *(FIG 10-45)*.

   3. Practice palpation consistently with a particular hand.
      ▪ It is sometimes useful to alternate intravaginal hands, using the right hand to palpate for left-sided pelvic masses and the left hand for right-sided masses.

   4. Apply lubricant.
      ▪ Either allow the gel to drop onto your gloved fingers *(FIG. 10-46),*
      ▪ Or place some gel onto a square of sterile gauze, then swab your fingers through it *(FIG. 10-47)*.
      ▪ *Never* allow your examining fingers to touch the tube opening *(FIG. 10-48)*.
         —This may cause contamination of the tube. If this happens, discard the tube.
         —Small, disposable, single-use tubes or packets are also available to avoid the contamination potential of multi-use tubes.

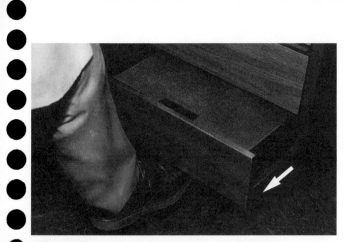
Fig. 10-45

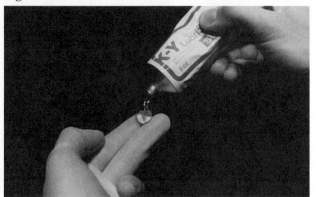
Fig. 10-46

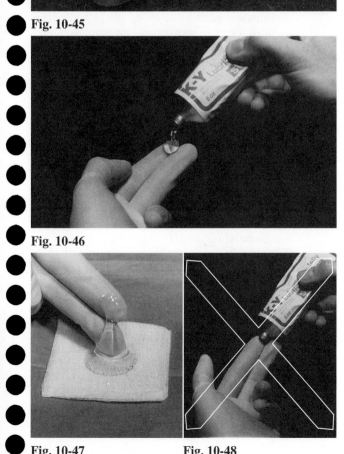
Fig. 10-47

Fig. 10-48

B. Finger Insertion.

1. Place the fingers into the obstetrical position, with: *(FIG. 10-49)*
   - Thumb abducted.
   - Index and middle fingers pressed together and extended. (If the introitus is small, use only one finger.)
   - Ring and little fingers flexed into the palm.

2. Hold the hand, wrist, and arm in a straight line.

3. Initiate contact by touching the patient's inner thigh, moving down towards the introitus in steps as described earlier. Again, before you touch the touch the genitalia, say "you'll feel my fingers."

4. Enter the introitus *(FIG. 10-50)*. Keep pressure posteriorly to avoid pressure on the sensitive clitoris and urethra.

5. As you enter, palpate the vaginal walls, feeling with the pads of the fingertips. Feel for nodularity or tenderness of the vaginal walls, including anteriorly.

6. When your fingers are fully inserted:
   - Place your leg on the step (same side as inserting hand) *(FIG. 10-51)*
   - Rest the weight of your arm on your thigh *(FIG. 10-52)*. This braces the examining hand and lessens pressure on the perineum and allows for more controlled hand movement.

7. Observe the patient's face during palpation, particularly bimanual. Watch for signs of discomfort.

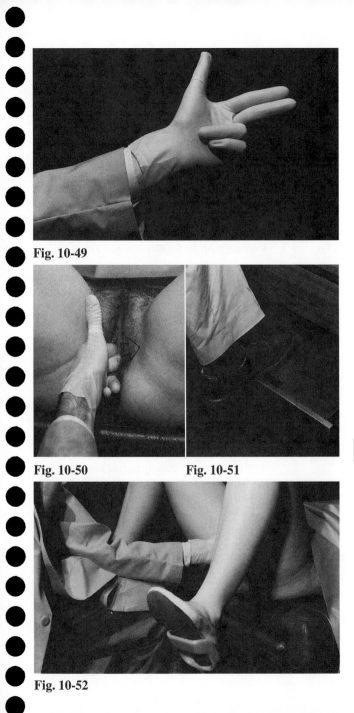

Fig. 10-49

Fig. 10-50   Fig. 10-51

Fig. 10-52

C. Palpate the Cervix.

1. Note its position *(FIG. 10-53).*
   - It usually points posteriorly from the top of the anterior vagina, indicating anteversion (1).
   - If the cervix lies directly in the same axis as the vagina, it indicates midposition of the uterus (2).
   - If it points anteriorly from the top of the posterior vagina, it indicates retroversion of the uterus (3).
   - It normally lies in the midline, pointing neither left nor right. Deviation may indicate a pelvic, uterine, or ovarian tumor, or inflammatory changes pushing the uterus to one side.

2. Note its consistency and shape *(FIG. 10-54).*
   - It is normally firm and feels similar to the tip of the nose. It may become hardened and irregular with advanced malignancy, or "bumpy" with nabothian cysts.
   - Its shape is normally round or conical.

3. Palpate the os (the outward opening of the cervical canal) *(FIG. 10-55).*
   - Gently insert a finger into the os and feel for dilation.
     —In the nonpregnant patient, the os will normally admit a finger to a depth of about 5 mm.
     —If material has recently passed through it or is about to (threatened or spontaneous abortion), the os may be softened and admit a finger further in.
     —After childbirth, a healed cervical laceration may be present. This produces a horizontal crease, often from the 3:00 to 9:00 o'clock positions on the cervix.

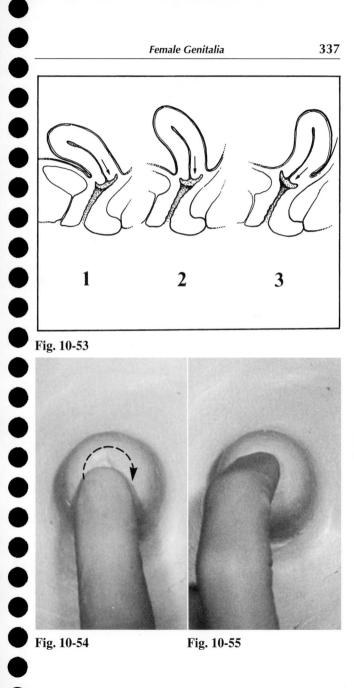

Fig. 10-53

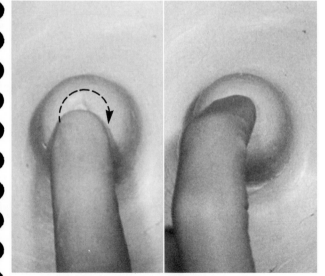

Fig. 10-54   Fig. 10-55

4. Palpate for lesions around the cervix.
   - Adjust your examining hand to feel with the pads of the fingertips in the: *(FIG. 10-56)*
     —Posterior (inferior) fornix (1).
     —Right lateral fornix (2).
     —Anterior (superior) fornix (3).
     —Left lateral fornix (4).

5. Assess mobility of the cervix.
   - Grasp the cervix with your two inserted fingers *(FIG. 10-57)*.
   - Move it from side to side 1 or 2 cm in each direction.
   - It should be freely movable and nontender.
     —This motion stretches the peritoneum in the lower pelvis.
     —In cases of pelvic peritonitis (as in acute salpingitis, pelvic inflammatory disease) it can cause marked tenderness.

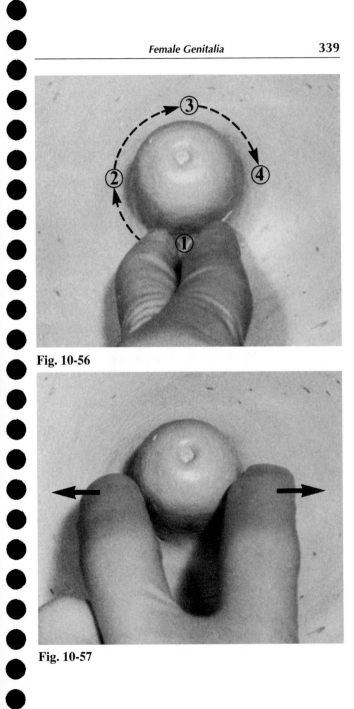

Fig. 10-56

Fig. 10-57

D. Palpate the Uterus.

1. Position the hands.

   - Place your free hand on the abdomen about mid-way between the umbilicus and symphysis pubis *(FIG. 10-58)*.

     —Position the hand palm down, fingers slightly flexed, and pointed toward the patient's head.

     —This hand will be used to press the abdominal and pelvic contents toward the intravaginal hand.

     —If the fingers are too close to the symphysis, the abdominal wall is pressed downward in front of the normally positioned uterus. This hinders palpation of pelvic structures.

   - Press downward toward the intravaginal hand *(FIG. 10-59)*.

     —When pressure is applied to the uterus (or other pelvic mass) it is felt by the vaginal hand.

     —The intravaginal hand maintains slight upward pressure to stabilize the uterus between the two hands.

   - Movement of both hands should be slow and firm.

     —If the patient becomes tense, stop palpation and allow the patient to take a few slow deep breaths to relax the abdominal and pelvic muscles.

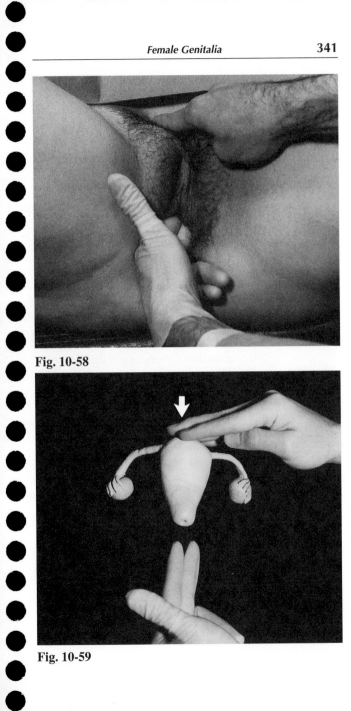

Fig. 10-58

Fig. 10-59

2. Note its size, shape, and consistency.
   - The uterus is normally about 8 to 10 cm long and is pear-shaped, narrowing toward the cervix.
   - Its consistency is normally firm and rubbery.
   - It is freely movable and can normally be displaced down and forward by the abdominal hand *(FIG. 10-60)*.
   - Note any:
     —Arterial pulsations, which may indicate ectopic pregnancy.
     —Softening between the uterine body and cervix (the isthmus), a sign of pregnancy (*always* confirm with a urine or serum pregnancy test).
     —Any masses attached to the uterus, such as uterine fibroids or other tumors.

3. Note its position.
   - Terminology:
     —"Version" means deflection of the long axis of the uterus from the long axis of the body *(FIG. 10-61)*.
       - If the axis of the uterus is deflected anteriorly, it is considered "anteverted," which is the most common presentation (1).
       - If roughly parallel, it is "midposition (2)."
       - And if deflected posterior, it is "retroverted (3)."
     —When the uterus is not straight, but is bent upon itself, the uterus is said to be flexed *(FIG. 10-62)*.
       - Forward flexion is termed *anteflexion* (1).
       - Backward flexion is termed *retroflexion* (2).

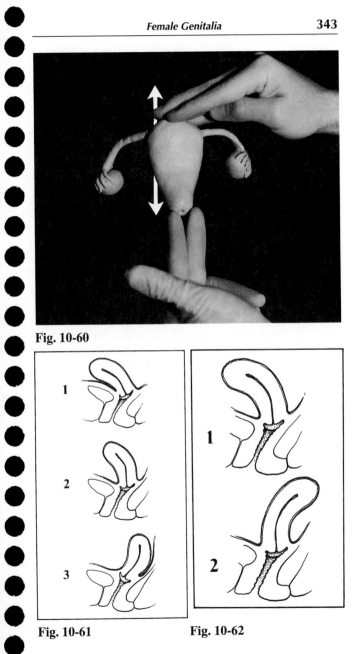

Fig. 10-60

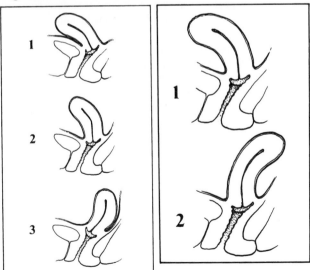

Fig. 10-61   Fig. 10-62

- To palpate:
  - —With the uterus in its usually (85%) anteverted position:
    - The abdominal hand rests on the uterine fundus, pushing it toward the vaginal fingers *(FIG. 10-63)*.
    - When the intravaginal fingers are placed in the anterior fornix, the uterine fundus will be palpable between the two hands.
  - —If the fundus is not felt, place the fingers in the posterior fornix and palpate again.
  - —With the uterus in retroversion:
    - The isthmus will be felt between the two hands.
    - The fundus will be felt with the backs of the intravaginal fingers.
    - More complete examination of the retro-displaced uterus is best done during the rectovaginal examination.
- Note its mobility. Fixation of the uterus in any position suggests peritoneal adhesions from infection, endometriosis, or malignancy.

4. Palpate the uterine surface.
   - In anteversion:
     - —Lift up on the cervix with the intravaginal fingers and palpate the contour of the uterus with the external hand *(FIG. 10-64)*. It should be small, round, and smooth.
     - —Then press in with the abdominal fingers *(FIG. 10-65)*.
       - Palpate the lower anterior surface through the anterior fornix.
       - Repeat on the posterior wall through the posterior fornix. This is easier via rectal examination.

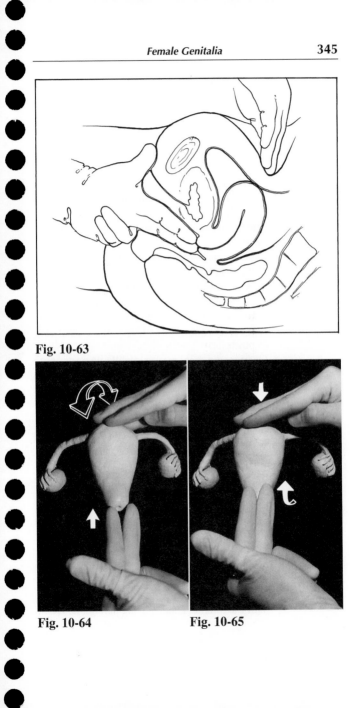

Fig. 10-63

Fig. 10-64   Fig. 10-65

E. Palpate the Adnexae (the ovaries and fallopian tubes).
  1. Anatomy.
   ▪ The normal ovaries are about 3×4 cm in size and freely movable.
     —Palpation of the ovaries normally produces an aching sensation, and the patient should be informed of this.
     —This aching sensation helps to distinguish the ovary from other nontender masses, such as stool.
   ▪ The fallopian tubes are soft and are not normally palpable.
     —Tenderness or a cordlike thickening between the ovary and uterus indicates tubal disease.
     —Another cordlike structure that may be palpated nearby is the round ligament. This structure arches anteriorly from the body of the uterus, whereas the ovaries and tubes curve posteriorly.
   ▪ Ovarian and tubal masses usually lie posterior to the uterus and tend to displace it forward within the pelvis.

  2. To palpate the left ovary:
   ▪ Place your right (external) hand low in the left lower quadrant *(FIG. 10-66)*.
     —This hand is most easily placed by palpating the uterine fundus and then moving your fingertips about 10 cm laterally.
   ▪ Place the vaginal fingers in the left lateral fornix, with the pads of the fingers aiming upward and outward *(FIG. 10-67)*.
     —You are pushing these fingers upward into the abdomen as far as they will go without patient discomfort.
     —The external hand should match the location of the internal hand, staying parallel above it.

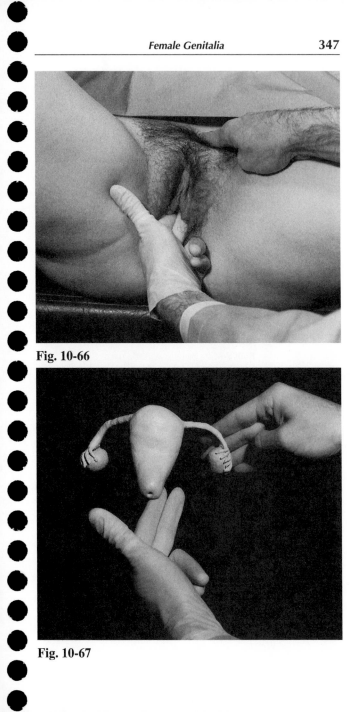

Fig. 10-66

Fig. 10-67

- Your hands are now positioned to "sandwich" the adnexa between them.
- Move the fingertips of each hand toward the other, gently compressing the tissues between *(FIG. 10-68).*
- Then, maintaining gently pressure, pull your hands inferiorly and medially.
  —Allow the tissues to slip between your two hands *(FIG. 10-69).*
  —The ovary will be felt as a small rubbery ovoid mass that catches between the fingers. (It is also normal, in some individuals, *not* to feel the ovaries.)
- Repeat this forward-compress-pull back motion at least once more to delineate the ovary.
  —Note its size, shape, consistency, mobility, and any tenderness.
  —Mobility would be affected by adhesions, either from infection, endometriosis, or malignancy.
  —Size would be affected by similar disorders, including cystic lesions.

3. Repeat on the left side.
   - If palpation is difficult with an intravaginal left hand, insert the right hand and use the left one on the abdomen.

4. After palpating for the adnexa, move the vaginal fingers to the posterior fornix and palpate for the uterosacral ligaments and any masses in the cul-de-sac.
   - Tenderness or nodularity here may indicate endometriosis.

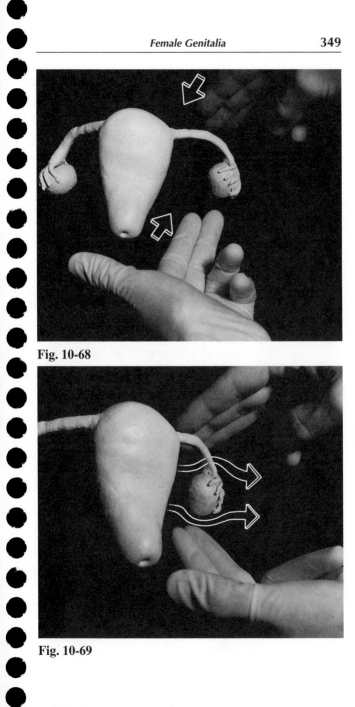

Fig. 10-68

Fig. 10-69

F. Rectovaginal Examination.

1. This is a uniquely informative portion of the examination.
   - It can be used in cases of a small introitus, where it is difficult to insert a finger far enough in or even at all.
   - It allows palpation of the rectovaginal septum.
   - It allows deeper palpation of other structures, such as:
     —A rectocoele.
     —An ovary not located by vaginal examination.
     —The posterior uterine wall.
     —Cul-de-sac masses.
     —Uterosacral and sacrococcygeal ligaments.
   - The deeper palpation is afforded by the intrarectal middle finger, which can insert more deeply than the intravaginal index finger.

2. Reglove and lubricate the examining fingers. This prevents the possible transfer of infection from vagina to rectum.

3. Ask the patient to bear down. This relaxes the anal sphincter.
   - Gently insert the distal half of the middle finger into the rectum and the index finger into the vagina *(FIG. 10-70).*
   - Inform her this may make her feel as if she has to move her bowels.

4. Feel the muscular perineal body between the two fingers. This is the outer third of the shelf. Feel in particular for thinning.
   - Weakness of the perineal body or anal sphincter can lead to fecal soiling. Ask the patient if this is a problem. This information is often not volunteered by the patient. It is sometimes a result of injury to these tissues during childbirth.

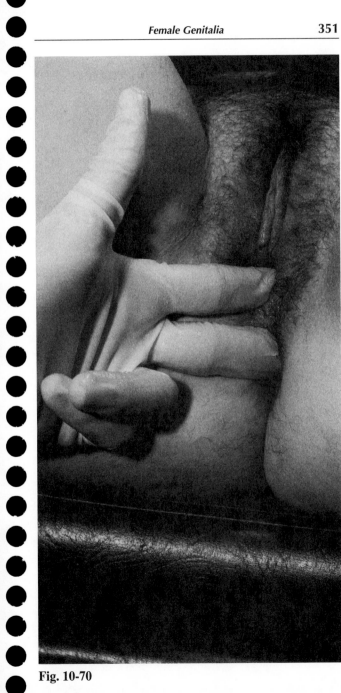

Fig. 10-70

5. Palpate the rectovaginal septum more deeply.
   - Fully insert the fingers *(FIG. 10-71).*
   - Sweep them from side to side *(FIG. 10-72).* Feel for tenderness, nodules (endometriosis), or thinning (rectocoele).

6. Repeat the steps of the bimanual examination.
   - The deeper internal finger and lack of restraining tissues often aid the rectal finger in palpating pelvic structures more accurately.
   - Palpate in turn the uterine fundus, cervix, and adnexae.

7. End by depressing the uterus downward.
   - Feel the region behind the cervix that may only be accessible to the rectal finger *(FIG. 10-73).*
   - Again, as the rectal finger penetrates farther in than does the vaginal one, palpate for:
     —The cul-de-sac.
     —The posterior uterine wall.
     —The uterine fundus in cases of retroversion or retroflexion.
     —The uterosacral ligaments, for nodules or tenderness.

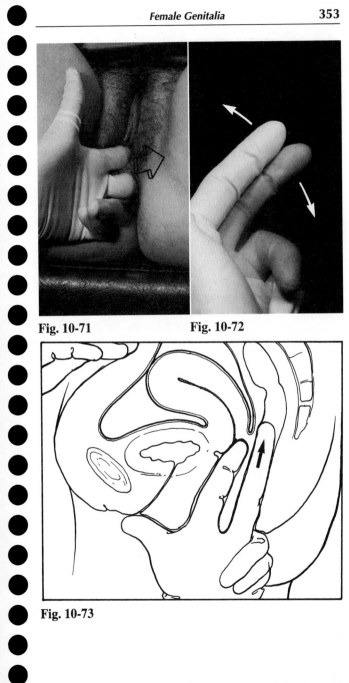

Fig. 10-71   Fig. 10-72

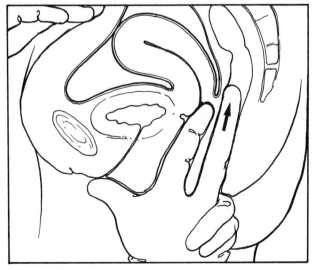

Fig. 10-73

G. **Rectal Examination:** You may wish to reglove, since the index finger is most often inserted.

  1. Inspection.

    ▪ Examine the skin around the anus *(FIG. 10-74).*

      —It is normally more pigmented and coarse than the surrounding skin, and is also moist and hairless.

      —Note any skin tags, external hemorrhoids, fistulas, or other lesions.

      —After informing the patient, gently stretch the anal skin with thumb and forefinger and look for an anal fissure.

        • This is a painful, narrow triangular split of the skin, usually located posteriorly.

        • If one is seen, perform further palpation very cautiously, as it can be painful.

    ▪ Have her bear down and inspect for rectal prolapse, fissures, or internal hemorrhoids.

    ▪ Describe any lesions as if on the face of a clock, *(FIG. 10-75)* with the 12:00 o'clock postition being directly superior.

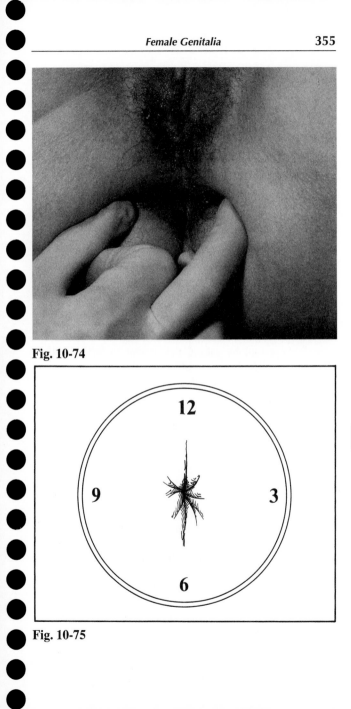

Fig. 10-74

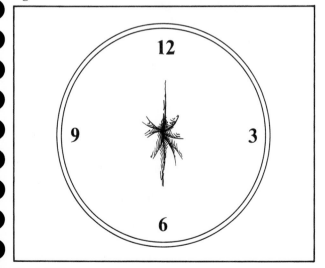

Fig. 10-75

2. Palpation.
   - Place a gloved finger at the anus *(FIG. 10-76).* This allows the patient to adapt to contact on such a sensitive area.
   - Have her bear down again, then reinsert the examining finger *(FIG. 10-77).* Note sphincter tone. Then ask her to tighten her muscles around your finger; this is a useful measure of sphincter strength.
   - Palpate the rectal walls, feeling in turn:
     —Anterior *(FIG. 10-78).*
     —Left lateral.
     —Posterior.
     —And right lateral rectal walls.
       • Be aware that the rectum between the 12:00 and 3:00 o'clock positions is hard to reach. You may need to turn slightly away from the patient to rotate your right index finger counter-clockwise enough.
   - End by asking the patient to strain. Palpate deeply for rectal lesions that are almost out of reach *(FIG. 10-79).*
     —Rectosigmoid carcinomas, felt as an induration in the rectal wall, are often located at this upper border of reach.
   - After removing the finger, check the rectal finger for stool color.
     —If not overtly bloody, check any fecal material for occult blood *(FIG. 10-80).*
   - Gently wipe the external genitalia with a tissue, or offer the patient a tissue to do it herself.
     —A discrete method is to place a box of tissues near the patient and encourage her to use them if she wishes. Then leave the room for her to redress.

H. **Let the Patient Dress Before Discussing Your Findings with Her.**
   1. This gives you an opportunity to check the wet preparation if one was taken.
   2. It also gives the patient a moment to relax from the stress of examination. In this way, she can benefit more from subsequent discussion with the examiner.

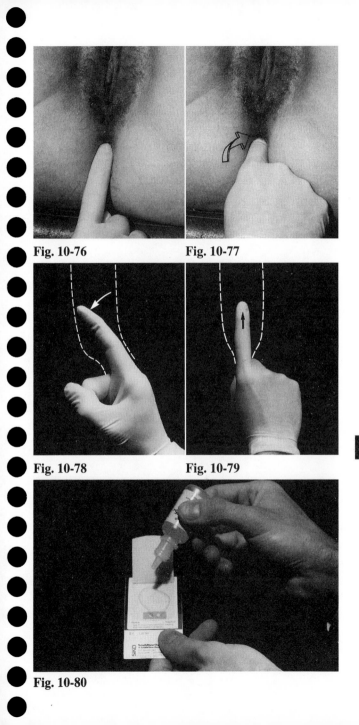

Fig. 10-76

Fig. 10-77

Fig. 10-78

Fig. 10-79

Fig. 10-80

11 Musculoskeletal Examination

WITH EVELYN V. HESS, M.D., F.A.C.P.

I. **INTRODUCTION: This examination is primarily an assessment of joints and related structures. It is particularly useful when searching for signs of rheumatic disease or to assess the severity of a traumatic or sports-related injury.**

  A. **Observation** plays a key role and begins the moment the patient enters the room.

   1. Note how he enters or is brought in, and the ease of motion involved with:
      - Sitting in interview chair, then getting up again.
      - Movement to the examination table.
      - Note use of assistive devices, such as a cane or walker.
      - (Further examination of gait is discussed in Chapter 12, Neurologic Examination.)

   2. At this time, the patient should undress to undergarments, shorts, or a swimsuit.

  B. **Be Aware That Many Systemic Diseases Can Cause Aches and Pains.**

   1. An overall assessment of the patient is as important as the study of individual joints.
      - Many illnesses cause these symptoms other than just the "rheumatic" diseases.
        —Hypothyroidism, for example, is a common and often hidden cause of diffuse aching and fatigue, particularly in the elderly.

   2. Visual signs of illness can often assist in the diagnosis.
      - Aches and pains form an enormous part of medicine.
        —It is easy to become lost in the mechanics of joint examination. To avoid this, begin with general observation, keeping in mind the many possible causative disorders.
      - Consider the patient's age and presenting complaint as you look for visual signs of illness that may relate to the patient's symptoms.
      - Although the range of possibilities is enormous, the initial assessment is visual and therefore very rapid.

C. **Screen Each Joint with a General Approach.**

1. Do the simple and general examination techniques first.
   - If they are normal, more detailed maneuvers may not be necessary.
     —Always perform the more detailed examination if joint involvement is seen or suspected (because of related signs or history of trauma).

2. Range of motion is not routinely measured in every joint; only on those with involvement or on suspicion of involvement.
   - If range of motion (ROM) is measured, record findings (in degrees) immediately in the chart. Do not attempt to memorize them.
   - The starting position for range of motion is usually considered the anatomic position of relaxed extension.

D. **In General:**

1. *Inspect* for:
   - Redness, particularly over joints.
   - Swelling over or near joints.
   - Limited joint motion.
   - Deformity.
   - The condition of overlying skin. Is it atrophic or scarred?

2. *Palpate* for:
   - Heat; feel with the backs of two fingers, touching lightly and briefly.
   - Tenderness; palpate gently, particularly if you see overlying redness or swelling.
   - Texture of the joint; is it hard, boggy, or fluid-filled?
   - Crepitus; a crackling or crunching sensation felt when the joint is moved through its range. Your fingers must be in contact with the joint to perceive this.
   - Instability and range of motion.
   - Muscle strength. This is reviewed in more detail in Chapter 12, Neurologic Examination.

3. Also note any symmetry of joint involvement.
  - Certain rheumatic diseases identify themselves by their relative symmetry of involvement, such as rheumatoid arthritis.

E. The Examination Progresses from Upper to Lower Extremities: going proximal to distal, and then to the spine. This order will vary among examiners.

F. When Dealing with a Person with Painful Joints, be gentle and allow the patient to move and change positions at his/her own pace.

G. To Speed the Recording of Your Findings, Consider Using:

1. A joint mannekin; to indicate which joints are involved *(FIG. 11-1)*. This is a schematic representation of the skeleton, allowing you to circle the involved joints.

2. A similar form showing range of motion for each joint (usually with a column showing normal range, and fill-in spaces for left and right sides).

II. UPPER EXTREMITY INSPECTION: Inspection and range of motion give an overall idea of which joints are involved, if any. The presence of any abnormalities prompts a more detailed testing of the affected areas than the simple screening examination described here.

A. Head and Neck.

1. Inspect for common signs of systemic diseases with joint manifestations:
   - Patchy baldness of lupus erythematosus.
   - Loss of lateral aspects of eyebrows with hypothyroidism.
   - Conjunctivitis or iritis of Reiters syndrome or other seronegative spondyloarthropathies.
   - Alterations in ear or nose cartilage of relapsing polychondritis.
   - Gouty tophi in rim of ear cartilage.
   - Swelling around the temporomandibular joints in rheumatoid arthritis and other illnesses.
   - Enlarged parotid glands or dry eyes of Sjogren's syndrome.
   - Wrinkling or skin tightening of scleroderma.
     —Pay close attention to wrinkling around the mouth and skin sclerosis on distal fingers.
   - Crusted lesions around the lip or nose (Stevens-Johnson syndrome) or urticarial/morbilliform rash of vasculitis.
   - Presence of goiter with hypothyroidism (and sometimes hyperthyroidism).
   - Psoriatic skin lesions, particularly on extensor skin surfaces.
   - Enlarged lymph nodes of infectious mononucleosis, particularly posterior cervical.

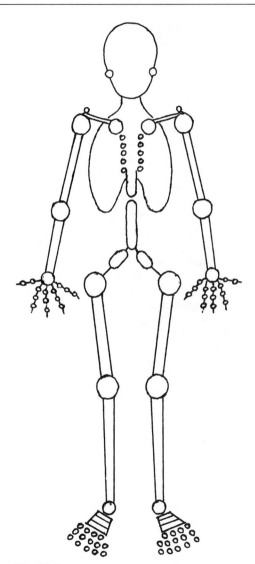

Fig. 11-1

2. Note alignment of the neck and shoulders. Are both shoulders level?

3. Screen for range of motion:
   - Temporomandibular joint as he opens his mouth as wide as possible, then closes it *(FIG. 11-2).*
     —Also have him protrude his jaw and move it from side to side.
   - Cervical spine range of motion as he:
     —Rolls his head around on the neck, keeping the shoulders straight *(FIG. 11-3).*
     —Extends and flexes his neck *(FIG. 11-4).* Ask him to touch his chin to his chest, then pull his head back as far as he can.
     —Laterally flexes to each side. Ask him to touch his ear to each shoulder as you hold his shoulders in place *(FIG. 11-5).*
       • This prevents shoulder lift at the extremes of motion, which can give a false impression of good neck mobility.
     —Rotates the neck by touching his chin to each shoulder.
   - For all range of motion testing, note the range of movement in degrees.

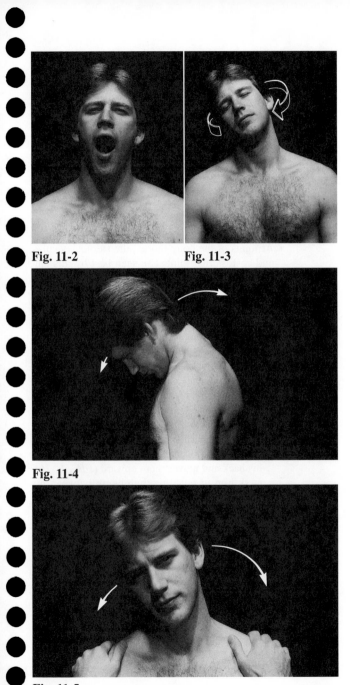

Fig. 11-2

Fig. 11-3

Fig. 11-4

Fig. 11-5

B. Shoulders and Thorax.

1. Inspect for alignment relative to the head and rest of the trunk. See if their level is symmetric.

2. Note soft tissue redness or swelling, and any deltoid atrophy *(FIG. 11-6)*.

3. Move to the side to check the shoulder for swelling: *(FIG. 11-7)*
   - Anteriorly and posteriorly. (1)
   - At the acromioclavicular joint. (2)
   - At joints of the bony thorax, the sternoclavicular, and costosternal joints (3), seen best by this tangential view:
     —Also check the skin surfaces and hair distributions on the chest and back.

4. Then screen for range of motion.
   - With his arms outstretched in front, palms down, observe:
     —Abduction, as he swings his arms laterally and moves them over head, palms touching *(FIG. 11-8)*.
     —External rotation, as he clasps his hands behind his neck and pulls the elbows back *(FIG. 11-9)*.
     —Internal rotation, as he places both hands behind his back and moves them upward *(FIG. 11-10)*. (Ask him to push his thumbs up between his shoulder blades.)
       - He should be able to reach to mid-back level (by scapular tip) *(FIG. 11-11)*.
   - Approximate normal ranges (in degrees):
     —Extension, 50 to 60.
     —Flexion, 160 to180.
     —Abduction, 170 to180.
     —Adduction, 50.
     —External and internal rotation, 90.

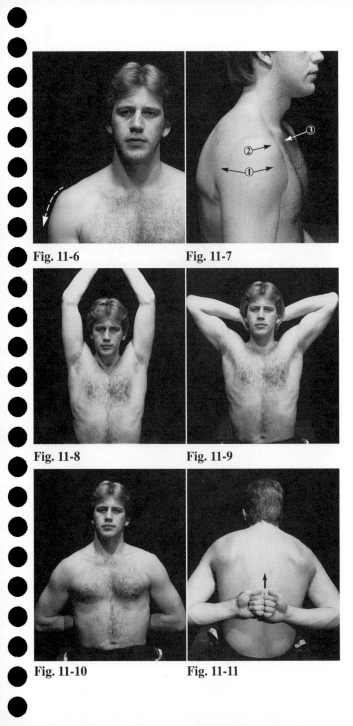

Fig. 11-6

Fig. 11-7

Fig. 11-8

Fig. 11-9

Fig. 11-10

Fig. 11-11

C. Elbows and Hands.

1. Screen elbow range of motion.
   - Have him extend his arms in pronation, then supination *(FIG. 11-12)*.
   - Then have him flex his elbows and raise them to the horizontal position. This makes the elbow tips easier to see *(FIG. 11-13)*.

2. Inspect the olecranon areas for bursal or joint swelling, and over the ulnar ridge for nodules.

3. Have him extend his arms again, palms down.
   - Inspect the wrists for redness or swelling.
   - Screen for range of motion at the wrist.
     —Note flexion and extension *(FIG. 11-14)*.
     —Note radial and ulnar deviation *(FIG. 11-15)*.
   - Inspect the fingers for inflammation.
     —Pay close attention over the metacarpophalangeal and interphalangeal joints.
   - Screen for range of motion.
     —Observe abduction (spreading the fingers), flexion (making a fist), and extension (*FIGS. 11-16 and 11-17*).
   - Approximate normal ranges (in degrees):
     —Elbow:
       - Flexion, 150 to 160.
       - Extension, 0.
       - Supination and pronation, 90.
     —Wrist:
       - Flexion, 70 to 90.
       - Extension, 70.
       - Radial deviation, 20.
       - Ulnar deviation, 50 to 55.
     —Fingers:
       - Metacarpophalangeal (MCP) flexion, 90; extension, 30.
       - Proximal interphalangeal (PIP) flexion, 120; extension, 0.
       - Distal interphalangeal (DIP) flexion, 80; extension, 10; abduction or adduction, 20.

4. Then perform palpation and watch for pain during joint motion.

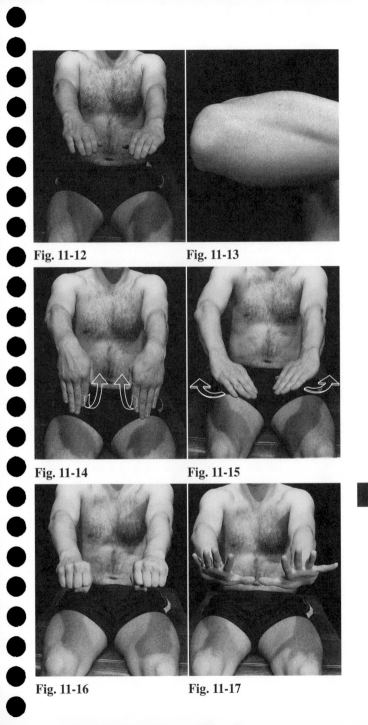

Fig. 11-12

Fig. 11-13

Fig. 11-14

Fig. 11-15

Fig. 11-16

Fig. 11-17

III. **UPPER EXTREMITY PALPATION: In all aspects of joint palpation it is extremely important to monitor the patient's reaction throughout the examination. Watch especially for signs of pain. Detailed palpation focuses on those joints with changes seen by inspection or suspected through the medical history.**

   A. **Temporomandibular Joints** (TMJ) (see *FIGS. 4-93* and *4-94*)

      1. Place your index fingers on each mandibular condyle, just anterior to the tragus, and apply light pressure.

      2. Feel for crepitus, tenderness, or palpable synovium as he opens and closes his mouth.
   - The finger will drop into the temporomandibular joint space as the mouth opens.
   - Some clicking may be heard or felt on TMJ motion and is normal.

   B. **Examination for Signs of Systemic Disease.** This is optional and may have already been performed during the head and neck exam.

      1. Face
   - Rub the pinnae of the ears, feeling for nodules.
   - Note hair texture (thyroid disease) and search for patchy baldness (lupus) or psoriatic lesions in the scalp, at the hairline or behind the neck.
   - Feel the skin of the cheeks and malar prominences for scarring (lupus).
   - Look for heliotrope (violet-colored) rash on eyelids as he closes his eyes (dermatomyositis).
   - Have him look up, check the inferior tarsal conjunctiva for redness (Reiter's syndrome) and degree of moisture (Sjogren's syndrome).
   - Palpate for parotid gland tenderness or enlargement (Sjogren's syndrome).

2. Mouth
   - Examine the teeth for gross deformities (congenital syndromes) and gums for infection (arthralgias from subacute bacterial endocarditis, seeded from infected gums).
   - Inspect the mucosal surfaces for mucocutaneous lesions (Reiters).
     —Look in particular at the tongue, buccal mucosa, palate, and underside of the lips.
   - Note the color and size of the tongue (amyloidosis, myxedema, anemia).

3. Neck
   - Briefly survey lymph node areas:
     —Postauricular and preauricular, submental, submaxillary, anterior and posterior cervical nodes.
   - Palpate thyroid gland if thyroid disease is suspected.
     —*Always* consider thyroid disease in the elderly. It is the great mimicker.

C. **Thorax:** brace one hand behind the patient on his mid-back.
   1. Sternoclavicular joint
      - Palpate on both sides with the index finger.
   2. Costosternal joints *(FIG. 11-18)*
      - Push on both sides simultaneously with the index and middle fingers.
      - Examine each pair in sequence, moving down to the xyphoid.
   3. Xyphoid process: apply gentle pressure, palpating for tenderness.
      - The xiphoid process varies widely in its size and prominence. Do not be alarmed by a large or even bifid (forked) xiphoid process.

D. **Shoulder.**
   1. Palpate for tenderness or deformities along the clavicle, moving outward to the acromioclavicular joint *(FIG. 11-19)*.
   2. Then feel around the top and sides of the shoulder joint for tenderness.
      - If tenderness is present, palpate for heat, using the backs of two fingers *(FIG. 11-20)*.
   3. Examine the subacromial bursa, which lies deep to the deltoid muscle *(FIG. 11-21)*.
      - It is about 3 cm across and separates the deltoid muscle from the joint capsule.
      - Press inward, feeling for tenderness.
   4. Palpate the insertion of the biceps tendon (long head), a tendinous cord that runs just medial to the greater tubercle of the humerus *(FIG. 11-22)*.
      - Locate it on the medial side of the upper arm, just below the shoulder joint, and slide your fingers over it, feeling it pop across.
        —Palpation here is aided by externally rotating the arm.
   5. Feel the muscle bulk of the upper arm, moving from proximal to distal *(FIG. 11-23)*. Note any atrophy.

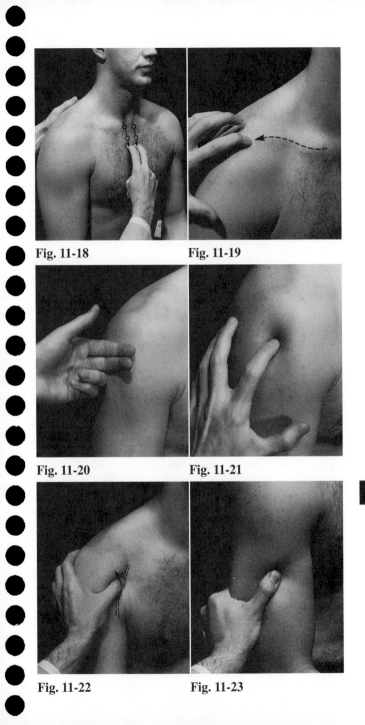

Fig. 11-18

Fig. 11-19

Fig. 11-20

Fig. 11-21

Fig. 11-22

Fig. 11-23

6. Palpate the scapula and surrounding muscle *(FIG. 11-24)*. Feel for localized tenderness.
7. Isolate motion of the glenohumeral joint (optional). This test is useful when limited shoulder motion is suspected, often secondary to rotator cuff tear or frozen shoulder.
   - Fix the scapular tip between the thumb and forefinger of your left hand.
   - Externally rotate and then abduct the arm *(FIG. 11-25)*.
   - Glenohumeral motion is complete when the scapula begins to move.
     —This maneuver helps you to confirm limited shoulder abduction, which can be masked by the compensatory movement of the scapula.

E. Elbows.

1. Grasp his wrist with your opposite hand, bending his elbow.
2. With your free hand, palpate in turn:
   - Any areas of described tenderness or over any visible redness or swelling.
   - The muscle mass around the elbow joint.
   - The olecranon bursa *(FIG. 11-26)*. Then pinch and roll it between your fingers, feeling for small nodules.
   - The epicondyles, for tenderness *(FIG. 11-27)*.
     —Tenderness over the lateral epicondyle occurs with *tennis elbow.*
   - The hollows on either side of the olecranon *(FIG. 11-28)*.
     —These are the best regions to palpate synovium of this joint.
     —Palpate in the hollows with thumb and forefinger. The synovium is normally not palpable.
3. Then place one hand behind the elbow and push it into hyperextension several times *(FIG. 11-29)*.
   - This checks for hypermobility, present with Ehler-Danlos or Marfan's syndromes.
   - In general, the elbow, wrist, and knee are the best areas to detect hypermobility.

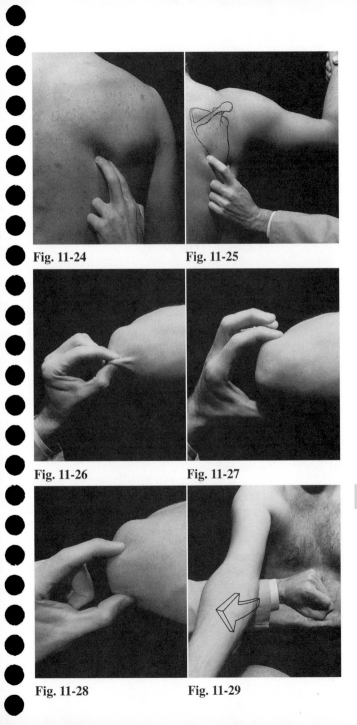

Fig. 11-24

Fig. 11-25

Fig. 11-26

Fig. 11-27

Fig. 11-28

Fig. 11-29

F. Wrists and Hands (Examined in detail, as they are of great diagnostic significance.)

1. Palpate across the wrist *(FIG. 11-30)*.
    - Pressing inward amongst the carpal bones with thumb and index finger on the ventral and dorsal sides. Feel for bogginess, tenderness, or swelling.
    - Then press inward around the radial and ulnar styloids, feeling for the same characteristics.
    - Then wrap your fingers around the wrist and squeeze laterally to check for pain. This opposes the carpal bones against each other and is a test of inflammation *(FIG. 11-31)*.

2. Examine the carpometacarpal joint of the thumb. This is an often overlooked joint, commonly affected by osteoarthritis.
    - It is located at the base of the thumb, just distal to the radial styloid.
    - Inspect for swelling.
    - Palpate by pressing the tip of your thumb into the joint space and moving the thumb with your free hand *(FIG. 11-32)*. In this way, you can feel the entire joint space.

3. Inspect and palpate the dorsal hand:
    - For extensor swelling or tenderness. This is often overlooked.
      —Sweep the tips of four fingers from proximal to distal over the tendons.
      —Begin at the retinaculum (visible crease) of the wrist, where swelling often originates *(FIG. 11-34)*.
    - For interosseous muscle atrophy, seen as grooves between the metacarpal bones *(FIG. 11-33)*.

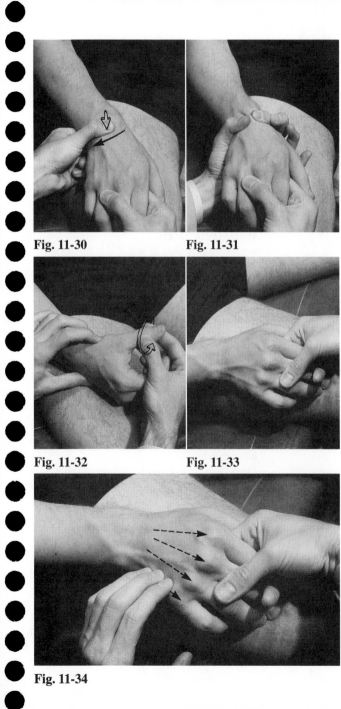

Fig. 11-30

Fig. 11-31

Fig. 11-32

Fig. 11-33

Fig. 11-34

4. Examine the fingers.
   ▪ Inspect for color (blanching or cyanosis), psoriatic changes, or vasculitis lesions (at the tip or near the nail).
   ▪ Compare the temperature of the fingers to that of the examining room. This is significant if the room is warm and the fingers are quite cool.
   ▪ Feel the pads and tips of the fingers for vasculitis lesions (lupus, etc.) and for the waxy stiffness of scleroderma.
      —Feel each nail, as psoriatic pitting may not be visible *(FIG. 11-35)*.
   ▪ Pinch the dorsal skin to see if it is bound down (scleroderma) *(FIG. 11-36)*.

5. Check the joints.
   ▪ Record synovial thickening or tenderness on a scale of 0 (absent) to 4.
   ▪ Follow a set pattern:
      —One method, used here, is to examine from distal to proximal, small finger to index.
      —This pattern varies among clinicians.
   ▪ Distal interphalangeal (DIP) joints.
      —Grasp the joint by the sides with thumb and index finger and fix it in slight flexion *(FIG. 11-37)*. This opens the joint space, making synovium more palpable.
      —Press perpendicularly downward into the joint space with the index finger of your free hand *(FIG. 11-38)*.
   ▪ The lateral fingers feel for bony swelling or tenderness.
   ▪ The index finger feels for synovium on either side of the extensor tendon.
   ▪ As a variant of this technique, place the thumb and forefinger of the free hand anteroposteriorly on the joint. Alternate pressure with the two hands, squeezing first laterally, then anteroposteriorly. This helps to feel spongy swelling of these small joints.
      —Repeat on the remaining fingers and thumb.

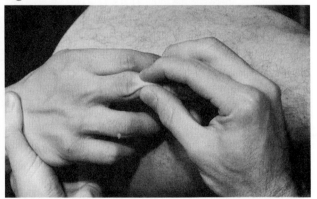

Fig. 11-35

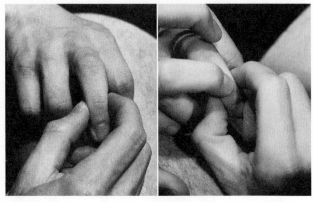

Fig. 11-36

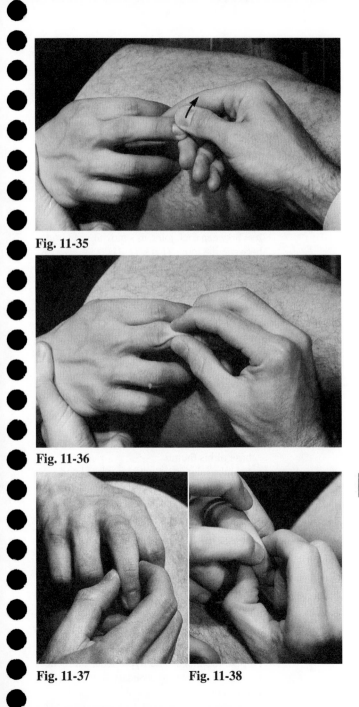

Fig. 11-37 Fig. 11-38

- Proximal interphalangeal (PIP) joints.
  —Repeat, small finger to index (the thumb has only one interphalangeal joint) *(FIG. 11-39)*.
  —Hard, sometimes tender nodules on the dorsal PIP joint are called *Bouchard's nodes,* a sign of osteoarthritis. On the DIP joints, they are called *Heberden's nodes.*
- Metacarpophalangeal (MCP) joints.
  —Best felt with the fingers in a loose fist *(FIG. 11-40).*
  —Palpate each joint, small finger to index. Then feel between each joint, as synovium can bridge between the joints *(FIG. 11-41).*
    • This is done by sweeping the pad of your index or middle finger up and down in the grooves between.
    • As an alternate method, grasp the patient's hand with both of yours and place your thumbs on either side of his MCP joint. Palpate for tenderness or swelling over each joint.
  —For the thumb MCP:
    • Place your index finger under the base of his thumb and grasp his distal phalanx with your remaining fingers *(FIG. 11-42).*
    • Lift up with your index finger, elevating the base of his thumb.
    • Feel the joint space with your free hand.

6. Examine the palm.
   - Inspect for swelling or flexion (Dupuytren's) contractures, as finger contractures may be from tendon involvement and not the joints themselves.
     —Also note any flushing of the palm.
   - Palpate each flexor tendon as you flex and extend each of his fingers.
   - Then sweep your thumb down his palmar fascia, feeling for nodules *(FIG. 11-43).*
     —Dupuytren's contractures are often felt as linear thickenings on the palmar surface over the MCP joints.
     —Palpate the thenar and hypothenar eminences for muscle atrophy, a secondary sign of wrist involvement.

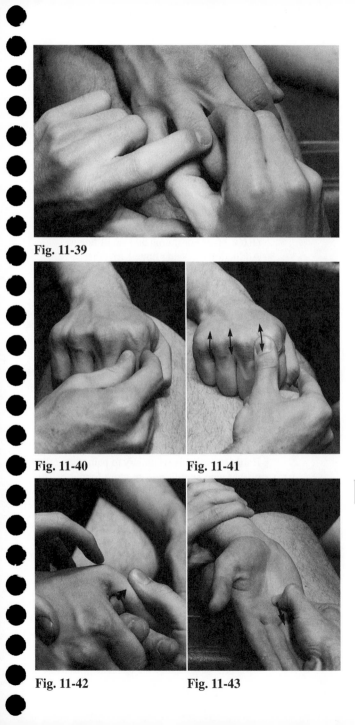

Fig. 11-39

Fig. 11-40

Fig. 11-41

Fig. 11-42

Fig. 11-43

7. Test the hand as a functional unit.
   - Watch for finger deviation during finger flexion (makes a fist) and extension (releases) *(FIG. 11-44)*. Observe this with the hand pronated.
     —Ulnar deviation is common with rheumatoid arthritis
   - Repeat flexion and extension with the hand in supination and watch for tightening in the palmar fascia *(FIG. 11-45)*.
   - Check basic finger motions:
     —Opposition, pinching thumb and index finger *(FIG. 11-46)* or thumb and small finger.
     —Adduction (pressing fingers together).
     —Abduction (if weakness is present). Have him spread his fingers while you resist with your inward pressure on his index and small fingers *(FIG. 11-47)*.
   - Check grip strength against resistance. Have him squeeze your index finger as you try to pull it out *(FIG. 11-48)*.
   - When motion is impaired, determine whether limitation is due to pain or true loss of (mechanical) function.
     —When limited motion is seen, ask the patient if that is the full extent of his motion, or if he is holding back because of pain.
     —If the limitation is secondary to pain, then relief of that pain should restore more function. This is written: "motion was limited (this much) and was limited by pain."

G. Before Continuing: *(FIG. 11-49)*
1. Palpate the lower thorax for rib pain.

2. Note any abdominal scars, indications of prior surgery, such as for inflammatory bowel disease.
   - Disorders such as ulcerative colitis and Crohn's disease are associated with arthritis patterns.

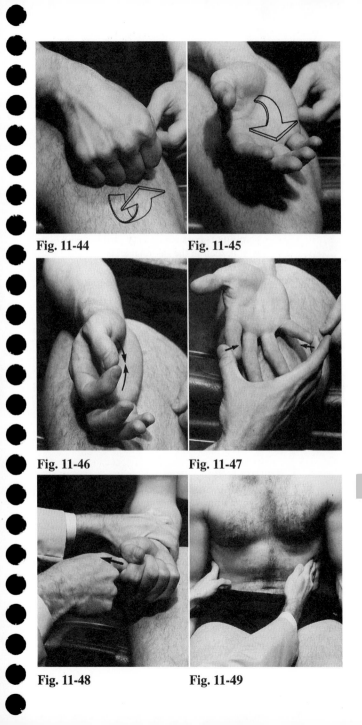

Fig. 11-44

Fig. 11-45

Fig. 11-46

Fig. 11-47

Fig. 11-48

Fig. 11-49

IV. **LOWER EXTREMITIES: Have the patient lie supine.
His movement to the examination table gives some
indication of lower extremity function. The order of
examination varies, again, with the clinician. Here, it
progresses from hips to legs to feet.**
   A. **Hips**
      1. Inspection.
         - Note any abnormal positioning of the legs *(FIG.
           11-50)*.
         - Inspect anteriorly for swelling or redness around
           the joint.
           —Swelling is not usually very visible, but when it
             is, it is seen in the inguinal area.
           —Inspect also for enlarged inguinal lymph nodes.
           —Also inspect laterally over the subtrochanteric
             bursa.

      2. Palpation.
         - Anteriorly, over the inguinal area for effusion
           (FIG. 11-51).
           —If present, it feels like a sense of resistance be-
             low the inguinal ligament. This is the anatomic
             location of the hip joint.
         - Laterally, over the subtrochanteric bursa (palpate
           near the greater trochanter for tenderness) *(FIG.
           11-52)*.

      3. Range of motion.
         - Roll each leg from side to side in internal and ex-
           ternal rotation.
           —This is a good screening test of intraarticular le-
             sions *(FIG. 11-53)*.
         • External rotation is often lost first in hip osteoarthritis.
           —Watch the patient's face carefully during this
             maneuver, since pain here prompts caution with
             further testing.

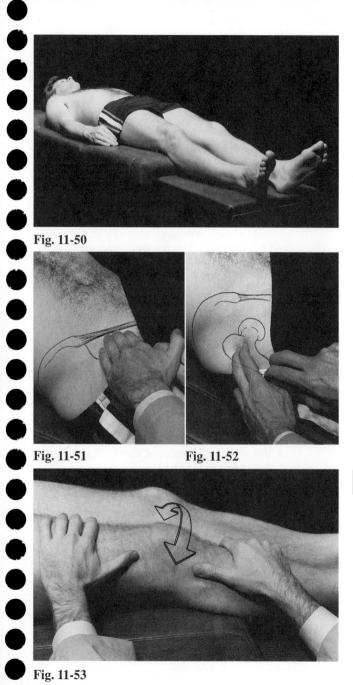

Fig. 11-50

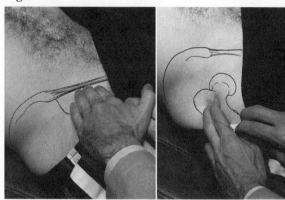

Fig. 11-51   Fig. 11-52

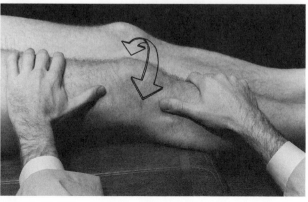

Fig. 11-53

- Check lateral motion.
  —Ask the patient to keep his untested leg in place. Make sure both legs are lined up straight.
  —Stand on the same side as the leg being tested.
    • Place your hand on that anterior illiac crest. In this way, you can tell the limit of hip joint motion when the pelvis itself begins to move.
  —Grasp the patient's ankle and move the leg through:
    • Full abduction *(FIG. 11-54).*
    • Full adduction *(FIG. 11-55).*
  —As always, note range of motion in degrees.
- Check rotation. This is a useful addition to simply rolling the legs.
  —Flex the knee to 90 degrees, holding the leg at the ankle and over the patella.
  —Rotate the leg internally and externally to its limits of motion *(FIG. 11-56).* Watch for signs of patient discomfort.
  —The leg acts as a pointer showing the angle of rotation.

4. Check for flexion contractures of the hips and knees *(FIG. 11-57).*
   - Have him sit up and reach for his toes. Watch for normal lumbar flexion.
   - If contractures are present, the hips and knees will flex as he bends forward.
   - As an alternate method, have the patient lay flat and ask him to flex one knee onto his chest, holding it in place with his arms. If the other hip has a contracture, it will flex.

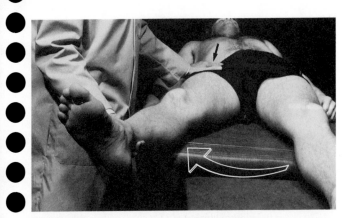

Fig. 11-54

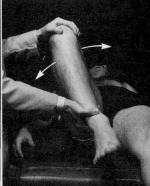

Fig. 11-55

Fig. 11-56

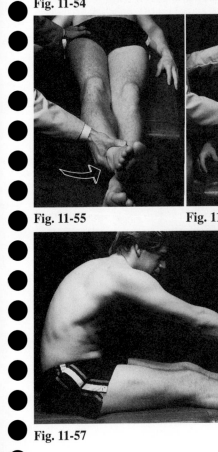

Fig. 11-57

- While he is sitting up:
  —Check the level of the posterior iliac crests for symmetry. Place your thumbs on the crests, watching for equal level *(FIG. 11-58)*.
  —Palpate over the lower sacrum and coccyx for rheumatoid nodules *(FIG. 11-59)*.

5. Approximate normal hip ranges (in degrees)
   - Knee straight:
     —Flexion, 90.
     —Extension, 0.
     —Hyperextension, 15.
   - Knee bent:
     —Flexion, 120.
     —Extension, 0.
     —Internal and external rotation, 40 to 45.
   - Abduction, 45 to 50; Adduction 30.

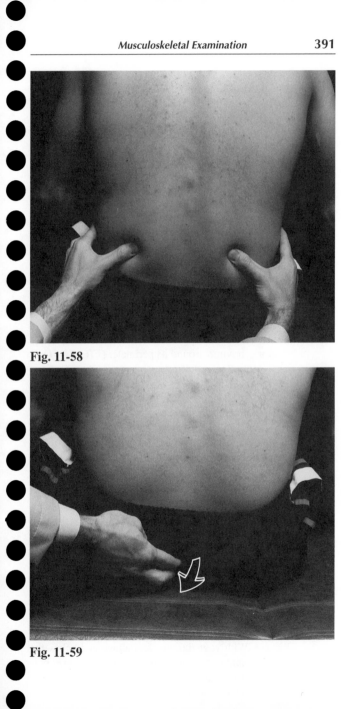

Fig. 11-58

Fig. 11-59

B. Knees.

    1. Inspection: with the patient supine, note.

- Any muscle atrophy, especially of the quadriceps *(FIG. 11-60).*

    —The vastus medialis forms a slight bulge on the medial aspect of the quadriceps. Loss of this bulge is often the first sign of quadriceps atrophy.

- The fossae above (medial and lateral) and below the knee. They should all be visible.

    —Joint effusion causes a general rounding of the knee, removing these depressions.

- The shape and size of the patella.

    —A soft bulging directly over the patella is usually a prepatellar bursitis with effusion.

- Any skin lesions, such as psoriasis.

    2. Palpation (flex the knee slightly).

- With hands on opposite sides of the patella, palpate for synovium around its perimeter *(FIG. 11-61).*
- Note bursal swelling, using a pinching motion: *(FIG. 11-62)*

    —Suprapatellar, above the patella.

    —Prepatellar, over the patella.

    —Infrapatellar, over the patellar tendon.

    —Anserine bursa, on the medial aspect of the proximal tibia, about 3 cm beneath the joint line *(FIG. 11-63).* Palpate over this area with the index and middle fingers.

- Palpate for tenderness:

    —Over the patella *(FIG. 11-64).*

    —On the tibial tuberosity, the inferior insertion of the patellar tendon.

        • Pain in this location is more common in young adolescents with Osgood-Schlatter disease, a local inflammation that occurs before the tuberosity has completely ossified.

    —Over the collateral ligaments, medial, and lateral *(FIG. 11-65).*

        • With your thumbs, feel above and below the joint line, which is usually near the lower border of the patella. It is easiest to locate near the patellar tendon.

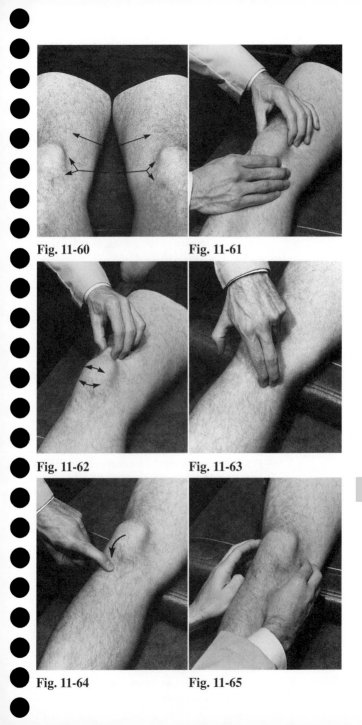

Fig. 11-60

Fig. 11-61

Fig. 11-62

Fig. 11-63

Fig. 11-64

Fig. 11-65

- If tenderness is present, feel for heat in several locations *(FIG. 11-66).* Tenderness at the joint line on one side, usually over the tibia, suggests a meniscus tear.
- Sweep four fingers through the popliteal space to feel for the swelling of a Baker's cyst *(FIG. 11-67).*
- If a small knee effusion is suspected, test for the bulge sign.
  —Adjust lighting to increase shadows in the medial fossae of the patella.
  —Sweep your fingers through the fossa on the upper medial aspect of the patella, then fix them against the patella *(FIG. 11-68).* This displaces any fluid into the lateral fossa.
  —Then, using your bent thumb, sweep firmly through the lateral fossa, attempting to push fluid back across.
    • If fluid is present, a small wave will fill the medial fossa and will remain there even as you release your thumb.
    • Other soft tissue such as fat, which can also cause a bulging, will retract as you remove your thumb.
  —The test can also be repeated in the fossae below the patella *(FIG. 11-69).*
- For a large effusion, test for ballottement.
  —Place your hand about 15 cm above the patella with thumb and fingers on opposite sides of the thigh. With moderate pressure, slide your hand downward until just above the patella. This will milk any fluid from the suprapatellar pouch into the joint itself.
  —With the free hand, tap the patella. When a large effusion is present, the patella will sink and land against the femur with a palpable bump. At the same time, the other hand will feel fluid returning to the pouch above.

3. Range of motion
- Flex each knee, then extend and raise it.
  —As it rises, view the joint, front and back, for swelling *(FIG. 11-70).*
  —Then raise the leg as far as it will go, watching for pain *(FIG. 11-71).*

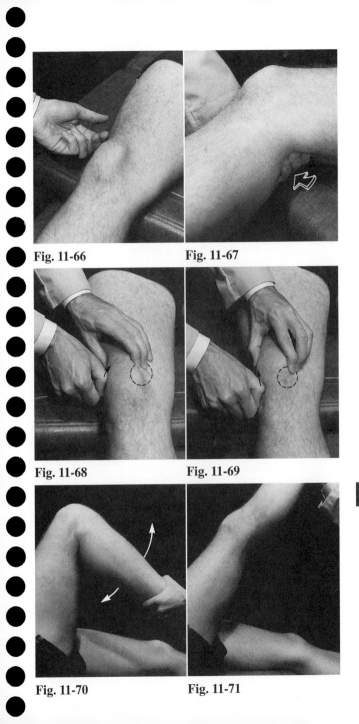

Fig. 11-66

Fig. 11-67

Fig. 11-68

Fig. 11-69

Fig. 11-70

Fig. 11-71

- This is the straight-leg raise test and is part of the spine examination.
- Place your hand under his lumbar spine; it will flatten when hip motion is completed.

4. Joint stability: performed in more detail later in "additional tests."
   - Anterior cruciate ligament *(FIG. 11-72)*.
     —Flex the knee to 90 degrees.
     —Place your left forearm under the joint and quickly lift upward several times.
     —Watch for forward motion of the tibia on the femur.
   - Collateral ligaments *(FIG. 11-73)*.
     —Hold the knee with one hand, his ankle with the other.
     —Apply a valgus (knee in, ankle out) and varus (knee out, ankle in) strain to the knee. Watch for laxity of the joint, seen by more than a few degrees of lateral and medial motion.
   - Gross capsule instability *(FIG. 11-74)*.
     —Straighten the leg somewhat (about 110 degrees of flexion) and place your hands above and below the joint.
     —Move your hands in opposition, attempting to move the femur and tibia across each other.
     —Repeat in full extension.
     —Normally, the joint is quite stable to lateral motion.
       - Stability should increase with the locked, extended position.
       - Any motion in this position indicates marked instability, which can occur in advanced rheumatoid arthritis.
   - Approximate normal ranges (in degrees).
     —Flexion, 130.
     —Extension, 0.
     —Hyperextension, 15.

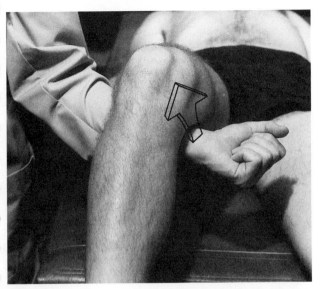

Fig. 11-72

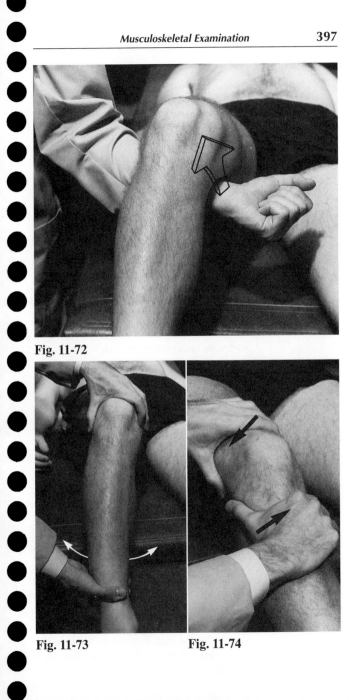

Fig. 11-73

Fig. 11-74

C. Ankles.
    1. Inspection.
- Check for swelling or redness.
  —In the gastroc-soleus complex *(FIG. 11-75)*.
  —All surfaces of the ankle joint.
  - Pay particular attention to any swelling around the malleoli.
  —Move the foot around to allow a tangential view of all surfaces; around the malleoli, above them, and by the extensor tendons *(FIG. 11-76)*.

    2. Palpation.
- For swelling in the gastroc-soleus complex.
  —If the swelling is acute, palpate gently. The calf is a high-risk area for deep venous thrombosis.
  —For bursal swelling.
  —Over the tips of the malleoli *(FIG. 11-77)*.
  —Over the insertion of the Achilles tendon into the heel *(FIG. 11-78)*.
  - Run your fingers from midcalf down the tendon to its insertion.
  - Probe in with fingers around the tendon insertion feeling for tenderness, nodules, or bony spurs.
- For synovial thickening.
  —Sweep both index fingers around each malleolus *(FIG. 11-79)*.
  —Feel also over the extensor tendons.
  - The retinaculum, like in the wrist, covers the flexion crease, and synovium can bulge out from underneath.
  - Probe over and between the tendons.
  - Palpate dorsally on either side of the retinaculum *(FIG. 11-80)*.
- For tenderness.
  —When an ankle sprain is suspected, palpate carefully around the malleoli. Try to locate the tenderness precisely.
  - The anterior talofibular ligament is most commonly affected in inversion-type ankle sprain. When this occurs, tenderness is maximal at the anterior-inferior lateral malleolus.

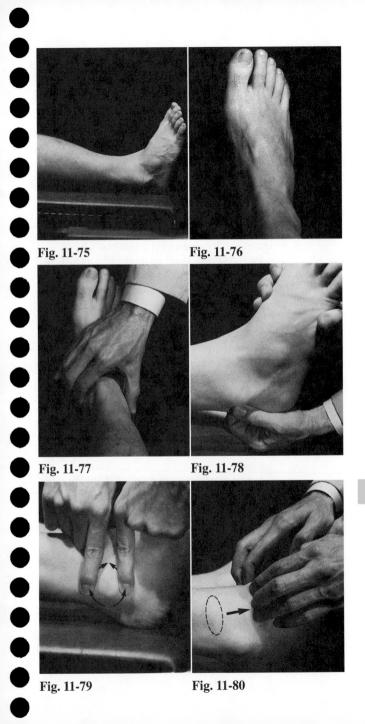

Fig. 11-75

Fig. 11-76

Fig. 11-77

Fig. 11-78

Fig. 11-79

Fig. 11-80

3. Range of motion.
   - Stabilize his ankle with one hand and observe:
     —Plantar and dorsal flexion (*FIGS. 11-81* and *11-82*).
     —Inversion and eversion (*FIGS. 11-83* and *11-84*).
     —Motion in a circle.
   - Test lateral motion within the ankle mortise (subtalar joint).
     —Grasp the malleoli with one hand and the heel with the other *(FIG. 11-85).*
     —Rock the heel from side to side. Only slight mobility is normal.
   - Test strength against your resistance.
     —Push down and pull up on the foot as he resists your motion *(FIG. 11-86).*
     —This tenses the tendons and may cause thickened synovium to bulge between them, making it more palpable.
       • When bulging is seen, palpate again dorsally and around malleoli.
     —Remember that the plantar and dorsal flexors of the foot are very strong. If weakness is suspected, they must be tested against full body weight.
   - If motion seems limited, check range passively.
     —Hold the foot above the ankle and by the toes.
     —Move the foot through extension, flexion, and rotation.
       • As with all range testing, see if motion is limited by pain or by loss of function (e.g., contractures).

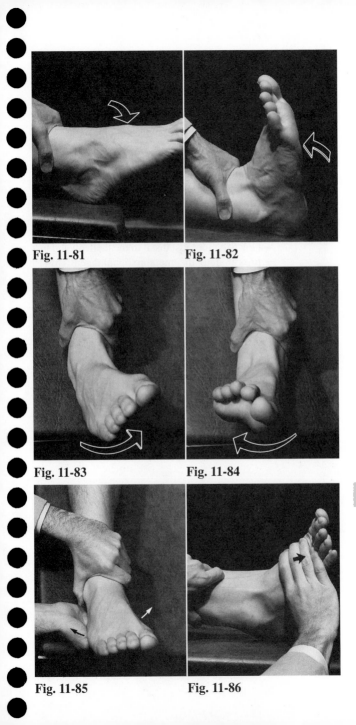

Fig. 11-81

Fig. 11-82

Fig. 11-83

Fig. 11-84

Fig. 11-85

Fig. 11-86

D. Feet.

  1. Midfoot.

    ▪ Inspection: for swelling and redness over the dorsal surface, including extensor tendons.

    ▪ Palpation.

      —Over the extensor tendons, using the same technique as for the hand *(FIG. 11-87).*

      —Over the intertarsal joints. Palpate with a squeezing motion of thumb and index finger over dorsum and sides of foot *(FIG. 11-88).*

    ▪ Range of motion of the intertarsal joint.

      —Grasp the foot just distal to the malleoli and just proximal to the metatarsophalangeal (MTP) joints.

      —Move your hands in opposition, letting the joint shift laterally back and forth between the fingers *(FIG. 11-89).*

      —Normal motion is slight, about 5 degrees. Note rigidity or hypermobility.

      —Another test is to apply a twisting motion with both hands *(FIG. 11-90).* These maneuvers will cause pain with rheumatoid arthritis.

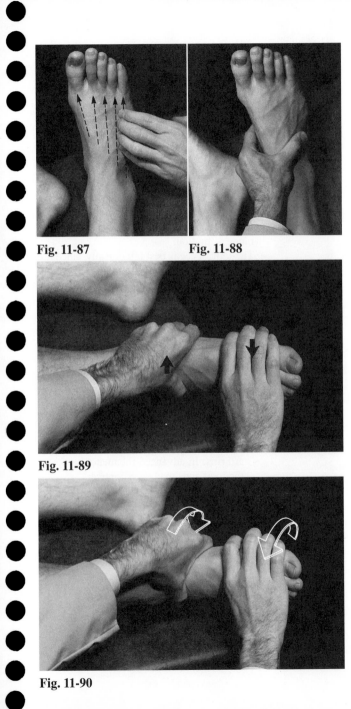

Fig. 11-87   Fig. 11-88

Fig. 11-89

Fig. 11-90

2. Toes.
   ▪ Inspection.
     —For inflammation, skin lesions, and characteris-
       tic lesions that affect the toes: such as corns and
       hallux valgus *(FIG. 11-91)*.
   ▪ Palpation.
     —Metatarsophalangeal joints.
       • Grasp the large toe with thumb and forefinger.
       • Feel the joint space with the other hand as you
         move the toe through extension, flexion, and
         rotation *(FIG. 11-92)*. This is also a test for
         range of motion.
       • The joint space is best felt dorsally, since it is
         obscured by the fatty pad ventrally.
       • Repeat this on the other toes *(FIG. 11-93)*.
       • Palpate for tenderness and synovial thicken-
         ing. The large toe is by far the easiest to feel.
         When acute swelling occurs in the large toe
         MTP joint, consider gout as a cause.
       • Then feel underneath for bony enlargement
         and for prominence of the metatarsal heads
         (hammer toes) *(FIG. 11-94)*.
       • If the metatarsal heads are "dropped down"
         with hammer toes, see if they can be pushed
         upward back into place.
         This is especially common with rheumatoid
           arthritis. In advanced rheumatoid arthritis,
           the joint ends may even contract.

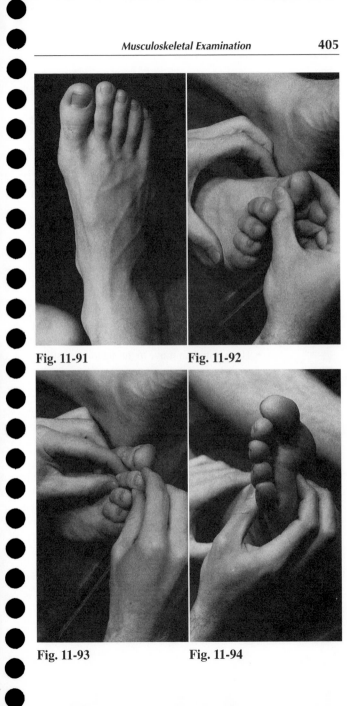

Fig. 11-91

Fig. 11-92

Fig. 11-93

Fig. 11-94

- Finish by opposing the MTP joints. Wrap fingers around this portion of the foot and squeeze, checking for pain *(FIG. 11-95)*.
  Pain here is often an early sign of rheumatoid arthritis.

—Interphalangeal joints.
  - Inspect and palpate as for the fingers *(FIG. 11-96)*.
  - Their motion is normally more limited than in the fingers.

—Plantar surface.
  - Inspect for skin lesions such as tinea pedis, psoriasis, keratoderma blenorrhagicum, gonococcal pustular lesions, and flushing.
  - Also check between the toes for the scaling and fissuring of tinea pedis (athelete's foot).
  - Palpate for nodules (contractions of plantar fascia) *(FIG. 11-97)*. Remember, the patient may be ticklish!
  - Have him then move to the standing position.

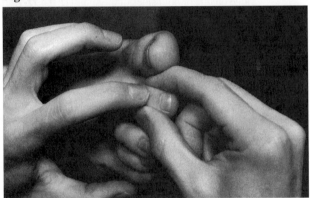

Fig. 11-95

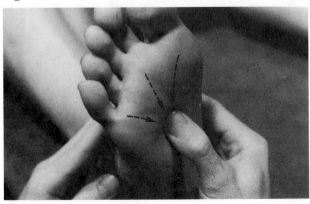

Fig. 11-96

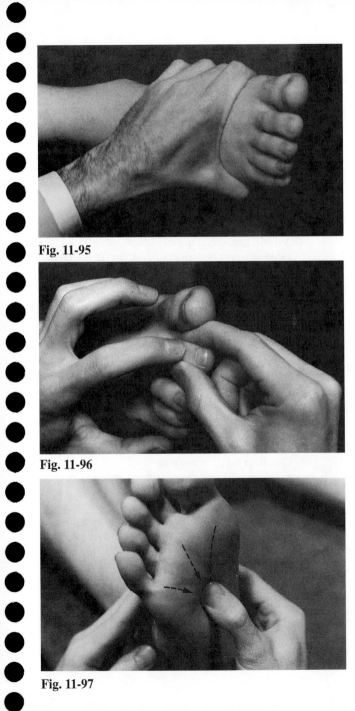

Fig. 11-97

V. SPINE.

  A. Note His Stance and Overall Posture, Including:

     1. Arches of his feet for high arch *(pes cavus)* or flattening *(pes planus)* *(FIG. 11-98).*

     2. Contour of leg musculature for atrophy, as with muscular dystrophy.

     3. Outward (valgus) or inward (varus) angling of the knees *(FIG. 11-99).*

     4. Visible paraspinal muscle spasm (seen as a raised ridge on one or both sides of the spine) *(FIG. 11-100).*

     5. Shoulder tilt.
       ▪ In scoliosis, one may be higher than the other.

  B. Note Normal Spinal Curvatures: Have him stand with feet together and knees locked. Move to the side to view the spine tangentially.

     1. Observe his cervical, thoracic, and lumbar curvatures *(FIG. 11-101).*
       ▪ Note any kyphosis, scoliosis, or lordosis.
       ▪ Refer to Chapter 6, Thorax and Lungs, for a more complete examination for scoliosis.

     2. Check for range of motion.
       ▪ Ask him to slowly bend forward, trying to touch his toes *(FIG. 11-102).*
       ▪ Watch for normal lumbar flexion.
       ▪ If there is limited motion or rigidity of the lumbar spine, measure the distance from his middle finger to the floor and record it *(FIG. 11-103).*
         —This limited motion occurs frequently in the patient with ankylosing spondylitis and is used for monitoring progression of the disease.

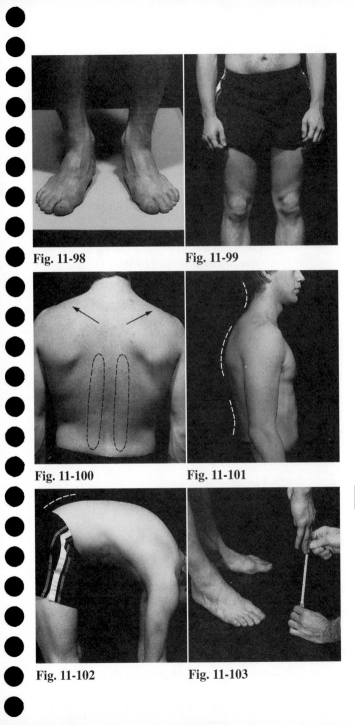

Fig. 11-98

Fig. 11-99

Fig. 11-100

Fig. 11-101

Fig. 11-102

Fig. 11-103

—Have him extend again and watch for return of normal lumbar lordosis *(FIG. 11-104)*.
- Assess lateral motion.
  —Move behind the patient.
  —Observe lateral bending left and right *(FIG. 11-105)*.
  —If motion is decreased:
    • Stabilize his right pelvis with your right hand (on his posterior illiac crest); have him slide his left hand down his left lateral thigh, causing lateral bending.
    • You can assist by gently pulling his left hand down further *(FIG. 11-106)*.
    • The pelvis will tilt at its limit of bending. (Check each side.)
    • Remember that limited motion may be caused by pain (muscle spasm) rather than spinal rigidity.
- Assess rotation.
  —Have him place his hands on his hips.
  —Watch rotation left and right. The elbow tips show the angle of rotation *(FIG. 11-107)*.
  —Again, if motion is decreased, stabilize his pelvis with your hands to isolate spinal rotation.
- Approximate normal ranges (in degrees).
  —Extension, 30.
  —Flexion, 75 to 90.
  —Lateral bending, 35.
  —Rotation, 30 (from lateral midline).

3. Palpate the spine.
   - Run your index and middle fingers down the spine. Feel for muscle spasm or minor degrees of scoliosis *(FIG. 11-108)*.
     —Paraspinal muscle spasm often produces tenderness to palpation. This occurs most commonly in the lower thoracic and lumbar area.
   - Brace the patient with one hand in front, and assess vertebral tenderness by percussing the spine every few inches with your fist *(FIG. 11-109)*.
     —Inform the patient before you do this.

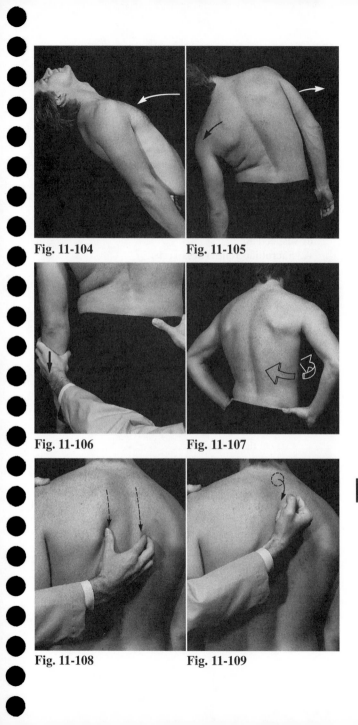

Fig. 11-104

Fig. 11-105

Fig. 11-106

Fig. 11-107

Fig. 11-108

Fig. 11-109

4. Perform the "three-point" test.
   - Have the patient stand against a wall.
   - Observe his points of contact. He should be touching at his occiput, buttocks, and the backs of his feet (*FIGS. 11-110* and *11-111*).
   - If any are not touching, measure their distance to the wall and record them. This may uncover kyphosis in osteoporosis or ankylosing spondylitis (AS) and the lumbar flattening of AS.

VI. **ADDITIONAL TESTS: Used if abnormalities are seen or suspected.**
   A. **Sacroiliac Tenderness Tests.**
      1. Sacroiliac push.
         - Position the patient prone on the examination table.
         - Place your hands, in CPR (cardiopulmonary resuscitation) fashion over the visible dimples of the posterior illiac spines *(FIG. 11-112).*
         - Inform the patient you will apply pressure, then apply a quick downward thrust. This may cause pain when sacroiliitis is present.

      2. Gaenslen's test.
         - Position the patient supine with his right side close to the table's edge.
         - Have him flex his left knee onto his chest, holding it in place with his arms *(FIG. 11-113).* This stabilizes the ilium.
         - Grasp his right leg and lower it over the edge of the exam table.
            —This extends the hip and causes a shearing force across the sacroiliac joints, which will cause pain on the involved side with sacroiliitis.

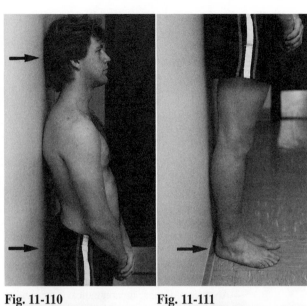

Fig. 11-110   Fig. 11-111

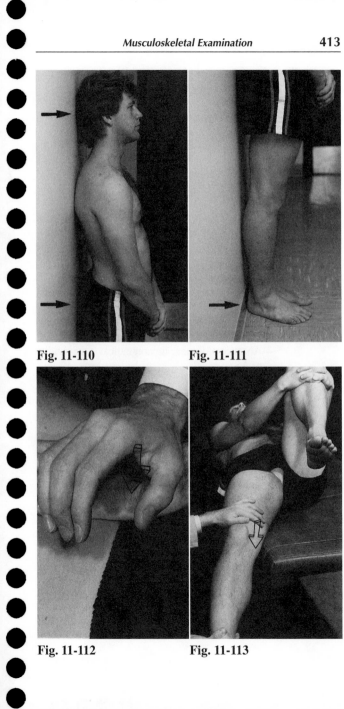

Fig. 11-112   Fig. 11-113

B. Tests for Joint Ankylosis (Rigidity); useful when ankylosing spondylitis (AS) is suspected.

    1. Schober's test.

- Mark the lumbar spine at the level of the posterior superior illiac spines.
   —There is a visible dimpling of the skin at this level, about L-4.
   —Mark the point at the line connecting these two dimples and another mark 10 cm directly above it *(FIG. 11-114)*.
- Have the patient fully bend forward and remeasure *(FIGS. 11-115* and *11-116)*.
   —It should increase at least 5 cm. With AS it may not increase at all.
- A less formal way to measure this is:
   —Place four fingers over the lumbar spine, pressing in with the fingertips.
   —Have him bend forward and watch for separation of the fingers with forward flexion.
   —Absence of lumbar flexion indicates the rigidity of AS.

    2. Chest expansion.

- Place a tape measure around his chest at nipple level *(FIG. 11-117)*. Placement of the tape may be easier with his arms raised over his head for a moment.
- Position the tape measure across itself so you can watch the measurement change relative to the zero point.
- Have him take a few practice breaths to make sure the tape moves easily.
- Then compare the measurement from full expiration to full inspiration. It should increase at least 5 cm but varies with age, sex, and body build *(FIG. 11-118)*.
   —Decreased expansion can occur with forms of arthritis that affect the joints of the thorax or by obstructive lung disease.

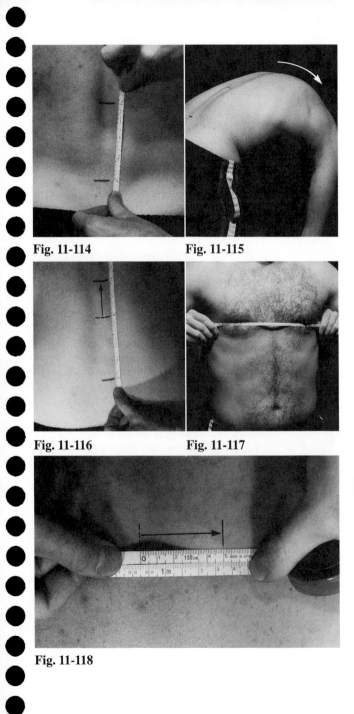

Fig. 11-114

Fig. 11-115

Fig. 11-116

Fig. 11-117

Fig. 11-118

C. **Use of the Goniometer:** simply, a pivoted, V-shaped device for more accurately measuring range of joint motion.
   1. Open the goniometer and place it over the patient's limbs, with the pivot lying over the joint.

   2. Measure zero as the point of relaxed extension *(FIG. 11-119)*.
      - From that point, move the limb into full flexion or hyperextension and read the angle directly off the goniometer.

   3. If possible, use a pocket version of this regularly during your training. If you do, you will eventually be able to visually approximate range of motion angles.

D. **Tests of Knee Ligament and Cartilage Integrity;** performed when joint instability is suspected by screening examination or prior history.
   1. Cruciate ligaments; there are two methods.
      - Drawer test.
        —With the patient supine, bend his knee to 90 degrees and stabilize the tibia by sitting on the tip of his foot.
        —Place your thumbs in the joint space with the fingers behind the tibia and rock the tibia repeatedly forward and backward *(FIG. 11-120)*.
        —Anterior pull stresses the anterior cruciate ligament (ACL), since it prevents anterior motion of the tibia on the femur.
          • Excessive forward sliding of the tibia, which occurs with an ACL tear, is called the "anterior drawer sign."
        —Posterior push stresses the posterior cruciate ligament (PCL), since it prevents posterior tibial motion.
          • Excessive posterior motion, which occurs with a PCL tear, is called a "posterior drawer sign."

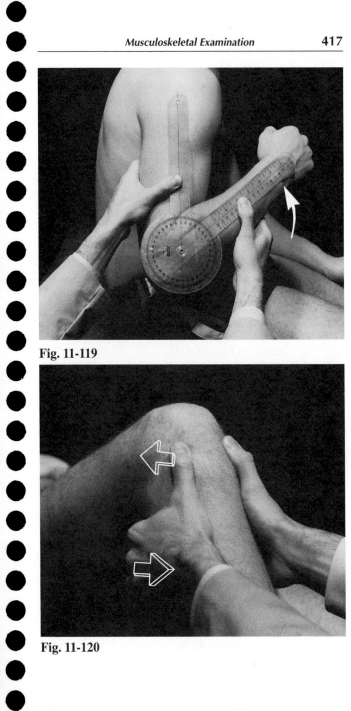

Fig. 11-119

Fig. 11-120

—Carefully compare the total forward and backward play of each knee, since up to 1 cm of total motion can occur and still be considered normal. Women normally have greater ligamentous laxity than men.

- Lachman's test (for ACL stability).

  —Lachman's test is more sensitive than the traditional "drawer" test, which is performed with the knee flexed to 90 degrees or more.

  —Flex the knee to 15 or 20 degrees. Grasp the proximal tibia in one hand and the distal femur in the other. Then jerk the distal femur forward against the tibia.

    • Any increased forward mobility of the tibia relative to the femur, compared with the uninjured knee, indicates significant damage to the anterior cruciate ligament.

2. Collateral ligaments: two methods: For each, stand on the same side of the table as the leg you wish to examine *(FIG. 11-121).*

   - Method one: Place his ankle inside your upper arm and press it firmly against your chest.

     —With one hand, apply an inward (valgus—medial collateral) or outward (varus—lateral collateral) strain *(FIGS. 11-122 and 11-123).*

       • Feel with your other hand in the joint space opposite to your pressure.
       Feel for opening of the joint space.
       A widening of more than a few millimeters is abnormal.

   - Method two: Hold the ankle as above, but cup the palm of the same hand posteriorly under his knee. For the right leg:

     —Place the fingers of your free hand in the medial joint space.

     —Press his ankle tightly against you with your elbow, then rotate your hips slightly clockwise.

       • This levers the knee across your waist, imparting a valgus strain.
       • Feel for widening of the joint space as before.

     —For the lateral collateral, move the leg so it is held by your left elbow, and rotate counterclockwise to apply a varus strain.

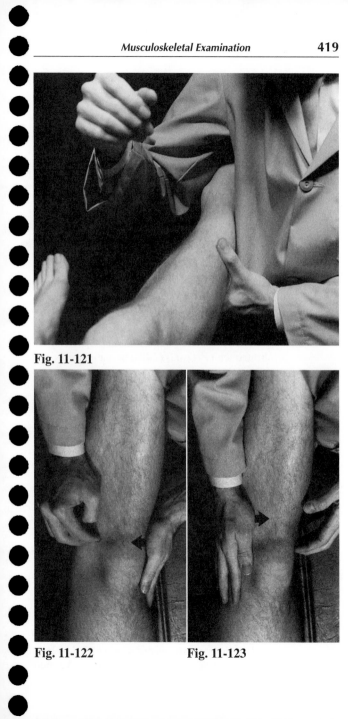

Fig. 11-121

Fig. 11-122   Fig. 11-123

- Perform both tests with the knee locked, then again at 30 degrees of flexion.
  —The posterior capsule can assist the collateral ligaments in stabilizing the knee.
  —The partially flexed position removes this added stability of the capsule. Instability of the flexed knee implies collateral ligament damage.

3. Menisci (cartilage): to test for a tear in the medial meniscus, especially its posterior portion, use the McMurray test. For the right leg:
   - With the patient supine, fully flex the knee.
   - Place your free hand over the knee with the fingers touching the medial joint line and the thumb on the lateral joint line.
   - Apply a valgus strain to the knee and rotate the leg externally.
   - Maintaining this motion, extend the knee slowly to over 90 degrees.
   - Feel in the medial joint line for a palpable or audible click *(FIG. 11-124)*. The patient may feel pain at the same time.
     —As the knee nears full extension, a clicking sensation is often felt over the patella and is not considered abnormal.
   - For the lateral meniscus, repeat the test by applying a varus strain and internally rotating the leg.

E. **Measurement of True Leg Length;** used when leg length seems unequal.
   1. With the patient supine, line up his legs as evenly as possible.
   2. Using a flexible tape, measure from the anterior-superior illiac spine to the distal point of the medial malleolus *(FIG. 11-125)*. The tape should cross the medial side of the knee joint. (Check each side.)

F. **Grip Strength:** Used to follow progression of hand disability, usually in patients with rheumatoid arthritis.
   1. Roll up a standard adult blood pressure cuff.
   2. Inflate to 30 mmHg.
   3. Have the patient grip it as hard as possible. Measure and record the rise in manometer pressure *(FIG. 11-126)*.
   4. This is useful because hand function may be more impaired than its appearance suggests.

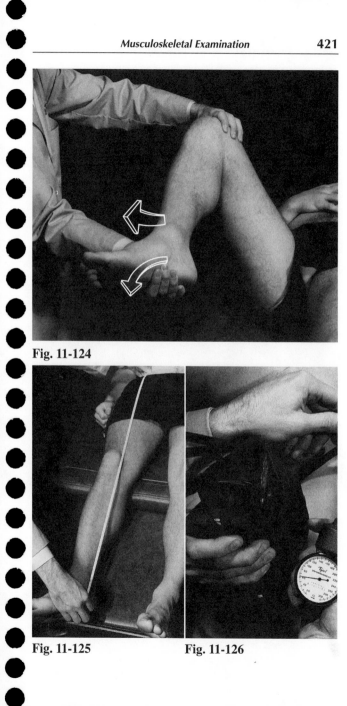

Fig. 11-124

Fig. 11-125   Fig. 11-126

12 Neurologic Examination

I. **INSTRUMENTS AND MATERIALS NEEDED.**
   A. **Three Sets of Screw-Top Test Tubes Filled with:**
      1. Tobacco, soap shavings, instant coffee.
      2. Warm and cool water.
      3. Mild solutions of sugar, salt, and vinegar, and a card with the words "sweet salty sour."

   B. **Tongue Blades, Cotton Balls, Cotton-Tipped Applicators, a Pencil, a Safety Pin.**

   C. **512 Hz Tuning Fork, a Pocket Flashlight (or Otoscope).**

   D. **Several Coins, a Cup of Water.**

   E. **A 20-ml Syringe and Butterfly Needle with Tubing (Optional).**

   F. **Reflex Hammer;** a heavier rubber head will improve the chances of seeing a reflex response.

   G. **Cotton Ball, Safety Pin, Tongue Blades.**

   H. **128 Hz Tuning Fork, a Key, Coins, a Paper Clip.**

II. SCREENING MENTAL STATUS CHECKLIST: Much of the mental status assessment is observed during the history taking. Observe:

A. General Appearance. Note:

1. The patient's dress, grooming and personal hygiene, and physique, compared to others of similar age and socioeconomic status.
   - Note condition of the skin, hair, nails, and teeth.
2. Compare one side of the patient's body with the other.
   - Certain disorders, such as stroke, can cause one-sided neglect.

B. Level of Consciousness. Is the patient in a state of:

1. Alertness.
2. Somnolence (can be fully aroused).
3. Semi-coma (can be only partially aroused).
   - Talk in a loud voice and gently shake the patient if necessary.
   - If no response, try a painful stimulus such as squeezing the nipple or pressing upward on the superior orbital ridge.
4. Coma (cannot be aroused).
   - Light: reflexes intact.
   - Deep: reflexes cannot be elicited.

C. Orientation of the Patient to:

1. Time (day, month, year, season).
2. Place (where he/she is).
3. Person (who he/she is, who examiner is, what examiner does).

D. Affect (Mood).

1. Type (anxiety, fear, sadness, anger).
2. Range:
   - Broad: with wide swings to either extreme.
   - Labile: quickly changeable.
   - Restricted: to one type.
   - Blunted or constricted: for all types.
   - Flat: no emotional response whatsoever.
3. Intensity and appropriateness of emotion.
Self-destructive, suicidal, or homicidal ideation?
4. Facial expression: (appropriate? absent?)
5. Verbally expressed emotion (as 1 to 3 above.)

E. Speech.
  1. Quantity: spontaneous, verbose, or silent.
  2. Rate (fast or slow) and volume (loud/soft).
  3. Articulation, rhythm, and inflection.
F. Thought Process: ability to be logical, coherent, relevant, and goal-directed in one's expression.
G. Thought Content: compulsions, obsessions, delusions, etc.
H. Insight: ability to perceive and understand oneself realistically.
I. Abnormal Perceptions: illusions, hallucinations, paranoid ideation, feelings of depersonalization, etc.
J. Cognitive Functions (see Mini-Mental State: Appendix B).
  1. Attention span.
  2. Memory:
     ▪ Immediate: repeat back series of numbers.
     ▪ Recent: remembrances within one hour.
     ▪ Remote: after hours, days, or years.
  3. Ability for new learning: give patient three or four unrelated words and have her repeat them back to you a few minutes later (ball, flag, tree).
  4. Calculation: count backwards from 100 by 3 or 7, or simple addition or multiplication.
  5. General knowledge: hobbies, current events.
  6. Vocabulary: as above, varies with education.
  7. Abstract reasoning.
     ▪ Proverbs: "a stitch in time saves nine."
     ▪ Similarities: "how are an orange and apple alike?"
K. Judgment (Social and Moral): "What would you do if you found a stamped, sealed envelope lying in the street?"
L. Constructional Ability.
  1. Draw two intersecting pentagons. Have the patient attempt to copy it. Or, ask the patient to draw the face of a clock.
  2. These actions are difficult with constructional apraxia, often with parietal lobe lesions.
M. If Abnormalities Are Suspected, Reexamine Each Area in Greater Detail.

III. **CRANIAL NERVES: Examine sequentially from I to XII. This tests the course of each nerve and the integrity of the brain stem.**

    A. **Cranial Nerve I: Olfactory.** Test sense of smell using common odors such as tobacco, soap shavings, and coffee powder. Avoid pungent odors such as perfume and ammonia, since they stimulate (irritate) the nasal mucosa, which is innervated by cranial nerve V (trigeminal).

        1. Make sure each nasal cavity is patent.
   - Have the patient compress one nostril at a time and sniff through the other.

        2. Have her close her eyes.

        3. Place an opened screw-top tube containing an odor substance close to one nostril; she should occlude the other side *(FIG. 12-1).* Have her sniff deeply.

        4. Ask if she can smell anything, and if so, can she identify it?

        5. Check the other nostril, having her occlude the one just tested.

        6. A unilateral loss is especially significant, whereas a bilateral decrease in sensitivity is normal with aging.

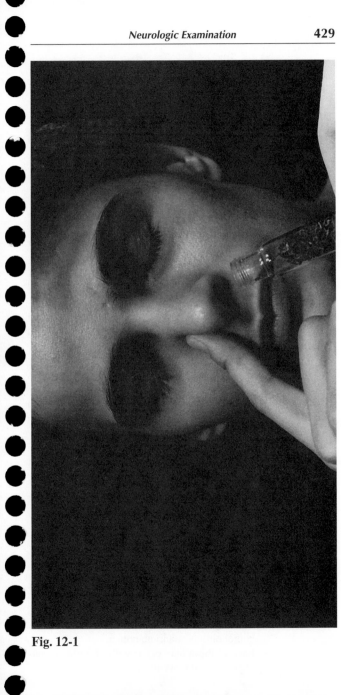

Fig. 12-1

B. Cranial Nerve II: Optic.

1. Visual acuity and examination of the optic disc are examined in Chapter 4, Head and Neck.

2. Determine visual fields by confrontation.
   - This is a rough clinical test for peripheral vision. If an abnormality is found, follow-up with perimetry or use of a tangent screen.
   - Stand 2 feet way from her at the same eye level.
     —Have her gently cover one eye.
     —Cover yours on the same side as you gaze directly at each other.
   - Bring a test object in from the periphery into her field of vision.
     —Have her say "yes" when she sees it.
       - Move slowly so she has time to respond *(FIG. 12-2)*.
       - If it is well within your vision and she still cannot see it, she probably has a visual field loss. Note its position.
     —Check in eight directions on each eye:
       - 3, 6, 9, and 12 o'clock positions and points halfway between *(FIG. 12-3)*.
       - In the temporal field, bring the object in from around her head, although it will stay within your vision.

3. In the uncooperative patient, move your hand toward her head and see if she jerks her eyes and head away from you.

4. If you find a visual loss, note its distribution:
   - In one eye: unilateral total blindness
   - In both eyes: *(FIG. 12-4)*
     —Missing both temporal fields: bitemporal hemianopsia.
     —Missing both right- or both left-sided fields: homonomous hemianopsia.
     —Missing the identical quadrant in each eye: homonomous quadrantanopsia
     —Each of these may occur with or without sparing of central (foveal) vision.

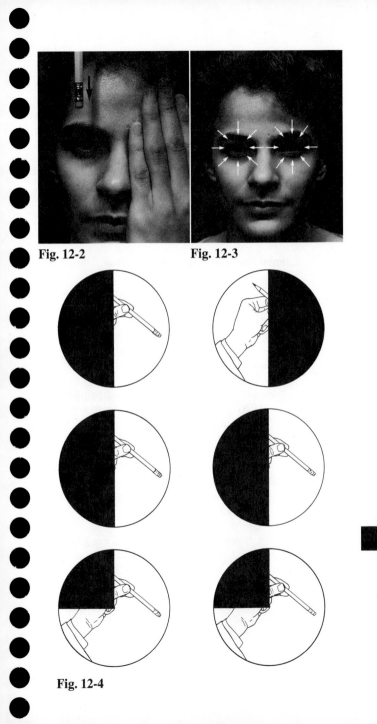

Fig. 12-2

Fig. 12-3

Fig. 12-4

- Enlarged blind spots and other smaller visual field defects are sensitive to the color red. Use a red-topped dropper bottle, pencil eraser, or pen cap and move it around in the patient's vision, looking for perceived dulling of the red color. Check one eye at a time.

C. **Cranial Nerves III, IV, and VI: Oculomotor, Abducens, and Trochlear.**
   1. Test for extraocular motion and pupillary responses. This is reviewed in Chapter 4, Head and Neck.

D. **Cranial Nerve V: Trigeminal.** Two functions are usually tested:
   1. Motor: Check strength in the muscles of mastication.
      - *Masseter:* place the tips of the fingers over each masseter muscle at the bite line *(FIG. 12-5)*.
        —Ask her to bite down.
        —Feel for symmetric contraction.
      - *Temporalis:* move your fingers to the hollow of each temple area.
        —Have her clench her teeth and palpate again *(FIG. 12-6)*. Feel for slight bulging as the muscles contract.
      - *Pterygoids:*
        —Check symmetry of pterygoid strength by having her protrude her jaw *(FIG. 12-7)*. It should stay in the midline.
        —Then check pterygoid strength individually *(FIG. 12-8)*.
          • Position her mouth slightly open.
          • Brace the patient's head with one hand.
          • Push on the jaw with the other hand, asking her to resist your motion. Check each side.

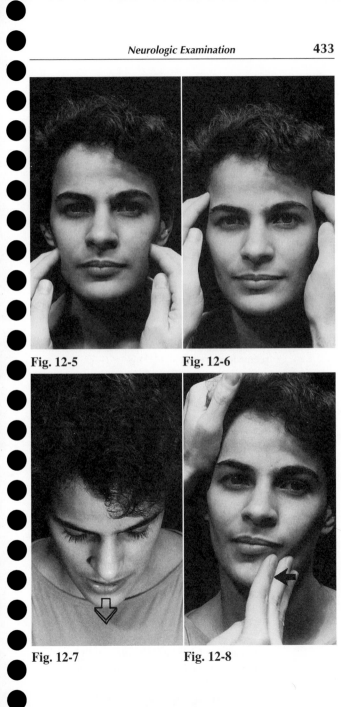

Fig. 12-5

Fig. 12-6

Fig. 12-7

Fig. 12-8

2. Sensory.
    - Check in the three trigeminal divisions: ophthalmic (upper), maxillary (middle) and mandibular (lower) *(FIG. 12-9)*. Have her close her eyes before you begin.
    - Pain sensation:
        —Demonstrate first on the wrist, using a safety pin, disposable needle, or broken tongue blade. Show both sharp sensation (the pointed tip) and dull sensation (the blunt end of the safety pin, etc.).
        • "Sharp" stimulates pain sensory fibers.
        • "Dull" checks the patient's reliability.
        —Check each side in the three divisions.
        • Alternate randomly between sharp and dull so the patient cannot predict the next stimulus *(FIG. 12-10)*.
        —To reduce the spread of infectious disease, dispose of the testing device after use with each patient.
    - Temperature sensation: tested when pain sensation seems impaired.
        —Use test tubes filled with warm and cool water (dry off the outside surfaces.)
        • Or use the side of a tuning fork for cool and the backs of two fingers for warm.
        —Demonstrate first.
        —Then test the three divisions alternating warm and cool at random *(FIG. 12-11)*.
    - Light touch:
        —Demonstrate on the wrist with a piece of cotton, then test over the three trigeminal divisions *(FIG. 12-12)*.
    - Check the corneal blink reflex. This is part of the ophthalmic division.
        —Roll out the tip of a cotton applicator to a fine wisp *(FIG. 12-13)*.
        —Have the patient remove any contact lenses. Their prior use may dull this response.
        —Have the patient look to her right.
        —From outside her field of vision, reach the applicator in from her left side and lightly touch the cornea *(FIG. 12-14)*. The patient will reflexively blink. Avoid touching the lashes or sclera. Reverse sides and check the left eye.

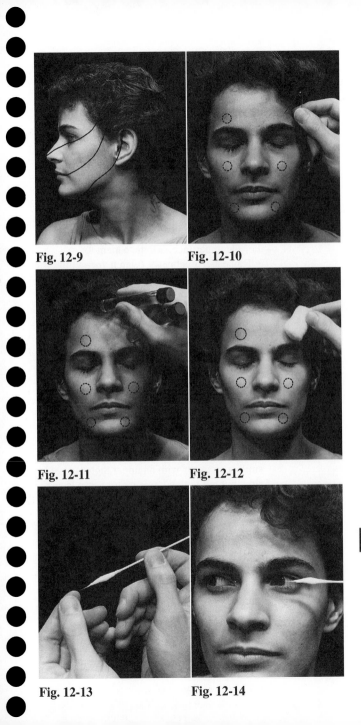

Fig. 12-9

Fig. 12-10

Fig. 12-11

Fig. 12-12

Fig. 12-13

Fig. 12-14

E. Cranial Nerve VII: Facial. Also tested for motor and sensory function.

1. Motor: Check muscles of facial expression.
   - Inspect the face both at rest and during conversation *(FIG. 12-15).*
     —Watch for symmetry of the lower lids, flattening of one nasolabial fold, or drooping at the corners of the mouth.
     —Note tics or other abnormal facial motions.
   - Check active muscle strength in the upper and lower face.
     —For the upper face, ask the patient to:
       - Raise her eyebrows (watch for symmetric wrinkling of the forehead) *(FIG. 12-16).*
       - Close her eyes as you attempt to open them (you normally cannot) *(FIG. 12-17).*
     —For the lower face, ask her to:
       - Show her teeth *(FIG. 12-18).*
       - Whistle (check with the patient, some normally cannot do this) *(FIG. 12-19).*
       - Puff out her cheeks as you apply pressure *(FIG. 12-20).*
   - While talking to the patient, watch for spontaneous expressions, such as smiling. One way to elicit such a response is to ask: "Know any funny stories?"
     —Involuntary expression, such as a spontaneous smile, can occur with an upper motor nerve lesion, but not with a lower motor nerve lesion.
   - If weakness is present, note if the entire side is involved, or only the lower face on that side.
     —A unilateral facial nerve (Bell's) palsy typically causes unilateral paralysis of both upper and lower facial muscles.
     —A cerebrovascular accident (CVA) more commonly causes unilateral lower face weakness (and also weakness of the ipsilateral arm or leg).

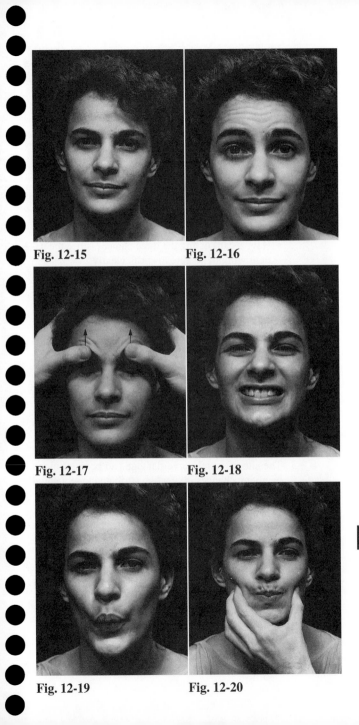

Fig. 12-15

Fig. 12-16

Fig. 12-17

Fig. 12-18

Fig. 12-19

Fig. 12-20

2. Sensation, check taste to the anterior two thirds of the tongue.
    - This test is usually performed as a follow-up to the discovery of facial nerve motor abnormalities.
    - Use mild solutions of:
      —Sugar for sweet.
      —Table salt for salty.
      —Dilute vinegar for sour.
      —Quinine (bitter) is not used here as it is perceived by the posterior one third of the tongue, innervated by cranial nerve IX.
    - Have a card listing the three choices, since the patient will not be able to speak clearly.
    - Have the patient extend her tongue.
      —Out of her vision, dip a cotton-tipped applicator into one solution *(FIG. 12-21).*
      —Streak it onto the lateral left or right side of her tongue *(FIG. 12-22).* Most tastebuds are clustered around the edge of the tongue, not on the top.
      —Have her point to the taste *(FIG. 12-23).*
    - Allow her to swallow.
    - Repeat on the other side of the tongue with a fresh applicator and a different solution. If there is any confusion of tastes, have her swish her mouth with water between tests.

3. The site of facial nerve damage can be determined by noting changes in function attributed to sequential branches of the facial nerve.
    - These functions branch off of the main nerve trunk one-by-one as the nerve travels from the brain stem to the face. The following functions are lost, in order:
      —Taste to the anterior two thirds of the tongue.
      —Hearing (becomes louder: hyperacusis) and ability of the eyes to tear (lacrimation).
      —Facial movements.

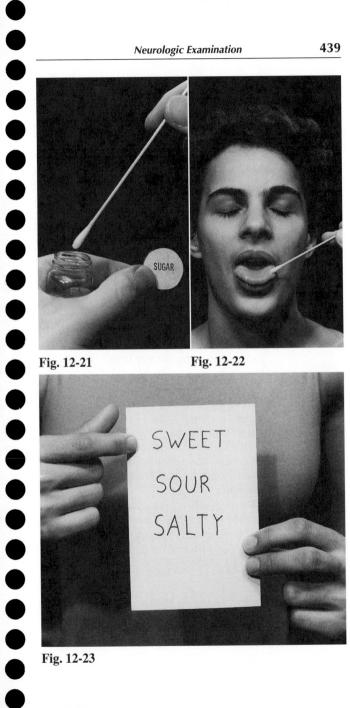

Fig. 12-21   **Fig. 12-22**

Fig. 12-23

F. Cranial Nerve VIII. The Acoustic (or Vestibular-Cochlear) Nerve. True to its name, it has two divisions, vestibular and cochlear.

1. Only its auditory (cochlear) functions are tested routinely.

   ▪ First assess hearing acuity to the spoken voice (a loss may first become apparent during the interview).

      —Assessment requires that one ear be tested at a time.

      • Have the patient cover one ear and look away, since lipreading can partially compensate for hearing loss *(FIG. 12-24)*.

      • Ask her to repeat after you.

      • Stand 2 feet away, exhale, then whisper "nine-four" or "five-one" (these all have soft consonants). Note her reply.

      • Check the other ear.

      —As you test, raise your voice as needed for her to hear, moving gradually from a whisper to a loud voice.

      —When you suspect one ear hears markedly better than the other:

      • Have her place a finger in one ear and wiggle it fast but gently.

      • This will mask hearing in that ear and allow the other one to be more accurately tested.

   ▪ Then check air and bone conduction.

      —Rinne test.

      • Use a 512 Hz or higher frequency tuning fork *(FIG. 12-25)*. Lower-frequency forks conduct vibration widely through the skull and cannot localize unilateral hearing loss as well.

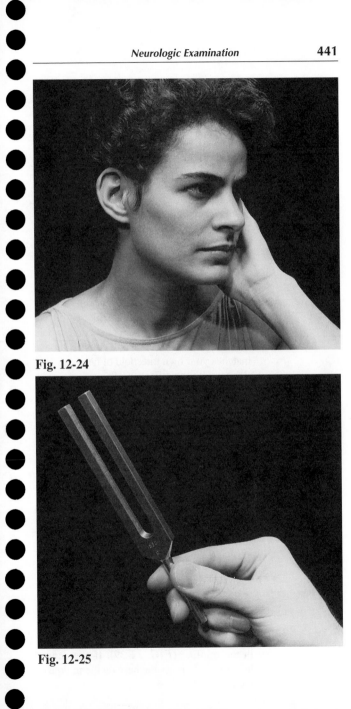

Fig. 12-24

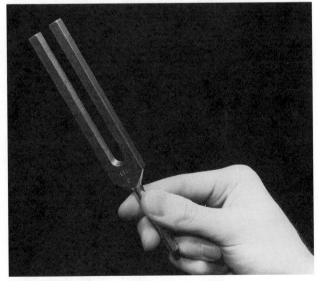

Fig. 12-25

- Hold the fork by its base *(FIG. 12-26)*.
- Strike it *gently* on the heel of your hand. Or, grasp the two tines with your thumb and fore-finger and pull off with a light snap.
- Place the base on her mastoid process, the bony ridge behind her ear *(FIG. 12-27)*.
- Ask if she can hear (not feel) the sound of the tuning fork. If she can, hold the fork there un-til she signals that the sound has faded away. At that point, move the fork as near to the ex-ternal ear canal as possible, sweeping away overlying hair if necessary *(FIG. 12-28)*. Hold one tine closer to her ear.
- Ask if she can again hear the tuning fork. If she can, have her indicate when she cannot.
- When she signals she can no longer hear it, lis-ten to the fork yourself. It should be barely au-dible. If so, this is normal conduction (where air conduction exceeds bone conduction and matches your own threshold of hearing).
- Repeat with the other ear.

—When you suspect an abnormality, watch for these two patterns:

- Air conduction loss, where only bone con-duction is audible, via the mastoid process. (The sound is heard with the tuning fork pressed to the mastoid, but not near the exter-nal ear.)
- Sensorineural conduction loss, where air con-duction exceeds bone conduction, but both are decreased relative to your normal hearing. (The tuning fork is heard in both locations, but when the patient can no longer hear it, it is loud and clear to you.)
- Hearing loss may occasionally be of mixed type.

—Weber test, which checks symmetry of hearing.

- Activate the fork.
- Press the base firmly on the apex of the skull in the midline *(FIG. 12-29)*. If she cannot hear the fork, press the base on the middle of the forehead.

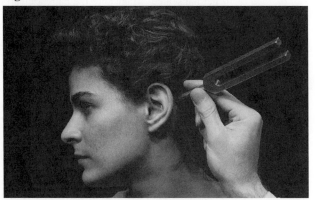

Fig. 12-26

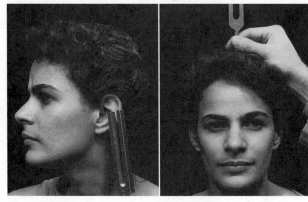

Fig. 12-27

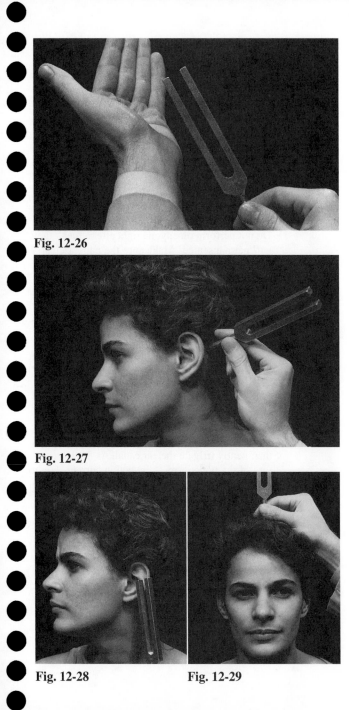

Fig. 12-28

Fig. 12-29

—Ask where she hears it. Normally, it is heard in the midline. Abnormally, it *lateralizes* to one side, either toward the side of air conduction loss or away from the side of bone conduction (sensorineural) loss.

—Initial impressions of hearing loss must be confirmed by audiometry. This is especially useful when hearing loss is partial or involves loss of only certain frequencies.

2. Optional vestibular tests: Caloric testing.

- Do not perform on anyone right after a meal; they *will* get nauseated! Make sure the patient clearly understands the temporary spinning sensation that will occur.
- Fill a 20-ml syringe with iced water. Attach a butterfly-type intravenous needle to the barrel and cut off the metal needle. This leaves you with a syringe with attached soft plastic tubing *(FIG. 12-30)*.
- For maximum effect, seat the patient and position her head 60 degrees backward (or supine with head 30 degrees elevated).
- Place a towel under the ear or use some form of basin to catch the water *(FIG. 12-31)*.
- Thread the tubing 1/2 inch into the ear.
- Warn the patient of the cold sensation to come, then gently irrigate the ear canal. As the temperature of the bone drops, convection currents begin in the endolymph of the semicircular canal. The brain interprets this as motion.
- Within 30 seconds, nystagmus will occur with:
  —The fast component directed away from the side of stimulation *(FIG. 12-32)*.
  —A sense of vertigo (or sense of leaning) away from the side of irrigation.
- The response should last, intensively, 60 to 90 seconds after irrigation, and faintly for several minutes longer.
- A lack of response indicates damage to the semicircular canals or to the vestibular nerve itself.

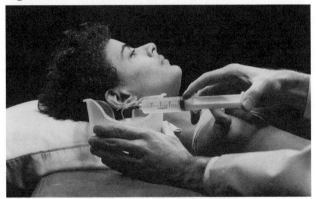

Fig. 12-30

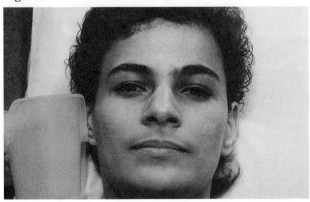

Fig. 12-31

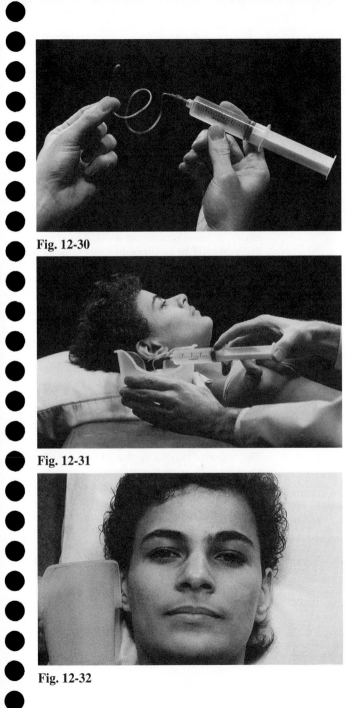

Fig. 12-32

G. **Cranial Nerves IX and X: Glossopharyngeal and Vagal.** They are clinically tested together, since they are anatomically and functionally closely related.
1. To test:
   - Inspect the soft palate for symmetry.
   - Have the patient say "ah . . ."
     —The uvula should rise in the midline (cranial nerve X) *(FIGS. 12-33* and *12-34).* In disease it will deviate *away* from the side of muscle paralysis.
     —The voice should be resonant and not hoarse, brassy, or nasal (cranial nerve X). Any abnormality should be confirmed by laryngoscopic examination.
   - Check for a gag response.
     —Using a tongueblade or cotton-tipped applicator, lightly touch each tonsil area *(FIG. 12-35).*
       • A light touch is all that is needed. With a slight stimulus, you will be able to see the reflex with minimal discomfort to the patient.
     —The uvula should jerk quickly upward in the midline and the posterior pharynx will sweep anteriorly. The sensation needed to gag is conducted through cranial nerve IX, and the motor response is mediated mostly through cranial nerve X.
     —The response may be decreased in those who wear dentures or are heavy smokers.
   - Further test by checking touch sensation to the posterior one third of the tongue (cranial nerve IX).
     —Use a cotton-tipped applicator. The tongue will move in response to each touch *(FIG. 12-36).*
     —See if the patient can easily swallow water (cranial nerve X). Retrograde passage through the nose indicates weakness of the soft palate *(FIG. 12-37).*
     —Check palatal paralysis by having her vocalize the "K" sound, as in "king."

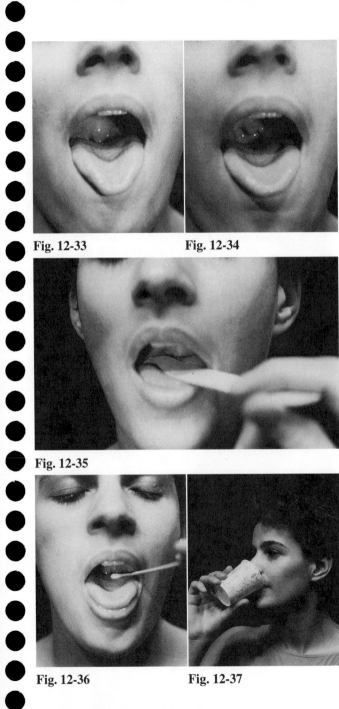

Fig. 12-33

Fig. 12-34

Fig. 12-35

Fig. 12-36

Fig. 12-37

H. Cranial Nerve XI: Spinal Accessory. Innervates two
muscles.

1. Inspect for symmetry and size of the sternomastoids
   (1) and trapezius muscles (2) *(FIG. 12-38).*
   - Trapezius atrophy shows as loss of the normal
     muscle contour between shoulder and neck.

2. Check strength of the:
   - Sternomastoids.
     —Both together: have her flex her chin while you
        try to resist *(FIG. 12-39).*
     —One at a time: have her keep her head in the
        midline as you try to push the chin to one side,
        then the other *(FIG. 12-40).*
        • When she resists you, the direction you are
           pushing points to the muscle you are testing.
           (i.e., if you push to the right, you are testing
           the right sternomastoid).
        • Watch for its bulging.
   - Upper trapezius *(FIG. 12-41).*
     —Have her attempt to shrug her shoulders upward
        against your resistance. Because of the large
        size of the trapezius muscles, most individuals
        can do this easily.

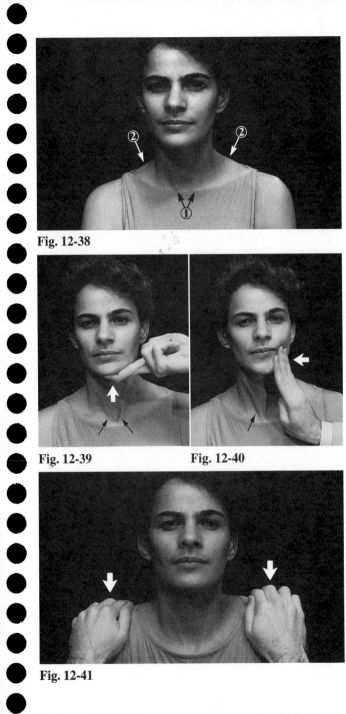

Fig. 12-38

Fig. 12-39

Fig. 12-40

Fig. 12-41

I. Cranial Nerve XII: Hypoglossal. Innervates muscles of the tongue.

  1. Inspect for atrophy or fasciculations *(FIG. 12-42)*. (The tongue is not protruded yet, but is resting in the mouth.)

- Atrophy shows as wrinkling or loss of bulk.
- Mild, intermittent twitching is normal. Fasciculations have a more undulating "bag of worms" appearance.

  2. Check symmetry of strength.

- Have her protrude her tongue *(FIG. 12-43)*. It should stay in the midline.
- In disease, it will deviate *toward* the side of muscle paralysis.

  3. Check tongue strength one side at a time.

- Have her push her tongue into one cheek as you push back with your fingers. You barely can displace the tongue normally *(FIG. 12-44)*.
- Repeat on the other side.

  4. Finally, check fine motor coordination.

- Use consonants that stress the tongue by having her repeat the phrase "no ifs, ands, or buts."
  —The consonants *n, d, and t* require tongue coordination.
  —The consonants *f, b, and p* stress the lips.
  —Tongue dysarthria produces thick "hot potato in the mouth" speech.
- Test rapid alternating motion.
  —Have her rapidly move her tongue side to side, in and out, and up and down.

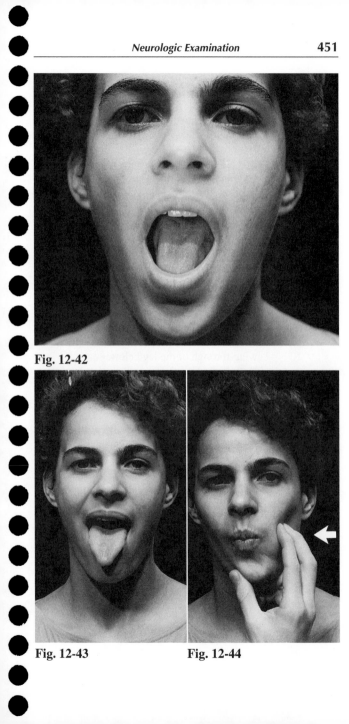

Fig. 12-42

Fig. 12-43

Fig. 12-44

IV. MOTOR SYSTEM.

A. Screening Examination: used when the history is uneventful.

   1. Gait: move to a hallway where the patient can build up some speed.

- Have the patient walk away, pivot, and return *(FIG. 12-45)*. Observe:
  - —The smooth, graceful quality of the walk: This is perhaps the first characteristic lost in early motor dysfunction.
  - —Imbalance with pivoting: This portion of walking requires the most coordination and may best reveal any unsteadiness.
  - —Alternate armswing: the arms should swing loosely, each arm moving with the opposite leg.
    - Loss of armswing is common with Parkinson's disease.
  - —The level of the hips: they should move with a gentle see-saw motion, each side rising with the swing-through of the leg below.
  - —The straight line of the walk or abnormal veering off to one side.
    - A *list* (veering off course) can occur with middle ear or cerebellar involvement.
- To bring out unsteadiness, have her walk heel-to-toe along a straight line *(FIG. 12-46)*.
  - —This is called tandem gait and will exaggerate ataxia, if present.
- To check for the ability of plantar flexion and dorsiflexion to support full body weight, have the patient walk a few steps on her heels, then her toes.
  - —This technique is particularly important because of the natural strength of these muscles. Even with weakness present, the patient can often still resist the examiner's efforts.

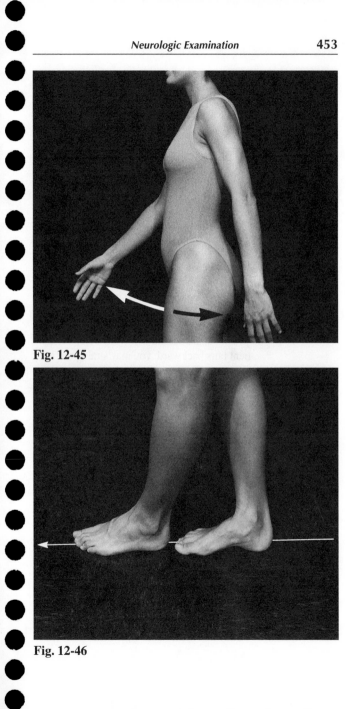

Fig. 12-45

Fig. 12-46

2. Station: the ability to stand. Evaluate with the Romberg test.
   - Have the patient stand with feet together, eyes open *(FIG. 12-47)*.
     —Note her posture for scoliosis, lordosis, or Parkinson's stance (stooped over, flexed neck, drooping shoulders, expressionless stare, decreased blinking, pill-rolling tremor in the hands).
     —Watch for obvious unsteadiness. If she remains stable, continue the test.
   - Move closer to the patient *(FIG. 12-48)*.
     —Place your hands on her shoulders.
     —Ask her to close her eyes.
     —Say "I won't let you fall."
     —Remove your hands to a few inches away, ready to catch her if necessary.
       - If the patient weighs considerably more than you do, stand behind her. Otherwise, if the patient falls backward, you may strain your back in your attempt to catch her.
   - Normally, she will waver slightly.
     —When balance is maintained, the Romberg test is considered negative.
     —If she sways enough to require shifting her feet to maintain balance, the test is positive.
   - Abnormalities:
     —Sensory ataxia: where loss of position sense causes unsteadiness when her eyes are closed. The patient may slap the feet down to gain a sense of position.
     —Cerebellar ataxia: where normal stance is difficult to maintain even with her eyes open. The patient may naturally stand with her legs more widely apart for better balance.

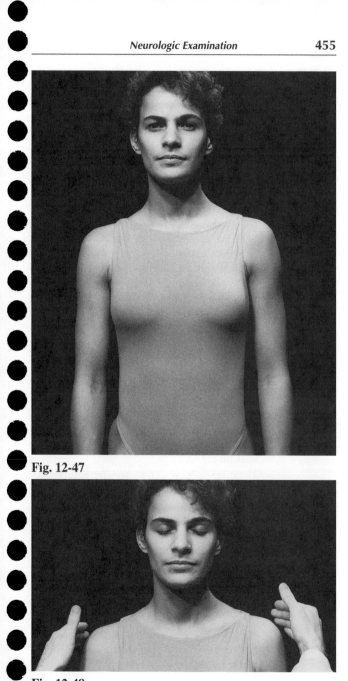

Fig. 12-47

Fig. 12-48

3. Screen for muscle strength in two upper and two lower extremity locations.
   - Proximal upper limbs.
     —Have her close her eyes and extend her arms palms up *(FIG. 12-49).* This is often performed after the Romberg test.
       • They should normally stay elevated.
       • In cases of mild hemiparesis, the weaker arm will slowly pronate and shift downward. This is called *pronator drift.*
   - Distal upper limbs.
     —Have her grip your index finger as hard as she can *(FIG. 12-50).*
       • You should have difficulty pulling it free. Use only one finger, otherwise you may be injured.
   - Proximal lower limbs *(FIG. 12-51).*
     —Have the patient stand and do a shallow knee bend one leg at a time. Do this only if the patient is fully ambulatory.
     —For elderly patients, if the above is difficult:
       • Have the patient rise from a chair without arm support, or step up onto a stool or the step of the examination table.
   - Distal lower limbs *(FIG. 12-52).*
     —Check plantar flexion by having the patient walk on tiptoes. Check dorsal flexion by having her walk on her heels.
     —These two tests are often incorporated into the assessment of gait.

4. Screen for coordination.
   - Check lower extremities.
     —Have her hop on one leg at a time. Check this only if the patient is ambulatory and is strong enough. See if she can maintain balance.
   - Check upper extremities.
     —Have her pick up several coins, one at a time, off of a smooth surface.
     —This tests independence of the thumb and forefinger versus flexion of the remaining fingers and is a sensitive test of early weakness.

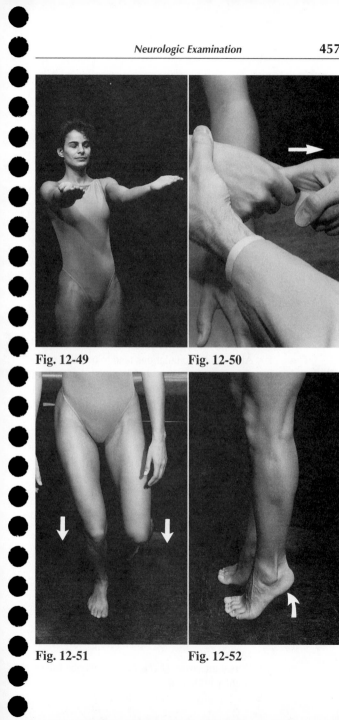

Fig. 12-49

Fig. 12-50

Fig. 12-51

Fig. 12-52

B. Detailed Motor Examination.

 1. Inspection.
 - Abnormal movements.
 —Tremor, especially of the head and hands.
 - Does the tremor occur at rest or only with motion?
 - If hand tremor is present, document it with a sample of handwriting. A useful test is to have the patient draw a spiral in the actual medical record. This can then be compared with future visits.
 —Fasciculations: seen as intermittent bursts of muscle twitching.
 - They are coarse in large muscles and fine in the hands and other small muscles.
 - They are more visible if the light is positioned to throw a partial shadow over the suspected muscle. Occasional twitching, as in the eyelid or thigh muscles, is normal.
 - Abnormal fasciculations tend to occur in multiple muscle groups and have an undulating "bag of worms" quality.
 —When abnormal movements are visible, note:
 - Their location, timing, rate, rhythm, and intensity.
 - Their relation to posture, activity, fatigue, or emotional stress.
 - Muscle atrophy.
 —Check for visible wasting (flattening). If present, palpate for its typical flaccid (limp) consistency.
 —Tap on atrophic muscles to see if they fasciculate.
 —Inspect in turn:
 - Anterior tibial muscles *(FIG. 12-53, white arrows).*
 - Quadriceps *(FIG. 12-53, black arrows).*
 - Deltoids *(FIG. 12-54).*
 - Thenar (by thumb) and hypothenar (by pinky) eminences *(FIG. 12-55).* Each should be full and round.
 - Dorsal interossei *(FIG. 12-56);* may be full or slightly hollowed.
 —Some atrophy is normal with aging.

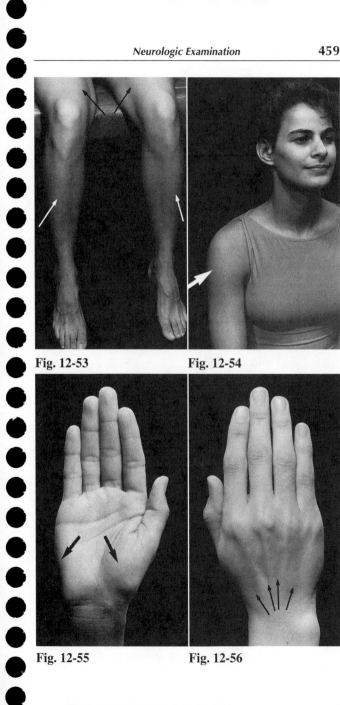

Fig. 12-53

Fig. 12-54

Fig. 12-55

Fig. 12-56

2. Muscle tone: felt as a mild resistance to passive stretching. The resistance is normally felt evenly thoughout the entire range of motion.
   - Palpate the muscle involved as you move each joint through its range of motion.
     —Support her limb so it can remain limp.
     —Move each joint, first slowly then quickly through flexion and extension.
     —Compare both sides for:
       - Fingers *(FIG. 12-57).*
       - Wrist *(FIG. 12-58).*
       - Elbow.
       - Shoulder *(FIG. 12-59).* Holding the forearm, move the shoulder through a continuous loop of flexion, abduction, extension, and finally adduction.
       - Ankle *(FIG. 12-60).*
       - Knee *(FIG. 12-61).*
   - Watch for abnormalities of tone:
     —Increased tone.
       - Spasticity: a rapid increase in resistance followed by suddenly giving way with continued stretch; from upper motor neuron lesions.
       - Rigidity: two types:
         "Lead-pipe," where a constant increased resistance is felt throughout the entire range of motion, like bending a stiff piece of wire.
         "Cog-wheel," resistance with a "rachet" sensation as the limb moves. This is particularly noticeable when flexing and extending the wrist of patients with Parkinson's disease.
       - Dystonia, a rubberband-like resistance that springs back to its former position when released.
     —Decreased tone: as a test, shake the limb. It should move freely but is not floppy *(FIG. 12-62).* This loss of tone is associated with lower motor neuron lesions.

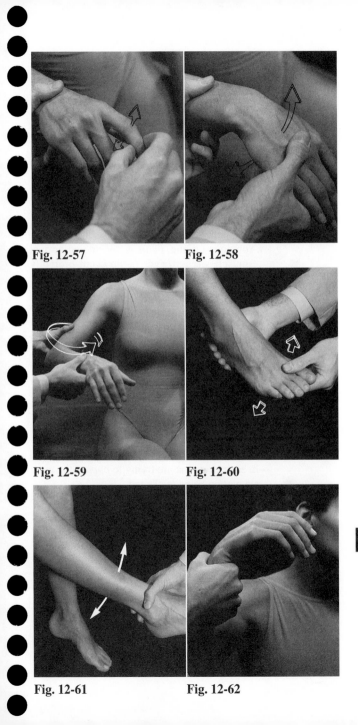

Fig. 12-57

Fig. 12-58

Fig. 12-59

Fig. 12-60

Fig. 12-61

Fig. 12-62

3. Muscle strength.
- Scale:
    —Graded 1 through 5:
      - 0 - no muscular contraction detected.
      - 1 - the barest detectable contraction is felt.
      - 2 - active movement of the body part with gravity eliminated (e.g., horizontal motion on the exam table surface).
      - 3 - active movement against gravity.
      - 4 - like (3) and against some resistance
      - 5 - like (3) and against full resistance without obvious fatigue. (This is considered normal muscle strength and should occur promptly and maximally.)
    —Adjust the scale for age, sex, and body build.
    —You must learn what to expect for each group (e.g., what is normal in an untrained individual may be considered significant weakness in an athlete or strenuous laborer).
    —Remember that small muscle groups may normally be too weak to overcome resistance, such as in the finger abductors and adductors.
- Technique:
    —The easiest method is to position the patient's limb to the desired posture. Then ask her to resist any motion on your part *(FIG. 12-63).*
    —In each case, you are trying to *oppose* the muscle motion being evaluated.
    —Compare the two sides: the dominant side is usually somewhat stronger.
      - The spinal nerves, peripheral nerves, or muscle involved for each muscle action are listed in parentheses.

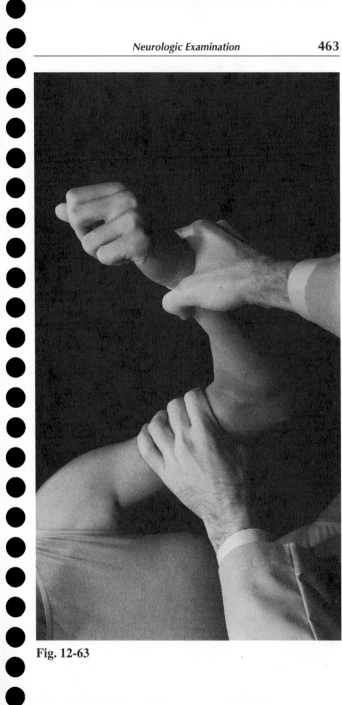

Fig. 12-63

- Upper extremities:
  —Hand: Support the patient's wrist with your hand.
  - Flexion (C7, C8, T1).
    Position the patient's fingers into flexion.
    Reach in your index finger and pull against all four fingers together *(FIG. 12-64).*
    Then test them one at a time.
    Also test grip strength, as mentioned in the screening examination.
  - Extension (C6, C7, C8).
    Position the fingers into arched extension.
    Resist as above *(FIG. 12-65).*
  - Abduction (C8, T1, ulnar nerve).
    Have the patient spread all four fingers.
    Try to squeeze together in pairs: *(FIG. 12-66).* Index and middle fingers; middle and ring; ring and pinky; index and pinky.
  - Adduction (C8, T1).
    Have her press all four fingers together *(FIG. 12-67).* Try to separate as above.
    Or, interlace your fingers with hers and try to pull them free.
    Another useful method is to place a slip of paper between each two fingers and try to pull it free.
  - Opposition of the thumb (C8, T1, median nerve).
    Have her firmly touch her thumb to her pinky.
    Hook your index finger through the loop and try to pull it free *(FIG. 12-68).*

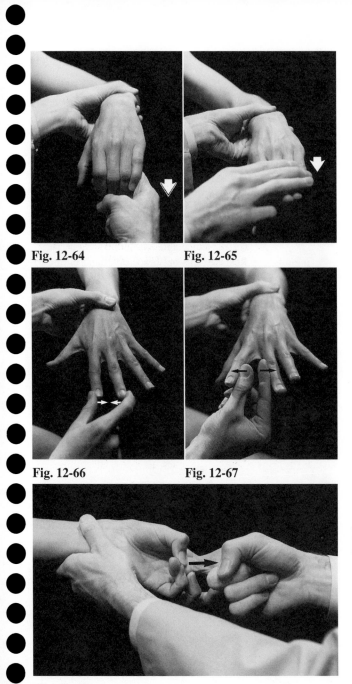

Fig. 12-64

Fig. 12-65

Fig. 12-66

Fig. 12-67

Fig. 12-68

—Wrist.
  • Place the wrist in neutral position.
  • Resist flexion by pushing up *(FIG. 12-69)* (C6, C7, median nerve).
  • Resist extension by pulling down *(FIG. 12-70)* (C6, C7, C8, radial nerve).
—Elbow.
  • Position the elbow to a 90 degree bend, palm up.
  • Resist flexion: brace one palm on the biceps, grasp her wrist, and pull *(FIG. 12-71)* (C5, C6, musculocutaneous nerve).
  • Resist extension: brace one hand on the triceps, grasp her wrist, and push *(FIG. 12-72)* (C6, C7, C8, radial nerve).
  • Test of supinator and pronator (optional). Have her make a fist, arm extended. Attempt to turn the fist into the supinated and pronated positions as she resists. Innervation for both is C6 and C7.
—Shoulder.
  • Let patient's arm hang at her side.
  • Resist adduction by attempting to pull her arm laterally *(FIG. 12-73)* (C5-T1).
  • Resist abduction by pushing her arm toward her trunk *(FIG. 12-74)* (C5, C6).

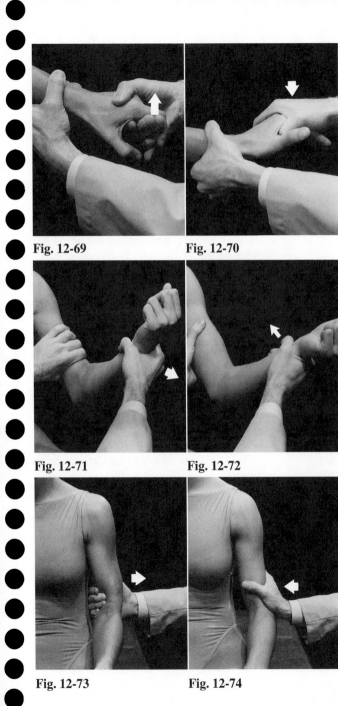

Fig. 12-69

Fig. 12-70

Fig. 12-71

Fig. 12-72

Fig. 12-73

Fig. 12-74

- Resist flexion by pushing posteriorly *(FIG. 12-75)* (C5-T1).
- Resist extension by pulling anteriorly *(FIG. 12-76)* (C5, C6, C7).
- Check deltoid strength (C5, C6).

—Stand posterior to the patient with her arm abducted laterally to full horizontal, palm up.

—Attempt to push downward on the upper arm *(FIG. 12-77)*.

—Watch the scapula for pronounced lifting of the medial edge. This is known as "winging" of the scapula (see serratus anterior test on p. 470).

—Neck.

- Check extensor strength (multiple spinal nerves).

  Position the patient's head tilted back 45 degrees.

  Brace her chest with one hand.

  Push on the occiput with the other hand, attempting to move the head anteriorly *(FIG. 12-78)*.

- Flexion has already been tested with cranial nerve XI.

- Back and abdomen: Have her lie prone on the exam table.

—Lower trapezius (Cranial nerve XI; C3, C4).

- Have her try to raise her shoulders and bring her scapulas closer together as you push downward on the shoulders *(FIG. 12-79)*.

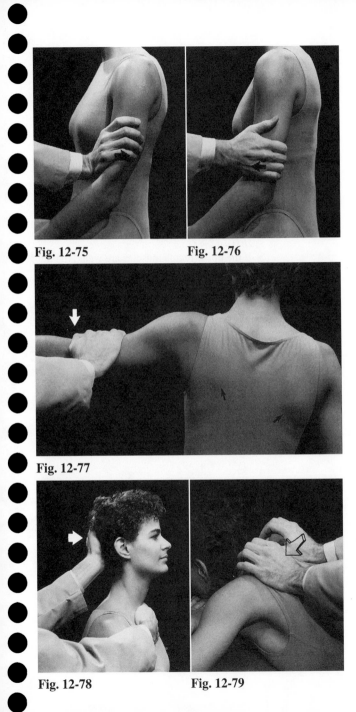

Fig. 12-75

Fig. 12-76

Fig. 12-77

Fig. 12-78

Fig. 12-79

—Back extensors (multiple spinal nerves).
  • Have her arch her back *(FIG. 12-80)*.
—At this time, check extension strength of the hips (S1, gluteus maximus).
  • Have her lie flat, then raise one leg and thigh off the table.
  • Apply downward pressure for resistance *(FIG. 12-81)*.
—Abdominal muscles (multiple intercostal and peripheral nerves).
  • Have her try to sit up without using her hands *(FIG. 12-82)*.
  • If the upper rectus muscles are weak, the umbilicus will slightly descend.
  • If the lower recti are weak, the umbilicus will rise slightly.
—Optional serratus anterior test (C5, C6, C7).
  • Have her stand, leaning toward a wall, pushing against it with both hands.
  • Weakness of these muscles will cause winging of the scapulas. This is seen as a lifting up and protrusion of the medial borders of the scapulas.

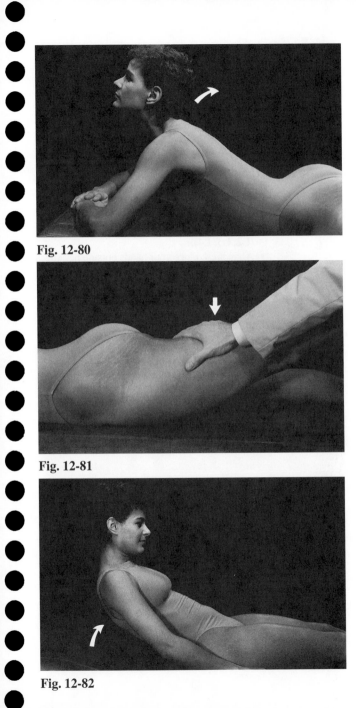

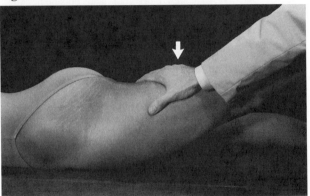

Fig. 12-80

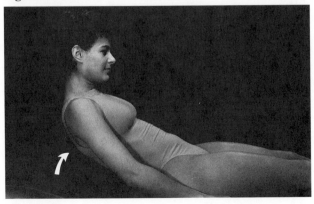

Fig. 12-81

Fig. 12-82

- Lower extremities: Have her sit on the exam table, legs dangling. Since these are strong muscles, you will need to make an effort to resist them.
  —Hips:
    - Resist flexion by having her raise her knee off the table as you push down *(FIG. 12-83)* (L2, L3, L4, iliopsoas muscle).
    - Extension was tested with the back and abdomen.
    - Adduction: place your hands between her knees and try to pull them apart *(FIG. 12-84)* (L2, L3, L4).
    - Abduction: place your hands outside her knees and try to push them together *(FIG. 12-85)* (L4, L5, S1, gluteus medius and minimus).
  —Knees: Position the knees to a 90 degree bend.
    - Resist flexion by pulling up on the lower leg *(FIG. 12-86)* (L4, L5, S1, hamstrings).
    - Resist extension by pushing down on the lower leg *(FIG. 12-87)* (L2, L3, L4, quadriceps muscle).

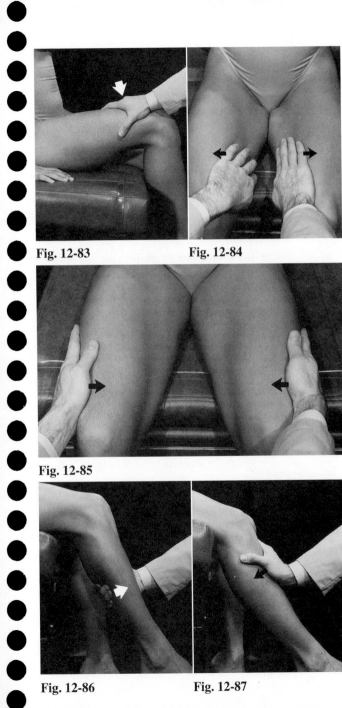

Fig. 12-83

Fig. 12-84

Fig. 12-85

Fig. 12-86

Fig. 12-87

—Ankle: Position yourself in front of the patient's feet. Place the ankle in neutral position (90 degree bend) and brace behind the lower leg with one hand. With the other hand:

- Resist plantar flexion by pushing up on the sole *(FIG. 12-88)* (L5, S1, S2, tibial nerve).
- Resist dorsiflexion by pulling down on the dorsal foot *(FIG. 12-89)* (L4, L5, deep peroneal nerve).
- Resist eversion by grasping the foot laterally and trying to invert it *(FIG. 12-90)* (L4, L5, deep peroneal nerve).
- Resist inversion by grasping the foot laterally and trying to evert it (the patient is countering each motion) *(FIG. 12-91)* (L4, L5, deep peroneal nerve).
- As mentioned earlier, because these are strong muscles, they may be weakened without your being physically able to resist them. Test for minimal weakness against the patient's full body weight:

  Have the patient stand on one leg (she may rest her hand lightly on the nearby exam table for balance).

  Observe as she plantar flexes and dorsiflexes ten times each.

  Watch for stepwise onset of fatigue.

—Toes.

- These are tested like the fingers, with flexion, extension, abduction, and adduction *(FIG. 12-92)*. In particular:

  Great toe extension: have the patient pull her great toe back. Resist by pressing down on the toenail (L4, L5, deep peroneal nerve).

  Great toe flexion: Have the patient curl down her toes, resist with your index finger, pulling upward (L5, S1, S2, tibial nerve).

- Adduction in the toes is difficult to assess separately from flexion.

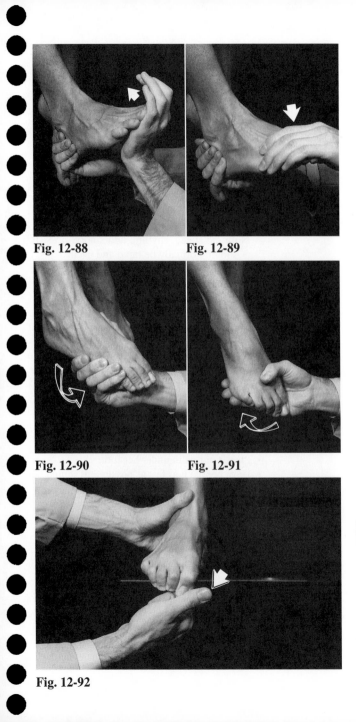

Fig. 12-88

Fig. 12-89

Fig. 12-90

Fig. 12-91

Fig. 12-92

4. Coordination: Remember to test each side.

- Rapid alternating motion, known as "diadochoki-nesia." An abnormality here is termed *dysdiado-chokinesia.*
- As you observe each motion, coax the patient on to perform it faster. This will serve to enhance any abnormality.

  —Upper extremities.
  - Hand patting.

    Have her pat her hands on her thighs as quickly as possible *(FIG. 12-93).*

    Note the speed, rhythm, and smoothness. It should normally be rapid and even.

    As a variation, have her perform a circular "polishing" motion on your palm.
  - Supination-pronation.

    Have her place her hands on her thighs and rapidly slap the palms, then the backs of her hands onto her thighs *(FIG. 12-94).*
  - Finger dexterity *(FIG. 12-95).*

    Have her touch the tip of her thumb to each of the four fingers, going back and forth as quickly as possible.

    The dominant hand will normally perform smoother and faster.

  —Lower extremities *(FIG. 12-96).*
  - Place your palm under her foot.
  - Have her pat it as fast as possible; it should be clumsier than the hands.

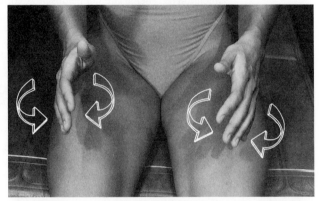

Fig. 12-93

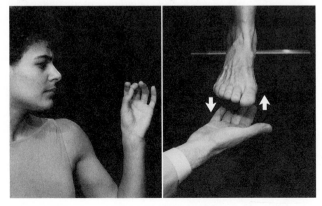

Fig. 12-94

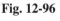

Fig. 12-95   Fig. 12-96

- Motion accuracy and intention tremor are assessed with point-to-point testing.
  —Upper extremities. Use the "finger-to-nose" test *(FIG. 12-97).*
  - Position your index finger 2 feet from her, at shoulder level.
  - Have her touch her index finger to yours, then to her nose, alternating back and forth several times.
  - Move your finger several times so she must accurately alter direction.
  - Watch for clumsiness or tremor:
    Intention (cerebellar) tremor begins after voluntary motion begins.
    It intensifies as the patient's finger reaches close to its goal (either your finger or her nose.)
    It may be associated with past pointing, where the finger completely misses its goal (called dysmetria.)
  - As a second test, have the patient extend her arms and hands straight in front, then close her eyes. Raise one arm about 30 degrees and ask her to return it to its former position. Check each side. This checks both cerebellar function and (with eyes closed) position sense (see *Fig. 12-142).*
    Watch for *past pointing* or oscillations.
    This can also be performed as part of the Romberg test.
  —Lower extremities *(FIG. 12-98):* Use the "heel-to-shin" test.
  - Have her run her heel up and down her opposite shin, moving from ankle to knee (and back) several times.
  - The foot should move in a straight line.
  - Watch for clumsiness or tremor.
    With cerebellar dysfunction, the heel rides in an S-shaped curve up and down the lower leg. Weakness resulting from aging may mimic this appearance.

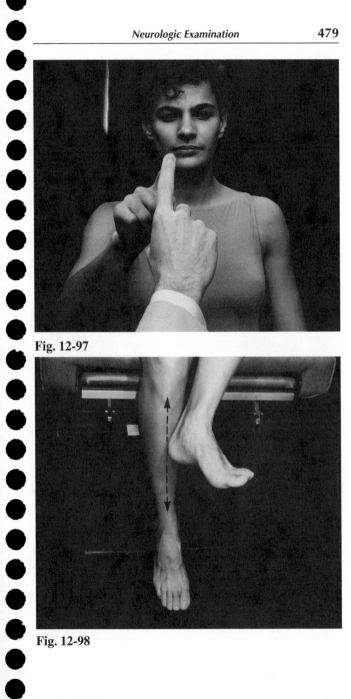

Fig. 12-97

Fig. 12-98

—In bedridden patients, check for truncal ataxia by
having the patient sit up.
- See if she fall consistently to one side. Midline
  lesions of the cerebellum may be overlooked if
  the patient is examined only while lying in bed.

V. **REFLEXES: These are involuntary responses to stimuli
and are typically divided into deep and superficial. A
third category, pathologic reflexes, are present only in
disease and are described later in "additional tests."**
A. **Deep Tendon Reflexes: Physiology.**
   1. The reflex arc:
      - The reflex hammer strikes the tendon, which causes
        a brief pull on the attached muscle, stretching it.
      - Muscle stretch receptors are activated, sending an
        impulse into its peripheral nerve through sensory
        fibers and up to the spinal cord.
      - The impulse enters the posterior root of the spinal
        cord on that side, traverses synaptic junctions, and
        exits via the anterior root (anterior horn) into its
        matching spinal and motor neuron. The impulse
        travels back down through motor fibers to the mus-
        cle.
      - The impulse crosses the neuromuscular junction
        and stimulates the muscle to contract.

   2. Influencing factors:
      - The intensity of the reflex response is tempered by
        its connections to the corticospinal (pyramidal)
        tract. When these connections are impaired, hyper-
        reflexia results. Recent stroke is a classic cause of
        hyperreflexia.
      - The reflex response is diminished or abolished by:
        —Interruption of the sensory (afferent) input from
          muscle to spinal cord.
        —Interruption of the motor (efferent) signal from
          spinal cord to muscle.
        —This dysfunction can occur at any point of
          synapse, or along the peripheral nerve.

3. Localization of a lesion.
   - Since each reflex arc involves only a few spinal cord segments:
     —Its function reflects on that particular segment of the spinal cord without implicating other segments.
     —Dysfunction in a reflex arc helps to localize the level of pathology, since each muscle group involves a particular set of spinal cord segments. The spinal cord segments involved are listed for each reflex.

4. Deep tendon reflexes are graded according to the intensity of the muscle response:
   - 0 - no response, even with a firm strike.
   - 1 - low normal, response is slightly diminished.
   - 2 - average.
   - 3 - response is brisker than normal, possibly but not necessarily pathologic.
   - 4 - very brisk response even from a light stimulus. Clonus is often present. This degree of hyperactivity often indicates disease.
   - Hyperreflexia indicates the sensitivity of the muscle stretch receptors to stimulation, not only how far the limb moves in response.

B. **Deep Tendon Reflexes:** technique (patient sitting).
   1. Reinforcement: used if reflexes are symmetrically decreased or absent. This is also called the *Jendrassik's* maneuver.
      - To increase reflex response in the legs:
        —Ask the patient to clench her teeth and, at the same time, lock her fingers together and try to pull them apart.
      - To increase upper extremity responses:
        —Ask the patient to clench her teeth and squeeze her thigh with the unused hand.
      - In both, have the patient tighten just before you strike the tendon.

2. Holding the reflex hammer *(FIG. 12-99).*
   - Hold the handle loosely in the fingers. A heavier re-
     flex hammer imparts more impact and can improve
     the chances of seeing a reflex response.
   - Keep the wrist relaxed so the hammer can swing
     freely in an arc.
   - Strike with a brisk, direct, but light, tapping motion.
     Since hyperactive reflexes respond to even a light
     tap, begin lightly and increase in intensity if no re-
     sponse occurs.
     —It is not necessary for the hammer to bounce off,
       as long as the tendon is stretched.

3. Biceps (C5-C6).
   - With the elbow slightly flexed and forearm resting
     in the lap (palm down), palpate the biceps tendon
     with your thumb and press in to produce moderate
     tension. (Removing the slack in the tendon allows
     the hammer's impulse to better stretch the muscle).
   - Stretch the tendon by striking your thumbnail *(FIG.
     12-100).* You will find up to three motions.
     —The limb may flex and pronate.
     —The belly of the muscle may visibly contract.
     —Or, if nothing else, the tendon will contract un-
       der your thumb.
   - Note the speed and intensity of each response.

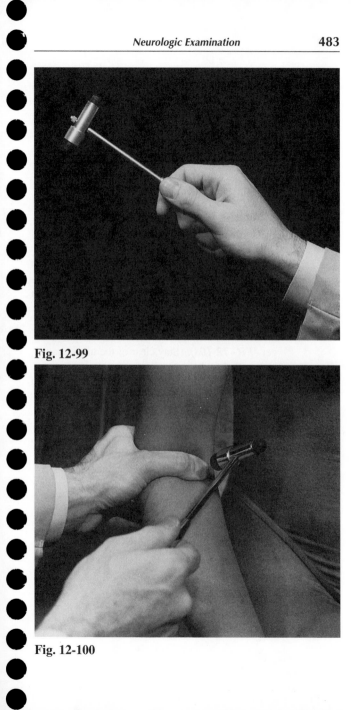

Fig. 12-99

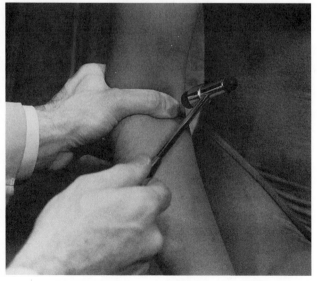

Fig. 12-100

4. Brachioradialis (C5-C6).

- Let the arm rest in the lap, elbow bent, forearm halfway between supination and pronation.
- Palpate the radial styloid (at the wrist by the base of the thumb) and move 2 inches proximally.
- Palpate the tendon over the radius.
- Stretch the tendon by striking your finger *(FIG. 12-101)*.
- Watch for flexion and supination of the forearm.

5. Triceps (C6-C7-C8).

- Position yourself posterior to the patient; her arms are still in her lap.
- Palpate the triceps tendon just above the olecranon *(FIG. 12-102)*.
   —If you have trouble locating the tendon, press on the tendon as she extends her arm against your resistance. The tendon will tighten and bulge.
- Strike the tendon directly, without an interposed finger *(FIG 12-103)*. (Stay clear of the ulnar groove, just medial to the tendon.)
- Watch for extension of the forearm or contraction of the muscle.
- If you don't get a response, try again:
   —With her hand on her hip *(FIG. 12-104)*,
   —Or supporting the upper arm with your hand so her forearm swings freely *(FIG. 12-105)*,
   —Or with her arms folded over her chest.

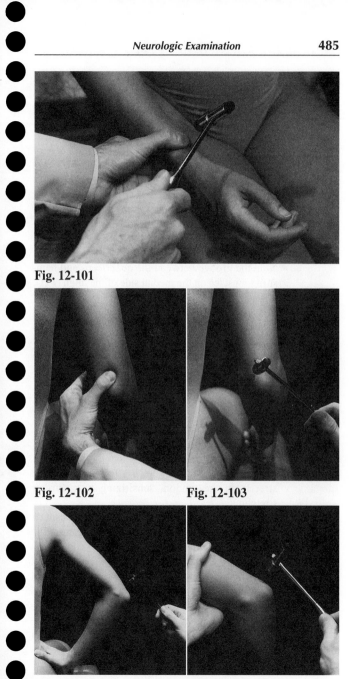

Fig. 12-101

Fig. 12-102

Fig. 12-103

Fig. 12-104

Fig. 12-105

6. Patellar (L2-L3-L4).
   - Position the patient with her legs dangling freely. Then, move to the side. You *can* get kicked!
   - Locate the tendon just inferior to the patella *(FIG. 12-106)*.
   - Tap briskly and observe extension of the knee, or contraction of the quadriceps muscle *(FIG. 12-107)*.
   - If you can't see a response, place your fingers on the quadriceps muscle just above the patella and feel for a contraction as you strike the patellar tendon.

7. Adductor reflex (also L2-L3-L4).
   - Note the groove between the quadriceps and hamstring muscles on the medial side of the thigh *(FIG. 12-108)*.
   - Palpate here just proximal to the knee. You will feel the cordlike adductor magnus tendon as it attaches to the bony knob of the adductor tubercle.
   - Strike the tendon either directly or with your thumb interposed *(FIG. 12-109)*. Watch for adduction of the thigh.
     —This response is usually less active than the patellar response.

8. Achilles (ankle) reflex (S1-S2).
   - With the legs still dangling, grasp the foot by the ball, and slightly dorsiflex it. This puts a slight stretch on the tendon, sensitizing it to further stretching.
   - Strike the tendon briskly *(FIG. 12-110)*. If using a reflex hammer with a narrow rubber head, strike with the handle instead.
   - Watch for the intensity of plantar flexion, and how quickly it relaxes afterward. Some illnesses, such as hypothyroidism, cause a delay before the foot returns to normal position.
   - If the patient is strong enough, the kneeling position allows you to compare both legs. Strike each achilles tendon in succession and compare the intensity of response.

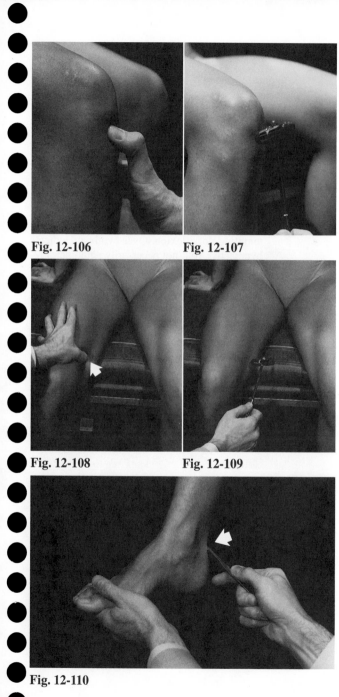

Fig. 12-106

Fig. 12-107

Fig. 12-108

Fig. 12-109

Fig. 12-110

9. Clonus: assessed if other lower limb reflexes are hyperactive.
   - Brace the leg with one hand over the achilles tendon.
   - Place the fingerpads of the other hand against the ball of the foot *(FIG. 12-111)*.
   - Very quickly dorsiflex the foot and maintain light pressure *(FIG. 12-112)*.
   - Note the response:
     —Normally, the foot will plantar flex once or twice.
     —This is often felt as "catches" while you are attempting dorsiflexion. Over two beats indicate hyperactive (but not necessarily pathologic) reflexes. A repetitive beating of clonus with continued pressure is pathologic.
   - Clonus can sometimes be elicited over the patella.
     —Extend the leg; it must be relaxed.
     —Grasp the patella with thumb and forefinger, then jerk it toward the foot.
     —Feel for repetitive contractions from the quadriceps muscle.

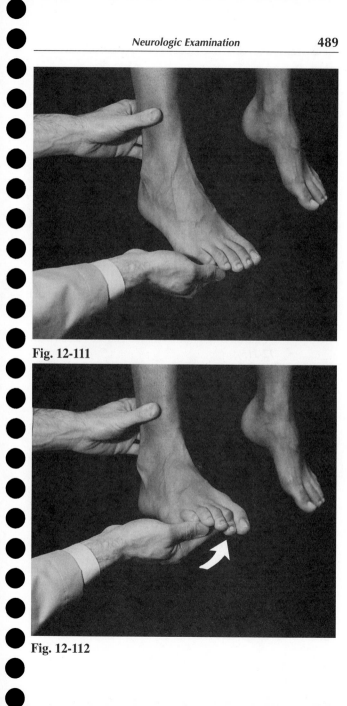

Fig. 12-111

Fig. 12-112

C. **Deep Tendon Reflexes:** technique (supine position). This is used when the patient is bedridden.

1. Biceps.
   - Flex the elbow to 90 degrees; place the hand in her lap *(FIG. 12-113)*.
   - Palpate the biceps tendon with one finger. Strike it with the reflex hammer.

2. Brachioradialis *(FIG. 12-114)*.
   - Position the arm as above.
   - Palpate the tendon and strike as before. It may be easier here to palpate with the forefinger rather than the thumb.

3. Triceps.
   - Stand behind the patient (or in front if you can hold the hammer in the left hand).
   - Grasp the wrist and pull the arm across the chest until the elbow is flush with the patient's side *(FIG. 12-115)*.
   - Strike the tendon as before.

4. Patellar.
   - Stand to one side near her knees.
   - Reach your left hand under her right knee and rest your palm on her left knee.
   - Lift up with your left forearm so the right knee rises to a roughly 145 degree bend *(FIG. 12-116)*.
   - Strike the tendon as described.
   - For the left knee, rest your forearm on the right knee and reach under the left, raising it as before.

5. Achilles *(FIG. 12-117)*.
   - Flex one leg at the knee and hip, and rotate it externally so the ankle rests across the opposite shin (the sole will be facing laterally).
   - Dorsiflex the foot and strike.

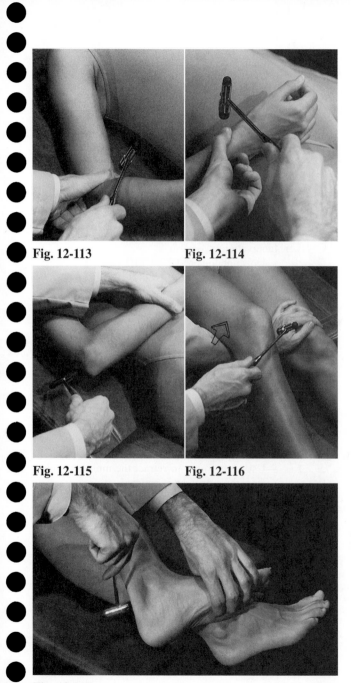

Fig. 12-113

Fig. 12-114

Fig. 12-115

Fig. 12-116

Fig. 12-117

D. Superficial Reflexes: These require cutaneous rather than muscle-stretch stimuli.

   1. Although deep tendon responses are inhibited by upper motor neuron pathways, the superficial reflexes must travel up and back down the cord for a response to occur. For this reason, whenever upper motor neuron pathways are impaired:
   - Deep tendon reflexes become *hyperactive.*
   - Superficial reflexes become *diminished.*

   2. Abdominal reflex.
   - Innervation:
     —Upper abdomen, T8-T9-T10.
     —Lower abdomen, T10-T11-T12.
   - Have the patient lie supine.
   - Using a pin or cotton-tipped applicator:
     —Stroke the skin in the four quadrants.
     —Each time, move from periphery toward the umbilicus *(FIG. 12-118).*
   - Normally, the umbilicus will jerk slightly toward each stimulus.
     —It may be decreased in the elderly or multiparous patient.
     —Watch especially for a unilateral decrease in response.
   - In an obese patient: *(FIG. 12-119).*
     —Use your finger to retract the umbilicus away from the side to be stimulated.
     —As you stroke, feel with the retracting finger for any abdominal muscle contraction.

   3. Cremasteric response *(FIG. 12-120)* (L1, L2).
   - With the patient standing, gently stroke the inner thigh with a pin or applicator stick (stroke upward).
     —Do this near the level of the scrotum.
     —Watch for slight elevation of the testicle on that side.

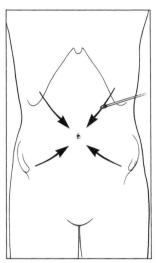

Fig. 12-118

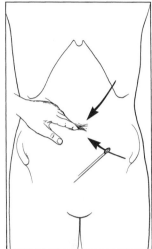

Fig. 12-119

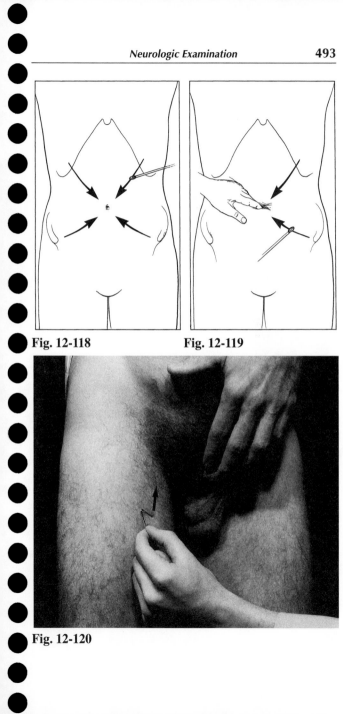

Fig. 12-120

4. Plantar response.
- It requires a moderately sharp object for stimulus.
    —Use a key, broken tongueblade, retracted pen, applicator stick, etc.
    —Use care in patients with fragile skin, especially those with diabetes mellitus or other vascular insufficiency.
- Hold the patient's ankle and stroke the plantar surface *(FIG. 12-121).*
    —Begin by the heel on the lateral side.
    —Continue upward to the ball (metatarsal heads).
    —Then curve medially over the ball to the large toe.
- You will normally see brief flexion of all toes *(FIG. 12-122).*

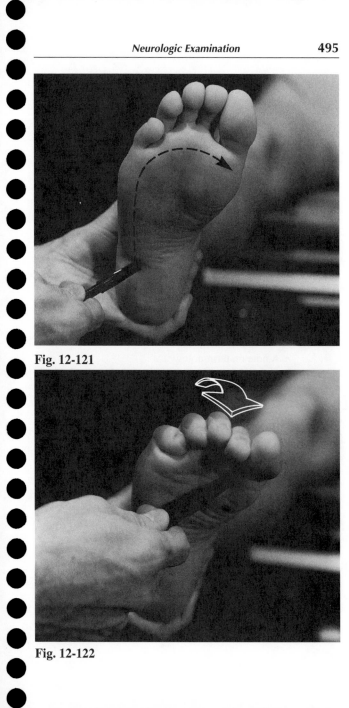

Fig. 12-121

Fig. 12-122

- If you don't get a response, try another maneuver:
  —"Chaddock": stimulate the lateral aspect of the dorsal foot, sweeping the stimulus under the lateral malleolus, and toward the toes *(FIG. 12-123)*.
  —"Oppenheimer": run your knuckles or pinched thumb and forefinger down the anterior edge of the tibia *(FIG. 12-124)*.
  —"Gordon": firmly squeeze the calf muscles *(FIG. 12-125)*.
  —"Schaeffer": firmly squeeze the achilles tendon *(FIG. 12-126)*.
- The positive response is called the *Babinski sign (FIG. 12-127)*.
  —A partial response is extension of the large toe.
  —A complete response is extension of the large toe plus fanning of the remaining toes.
    - It can be accompanied by withdrawal of the foot and leg (but withdrawal alone may be only due to ticklishness).
- A note on terminology:
  —An abnormal response is recorded as "Babinski sign is present."
  —A normal response is "plantar reflex shows downgoing toes." There is no such thing as a negative Babinski sign.

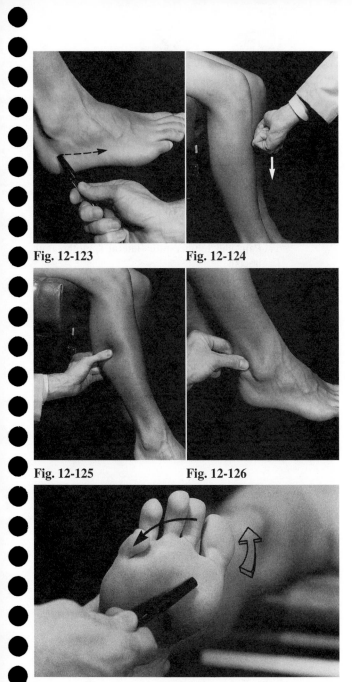

Fig. 12-123

Fig. 12-124

Fig. 12-125

Fig. 12-126

Fig. 12-127

VI. SENSORY FUNCTIONS: When patterns of sensory loss are correlated with motor findings, this aids in localizing the site of cerebral or peripheral dysfunction. Fatigue produces inaccuracy in sensory testing. Postpone this portion of the examination if you or your patient are overly tired.

A. **Functional Anatomy.**

    1. Sensory testing evaluates two aspects of sensation:

        ▪ The modality indicates regions of the cord that conduct sensation for:

            —Position and vibration (posterior columns).

            —Pain and temperature (lateral spinothalamic tracts).

            —Crude touch (anterior spinothalamic tracts).

                • Also known as light touch.

        ▪ The distribution of a sensory loss can be mapped on the skin according to the peripheral or spinal sensory nerves supplying each region *(FIG. 12-128).*

            —These regions are called "dermatomes."

            —Only a few spinal nerve dermatomes are routinely tested:

                • On the hand: C6, C7, and C8.

                • On the trunk: C3, T4, T10, and T12.

                • On the legs: L3, L4, L5, and S1.

        ▪ Test each sensory modality in at least these selected dermatomes.

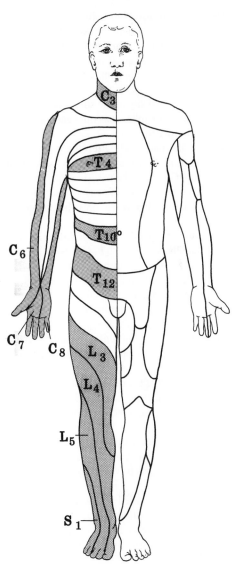

Fig. 12-128

B. Overall Technique Guidelines.

1. Test sensations with the patient's eyes closed.
2. Begin sensory testing on the fingers and toes. Check more proximal areas *only* if distal sensation is impaired, or if the patient has other signs of neurologic disease.
3. Increase intensity of the stimulus as needed for her to feel it. Remember that thickened skin is less sensitive normally.
4. Vary the pace and pattern of your stimulus so she cannot predict the quality or location of the next touch. Compare the two sides for symmetry.
5. If you find an area of sensory change:
   - Note whether sensation is heightened, decreased, or absent.
   - Move outward in several directions and try to locate its boundaries *(FIG. 12-129).*
     —The patient can more easily tell when a sensation is returning rather than fading.
     —Note whether the transition from normal to abnormal is abrupt or gradual.

C. Begin By Testing for Pain Sensation *(FIG. 12-130);*
use a safety pin or other stimulus as described in cranial nerves.

1. Check each of the dermatomal areas described above on the head, arms, chest, and legs. Check the back if sensation is impaired anteriorly.

D. Temperature Sensation *(FIG. 12-131).*

1. This is usually checked if pain sensation is impaired (both sensations travel through lateral spinothalamic tracts).
2. Use test tubes filled with warm and cool water; follow the same pattern as for pain sensation.
   - Again, as an alternate method, use the side of a tuning fork for cool and the backs of two fingers for warm.

E. Light Touch *(FIG. 12-132).*

1. Use a soft brush or cotton ball and have the patient respond yes whenever she feels it.

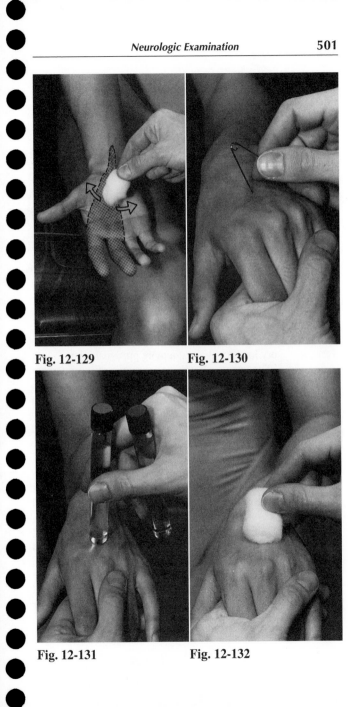

Fig. 12-129

Fig. 12-130

Fig. 12-131

Fig. 12-132

F. Vibratory Sensation.
1. Use a low-pitched tuning fork, preferably 128 Hz.
2. Hold it near its base and activate it by tapping it on the heel of your hand.
3. Always press the base to a bony prominence.
   - Ask if she can feel the buzzing and when it goes away. If you still can feel it when she cannot, she may have a sensory loss.
   - To make the test more objective, occasionally stop the fork prematurely to ensure she is responding accurately.
   - As decreased vibratory sense is normal with aging, check for asymmetry from right to left.
     —A unilateral sensory loss is more suggestive of a peripheral neuropathy.
     —A diffuse bilateral loss can be caused by a peripheral polyneuropathy, such as with diabetes, alcoholism, or vitamin B_{12} deficiency.
4. Begin with the most distal joint. If you find a sensory loss, try again at a more proximal joint.
   - The upper extremity sequence is: distal interphalangeal or metacarpophalangeal joint of fingers, wrist (radial or ulnar styloid), elbow, and sternum *(FIGS. 12-133 to 12-135)*.
   - The lower extremity sequence is: interphalangeal joint of large toe, ankle (malleolus), knee, and iliac crest *(FIGS. 12-136 to 12-138)*.
     —If vibratory sense is grossly absent, try to determine a sensory level by touching the tuning fork to each posterior spinous process, going upward one at a time.
     —If you are unsure if the patient is truly sensing vibration, ask her to tell you when it stops, and then stop the vibrating fork with your finger.
5. If you do not have your tuning fork, but you are wearing a beeper, turn it to its "vibrate" setting, and apply it firmly to the bony prominence. The beeper will vibrate for a few seconds each time you switch settings. Proceed sequentially as for the tuning fork.

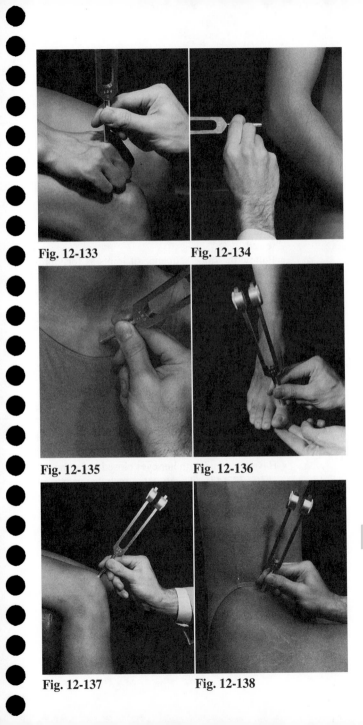

Fig. 12-133

Fig. 12-134

Fig. 12-135

Fig. 12-136

Fig. 12-137

Fig. 12-138

G. Position Sense *(FIG 12-139)*.

  1. Grasp the large toe by the sides.
  - To avoid confusion, demonstrate up and down motions with the patient's eyes open. The joint must be completely relaxed.

  2. Then, with the patient's eyes closed.
  - Move in large motions at first. She should respond "up," "down," or "I don't know."
  - Let the motions become smaller and smaller. Normally motion as small as 1 to 2 mm can be detected.
  - Follow the same sequence of joints as for vibration *(FIG. 12-140)*.
    —Make sure to move randomly up and down so she cannot predict your next direction.
    —Test more proximally if distal sensation is impaired.

  3. Two additional methods for testing upper extremity position sense:
  - Repeat finger-to-nose testing as if checking coordination. Then have her close her eyes (and continue) *(FIG. 12-141)*.
    —Her continued accuracy depends on position sense.
  - Have her stand with her eyes closed and arms out *(FIG. 12-142)*. (This is often included as part of the Romberg test.)
    —Move one arm a few inches upward and ask her to put it back where it was.
    —She should be able to return it to its former position.

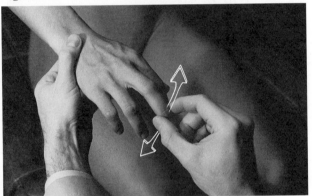

Fig. 12-139

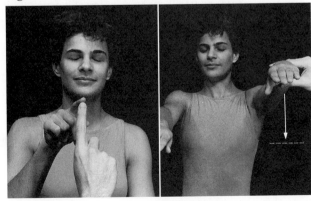

Fig. 12-140

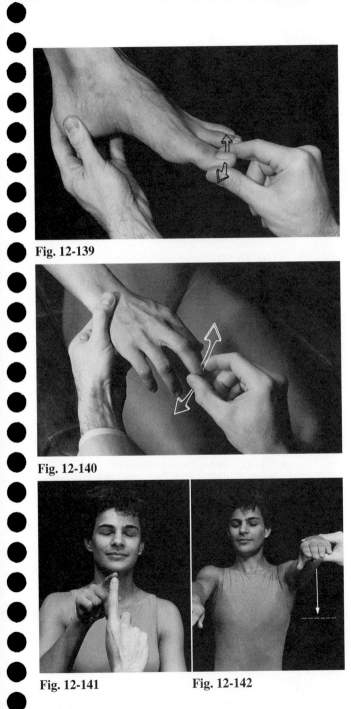

Fig. 12-141   **Fig. 12-142**

H. Sensory Discrimination Tests.

1. Physiology.
   - These test the ability of the contralateral cerebral cortex (especially the parietal lobe) to analyze and interpret sensations.
     —They require intact sensory functions, particularly in the posterior columns of the cord (which transmit the sense of position and vibration).
   - These tests ask "if everything is intact below, is everything okay above?"

2. Stereognosis: the ability to identify objects by touch *(FIG. 12-143)*.
   - This is used as the screening test for this group. If the response is abnormal, the remaining tests are used.
   - With her eyes closed, place a familiar object in one of her hands. Use a universally familiar object, such as a key, coin, paper clip, or pencil.
   - She should be able to identify it correctly. Check each side.

3. Graphesthesia: the ability to identify objects drawn on the skin.
   - This test is especially useful when paralysis prevents testing for stereognosis.
   - Use the blunt end of a pen or pencil. Draw a number from 0 to 9 on the palm (draw it upright as if she were to read it) *(FIG. 12-144)*.
   - She should be able to identify it correctly. Inability suggests parietal lobe disease.
   - This can also be tested on the back and on the sole of the foot.

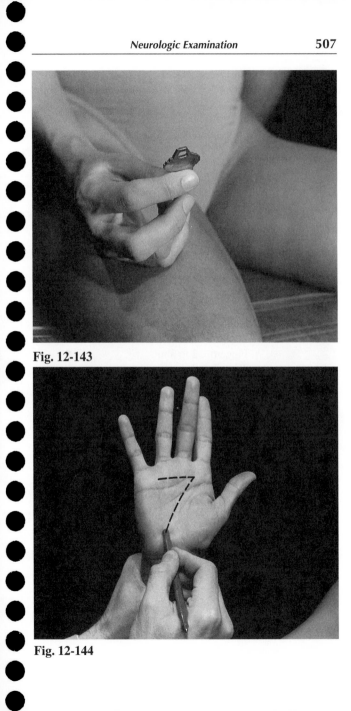

Fig. 12-143

Fig. 12-144

4. Two-point discrimination.
- Use two pins, a paperclip unbent to a 'U', or a dull compass.
- Demonstrate one and two points to the patient. Then note the minimal gap where she still feels two points *(FIG. 12-145):*
  —Make sure to touch the two points at the same time. Keep the two points side-by-side, rather than along the long axis of the limb or finger.
  —Begin on the pads of the fingertips or toes.
  —Alternate randomly between one and two points.
  —Move more proximally when the threshold is wider than expected.
     • Be aware that the threshold will normally widen as you move proximally.
     • The average minimal distances where two points are still felt are:
       Tongue, 1 mm
       Fingertip, 2 to 3 mm
       Toes, 3 to 8 mm
       Palm, 1 cm
       Forearm/chest, 4 cm
       Back, 4 to 7 cm
- Compare right to left, upper and lower extremities. Begin distally each time.

5. Point localization.
- With her eyes closed, brush a pin or cotton ball on the skin *(FIG. 12-146).*
- She should be able to point to and tell you almost exactly (within 2 to 3 cm) where you have touched.
- Test both sides on the face, arms, and legs.
- Disorders of the sensory cortex will impair the ability to accurately localize points.
  —With contralateral parietal lobe dysfunction, she will describe the touch as more proximal than it was.

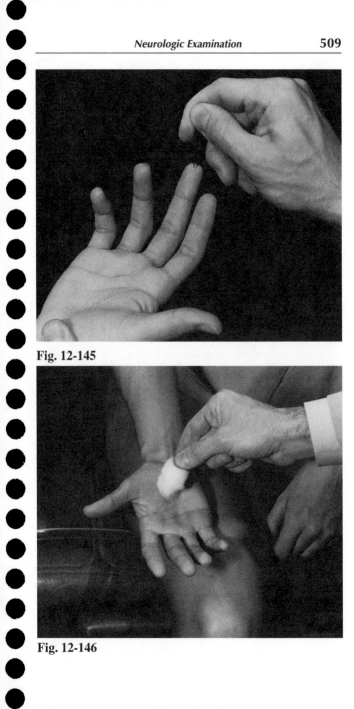

Fig. 12-145

Fig. 12-146

6. Extinction.
   - Perform as for point localization, but touch both sides simultaneously *(FIG. 12-147)*. She should be able to feel both sides.
   - When extinction is present, she will feel only one side *(FIG. 12-148)*.
     —For example: if the *left* parietal lobe is compromised, she will not feel the *right*-sided stimulus.
   - Visual extinction is checked by wiggling a finger in both upper-temporal or lower-temporal fields simultaneously.

7. Other discrimination tests include:
   - Baresthesia: the ability to discriminate the weight of objects.
     —Use two objects of different weight but similar texture *(FIG. 12-149)*. Place one in each of the patient's hands.
     —With her eyes closed, she should be able to tell which one is heavier.
   - Identification of body parts.
     —Ask her to hold up or point to her ring, middle, and index finger *(FIG. 12-150)*.
     • Extreme damage must occur before she loses identification of the thumb.
     —Inability to identify indicates damage to the functionally dominant parietal lobe.
   - Praxis: the ability to perform a planned motor act in the absense of paralysis of those muscles normally needed.
     —The patient is asked to demonstrate how she would:
     • Strike a match.
     • Use a scissors.
     • Clean her teeth.
     —Then have her construct a simple geometric figure from matches, such as a five-point star.
     —Inability to perform these tasks suggest deep frontal lobe damage.

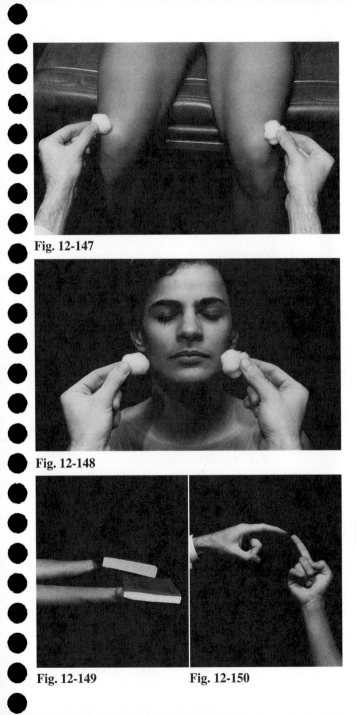

Fig. 12-147

Fig. 12-148

Fig. 12-149   Fig. 12-150

VII. ADDITIONAL TESTS.
A. For Coordination.
1. Overshoot.
   - Have her close her eyes and extend her arms *(FIG. 12-151)*.
     —Forewarn her of what you will do.
     —Tap sharply downward on one hand. It should rapidly bounce up to its original position.
   - In cerebellar disease the arm will oscillate (overshoot) several times before reaching the original resting position.

2. Blocking maneuver.
   - With the patient seated, eyes open, have her flex one arm, with her fist at the level of her neck.
   - Place your hand between her fist and body, to act as a guard.
   - Ask her to resist as you:
     —Pull hard on her arm *(FIG. 12-152)*. Then, suddenly let go.
       • Normally, she can check her motion and the arm will quickly stop.
       • This is actually a test of ability to rapidly alternate motion.
   - With a cerebellar lesion, her arm will fling toward her face and would be stopped only by your hand *(FIG. 12-153)*.

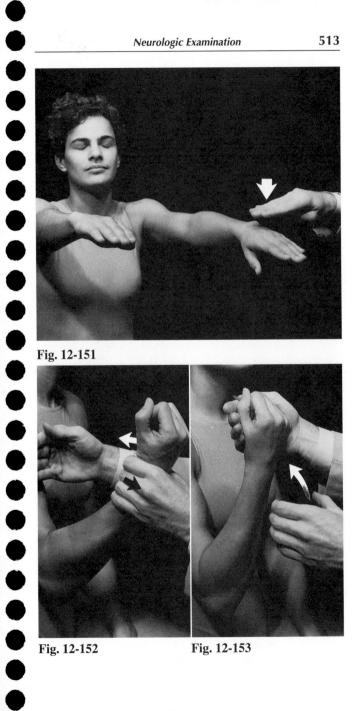

Fig. 12-151

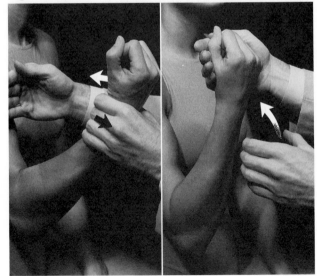

Fig. 12-152   Fig. 12-153

B. Frontal Release Signs: Reflexes normally present in infancy but supressed soon after. They may reappear with diffuse brain disease, especially in the frontal lobes. Test for these when dementia or widespread neurologic abnormalities are found.

1. Blink (glabella) reflex *(FIG. 12-154)*.
   - Using a reflex hammer, tap lightly and repeatedly between the patient's eyes. They will blink at first but soon adapt.
   - With *frontal release* (removal of the normal frontal lobe inhibition): the blinking continues without adaptation.

2. Snout reflex *(FIG. 12-155)*.
   - Tap lightly above the lips. There is normally minimal or no response.
   - With frontal release:
     —The lips will pucker with each tap.
     —In an extreme case, the face will grimace.

3. Sucking reflex *(FIG. 12-156)*.
   - Gently stroke the lips with a tongueblade. There is normally no response.
   - With frontal release, the patient will display sucking movements of the lips, tongue, and jaw. She may even follow the tongueblade, much as would a newborn baby (rooting response).

4. Grasp reflex *(FIG. 12-157)*.
   - Hold the patient's hand by her wrist.
   - Stroke her palm with your fingers. There is normally no response.
   - With frontal release, the fingers will flex. The harder you pull, the greater is her flexion response *(FIG. 12-158)*.
     —Although it appears natural, it *is* involuntary.

5. Jaw jerk.
   - With the jaw half open, tap each half of the mandible with the reflex hammer. This stretches the masseter and temporalis muscles.
   - In frontal lobe lesions or cortical damage, the jaw snaps closed. This is a sign of hyperreflexia.

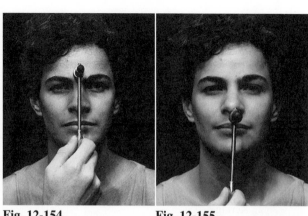

Fig. 12-154

Fig. 12-155

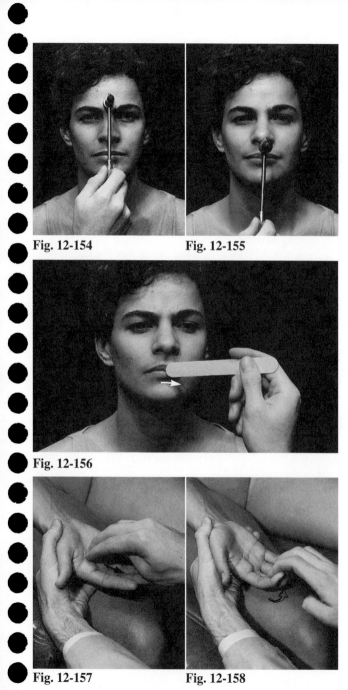
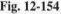

Fig. 12-156

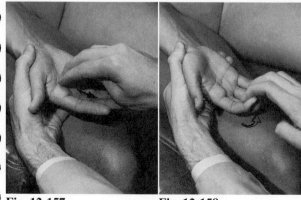

Fig. 12-157

Fig. 12-158

C. **Meningeal Signs.**
  1. Brudzinski's sign.
     - With the patient supine, attempt to flex the neck *(FIG. 12-159)*. There is normally no response.
     - With meningeal irritation:
       —The neck is stiff and will not flex well.
       —The patient may express pain and flex the knees and hips in response *(FIG. 12-160)*.
         • This is an unconscious effort to relieve tension on the spinal cord induced by neck flexion.

  2. Kernig's sign.
     - With the patient still supine, flex one knee and hip to a 90 degree bend *(FIG. 12-161)*. Then attempt to extend that knee.
     - With meningeal inflammation:
       —The patient will resist and complain of pain *(FIG. 12-162)*.
       —Extension of the knee places tension on the lumbosacral nerve roots and, in turn, pulls on the cord.
       —A patient with hamstring muscle tightness will also have limited extension of the knee, but not the marked pain.

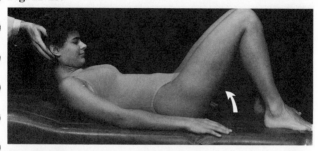

Fig. 12-159

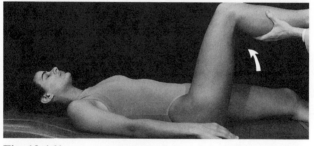

Fig. 12-160

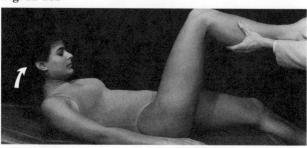

Fig. 12-161

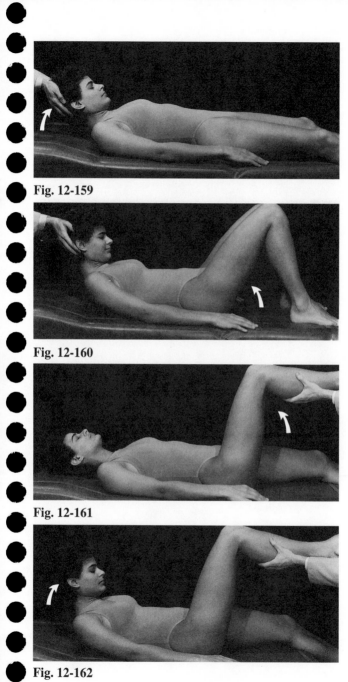

Fig. 12-162

13 *Integrated Screening Examination*

This approach is one used for the initial complete physical examination and examines the body region by region, posturally based, rather than by organ system. Additional techniques and more detailed examination can be added as clinical suspicion dictates. (Refer to each chapter for specifics on technique.) Although this description seems detailed, with practice the examination moves quite quickly.

I. PATIENT MOVES TO THE EXAMINATION TABLE.
A. General Assessment.
1. Observe how the patient enters the room. Note gait, posture, dress, body type, deformities, appearance of chronic illness, mood, apparent age, personal hygiene, and odor.
   - Note use of assistive devices, such as a cane or walker.
   - In addition, watch for facial flushing, dyspnea with exertion, audible or pursed-lip breathing.

B. Vital Signs, performed with the patient sitting.
1. Take pulse and respirations with the hand on the patient's wrist.

2. Check blood pressure. Be sure to use the right-sized cuff for the arm. If blood pressure is elevated, repeat at the end of the examination.

3. Check temperature, usually from the nurse's record. If not a recent reading, it can be repeated.

4. Note height and weight, recorded before patient entered the examination room.

II. PATIENT SITTING ON THE EXAMINATION TABLE, UNDRESSED, AND GOWNED. You stand in front of the patient.

A. Check Upper Extremities.

1. Hands.
   - Palms up.
     —Examine the hands for thenar, hypothenar, and dorsal interosseus muscle atrophy.
     —Check the palms for erythema or contractures. Note color of the digits for pallor or cyanosis.
   - Palms down.
     —Examine the DIP, PIP, and MCP joints for redness or swelling.
     —Palpate joints that are enlarged or mentioned by the patient. Note telangiectasia or sclerodactyly.
     —Note any tremor.
2. Wrists.
   - Inspect for swelling. Palpate as above.
3. Elbows.
   - Inspect for swelling. In particular, note any olecranon bursa enlargement or nodules on the ulnar ridge. Palpate as above.
   - Check biceps, triceps, and brachioradialis reflexes.
4. Shoulder: Move the shoulder through its standard range of motion by:
   - Arms over head, elbows touching ears.
   - Hands clasped behind head, elbows pulled back.
   - Hands behind back, push thumbs up between shoulder blades.

B. Move Your Attention to the Head.

1. Discretely observe facies for signs of illness (e.g., hypothyroidism).
2. Check the scalp for skin lesions and hair distribution. Note facial rashes or skin lesions. Remove wig or hairpiece if necessary.

C. Examine the Eyes.

1. Inspect the external eyes.
   - Check visual acuity with the pocket Snellen chart.
     —Make sure the patient has his/her glasses if needed, and use good lighting.
   - Compare the eyes for prominence.

- Examine the eyelids, conjunctiva, cornea, and iris.
  —Note scleral jaundice or conjunctival pallor.
  —Have the patient raise the eyebrows and shut the eyes tightly (cranial nerve VII).
- Check extraocular motion (cranial nerves III, IV, and VI).

2. Check visual fields by confrontation (cranial nerve II).
3. Dim the lights (if possible) and perform ophthalmoscopy.
   - First, check pupillary responses to light and accommodation (cranial nerve II).
   - Using the ophthalmoscope, check the red reflex, the disc, vessels, background, and macula.
4. Return the lights to normal brightness.

D. Move Your Attention to the Ears.
1. Rub your fingers lightly together next to each ear, as a screen for hearing loss.
   - If background noise is considerable, postpone this portion for a quieter environment.
2. Examine the external ear, including postauricular skin.
3. Check the Rinne and Weber tests (cranial nerve VIII).
4. Using the otoscope, check the ear canal and tympanic membrane.

E. Move Your Attention to the Nose.
1. Inspect the external nose.
2. Have the patient sniff through one nostril at a time, to check for patency.
3. Using the otoscope, examine the septum, turbinates, and nasal airway.
4. If there are complaints of sinus congestion, palpate the frontal and maxillary sinus areas for tenderness.

F. Move Your Attention to the Mouth.
1. Ask the patient to show his/her teeth (cranial nerve VII).
2. Have the patient stick out his/her tongue (cranial nerve XII).
3. Note jaw mobility as he/she opens his/her mouth wide.
   —Palpate the temporomandibular joints at the same time.

4. Using a tongueblade and light source, examine lips, teeth, gums, buccal mucosa, tongue (top and bottom), and pharynx.
   - Have the patient say "Ah" and watch for uvula rise and a clear voice (cranial nerves IX and X).

5. Test masseter and temporalis strength with your fingertips (cranial nerve V).
   - In addition, screen for sensation with a light brush of your fingertips simultaneously on each side of the face, in the ophthalmic, maxillary, and mandibular distributions.

G. Move Your Attention to the Neck.

1. Inspect for visible masses or an enlarged thyroid gland.
   - In addition, see if the patient uses accessory muscles during inspiration.

2. Note any jugular venous distention.

3. Check range of motion as he/she flexes, extends, lateral bends, and rotates the neck, both to the right and left.

4. Palpate for regional lymph nodes, feeling in turn preauricular, postauricular, occipital, submental, submandibular, anterior and posterior cervical nodes, and supraclavicular nodes.
   - Then palpate the carotid pulses one at a time.
   - Then auscultate both carotids for bruit, using the stethoscope bell.

5. Palpate tracheal position.

6. Have the patient shrug the shoulders upward against your resistance (cranial nerve XI).

III. **MOVE YOUR ATTENTION TO THE CHEST. The patient should be undraped from the waist up.**
   A. **Check the Shoulders for Equal Level.**

   B. **For Female Patients, Inspect the Breasts for Retractions as She:**
      1. Raises her hands over her head.

      2. Presses her hands to her hips.

      3. If breasts are pendulous, have her lean toward you. Observe the breasts for retractions and skin changes.

   C. **Have the Patient Take a Deep Breath.**
      1. Note any inspiratory retractions. Watch for symmetric chest expansion. Look for barrel chest configuration.

   D. **Check Tactile Fremitus on the Anterior Chest,** using the across-and-down pattern. Also compare the lateral chest; right to left.

   E. **Percuss the Anterior Chest Using the Across-and-Down Pattern.**

   F. **Auscultate the Heart in Its Four Auscultation Areas.**
      1. Note rate and rhythm, S_1 and S_2, splitting, any extra sounds or murmurs.

      2. Use both the diaphragm and the bell.

   G. **Auscultate the Lungs Using the Across-and-Down Pattern.**

   H. **Palpate for Axillary Lymph Nodes on Each Side.**

IV. **MOVE BEHIND THE PATIENT, WHO IS STILL SITTING.**
   A. **Observe the Back for Skin Lesions.**
   B. **Palpate the Thyroid Gland with Both Hands.** (Use the anterior approach only if the patient cannot sit up.)
   C. **Check Tactile Fremitus on the Posterior Chest, Using the Across-and-Down Pattern.**
   D. **Percuss the Posterior Chest Using the Across-and-Down Pattern.**
   E. **Auscultate the Lungs Using the Across-and-Down Pattern.**
   F. **Palpate the Spine for Muscle Spasm or Minor Degrees of Scoliosis.**
      1. Then, bracing the patient with one hand in front, percuss the spine every few inches with your fist, checking for tenderness.
         ▪ Check for costovertebral angle tenderness.
      2. Redrape the patient.

V. **SIT ON A STOOL NEAR THE PATIENT'S LEGS (or elevate the patient's legs).**
   A. **Inspect the Thighs and Legs for Muscle Atrophy.**
   B. **Note Any Skin Lesions:**
      1. On the anterior tibias.
      2. Any varicose veins, vascular collections, or pigment changes near the malleoli.
      3. Varicose veins in the thighs or lower legs.
   C. **Elicit the Patellar and Achilles Reflexes. Check for Clonus.**
      1. Check for a Babinski sign, if suspected.
   D. **Palpate the Dorsalis Pedis and Posterior Tibial Pulses.**
      1. If absent, when the patient is supine, check for popliteal and femoral pulses.
   E. **Note Pedal Edema,** and if present, how high it extends up the anterior tibia.
      1. See if the edema is pitting or non-pitting.
   F. **Examine the Toes** for Bunions, Hammer Toes, and Tinea Pedis. Note any onychomychosis (fungal nail).
      1. Check for signs of vascular disease, such as shiny, hairless skin, dystrophic nails, and prolonged capillary refill.

VI. IF HEART DISEASE IS SUSPECTED, move the patient to about 45 degrees of inclination. Check the jugular veins for distension and pulsations.

VII. HAVE THE PATIENT LIE SUPINE. The chest and pubic areas may remain draped until examined.

    A. Examine the Breasts (Both Sexes). Position the patient's arm as necessary.

        1. Inspect for skin changes or retractions.

        2. Palpate each breast systematically, including the tail.

    B. Examine the Heart. Stand to the patient's right side.

        1. Inspect for the apical impulse.

        2. Palpate the apical impulse, then check the remaining precordium for impulses or vibratory thrills.

        3. If the apical impulse cannot be seen or palpated, percuss the lateral heart border.

        4. Auscultate the heart in its four auscultation areas.

          ■ Note rate and rhythm, S_1 and S_2, splitting, any extra sounds, or murmurs. (Listening in both sitting and supine positions helps to identify murmurs.)

          ■ Use both the diaphragm and the bell.

    C. Examine the Abdomen.

        1. Inspect the skin and note abdominal contour. Note incisional scars or hernias.

        2. Auscultate for peristalsis frequency and pitch.

          ■ Then auscultate for bruits over the aorta, renal, and iliac vessels.

        3. Percuss for tympany pattern, liver, and splenic enlargement.

        4. Lightly palpate to localize any areas of tenderness. Note abdominal wall tone.

        5. Palpate for liver, spleen, and aorta.

          ■ Then do a general survey for masses.

        6. Palpate inguinal lymph nodes.

        7. Some clinicians prefer to examine male genitalia at this time (see below).

          ■ Following this, redrape the abdomen.

D. Check Lower Extremity Range of Motion.
   1. Roll each leg into full internal and external rotation, checking for pain or limitation.
   2. Fully flex each knee up to the abdomen. In full flexion, check internal and external rotation of the hips again.

VIII. HAVE THE PATIENT STAND. If the patient is wearing a paper gown, you may wish to secure the open parts with a piece of tape.

A. Recheck Pulse and Blood Pressure if Desired.

B. Move Your Attention to the Spine.
   1. Note kyphosis or scoliosis.
   2. Have the patient bend forward to touch his/her toes. Note flexibility.

C. For Men:
   1. Examine external genitalia.
      - Inform him you will examine his genitalia and check for hernia. Have him stand before you as you sit on a stool. Put on disposable gloves.
        —If patient has a latex allergy, use vinyl gloves.
      - Inspect the penis. Retract the foreskin if necessary. Look for skin lesions.
      - Gently palpate the testes.
      - Examine each side for hernia.
   2. Perform a rectal examination.
      - Have lubricant and stool occult blood test ready.
      - Have the patient bend over the exam table, supported by both of his elbows.
      - Perform a digital rectal examination including the prostate.
      - Test stool for occult blood.
   3. Provide a box of tissues. Let the patient redress before returning to discuss the examination.
   4. After the patient is dressed and settled, repeat blood pressure measurement if elevated before.

IX. FOR WOMEN, PERFORM A PELVIC EXAMINATION.

A. Inform Her You Will Perform a Pelvic Examination. She may wish to empty her bladder to make the examination more comfortable.

   1. When the practitioner is male, patients often prefer to have a female nurse or assistant in the room.

   2. Assist the patient into the lithotomy position. Put on disposable gloves.

   ▪ If patient has a latex allergy, use vinyl gloves.

B. Inspect External Genitalia.

C. Palpate External Structures and Check Muscle Tone.

D. Insert the Speculum and Perform a Pap Test. Take GC/chlamydia samples and KOH/saline preparation as necessary.

E. Inspect the Vagina as You Remove the Speculum.

F. Perform Bimanual Palpation of the Uterus and Adnexae.

G. Perform a Rectovaginal and/or Rectal Examination. Change gloves as necessary.

   1. Test stool for occult blood.

H. Provide a Box of Tissues. Let the patient redress before returning to discuss the examination.

I. After the Patient Is Dressed and Settled, Repeat Blood Pressure Measurement if Elevated Before.

14 *Pediatric Examination Checklist*

This outline provides tips and suggestions to make the pediatric examination easier. It applies to infants and children, but not to newborns.

I. SETTING.

   A. A Comfortably Warm Room with Pictures and Familiar-Looking Furniture Serve to Reassure the Small Child, who Is in an Unfamiliar Environment.

   B. Pastel "Playroom" Colored Walls Are More Familiar to the Child than Hospital White.

II. APPROACH.

   A. Some Familiarity Needs to be Established with Both the Child and the Parents.

   1. Let the child explore the examining room while the history is taken.

   2. Talk to the child, asking him/her simple questions about how he/she is feeling. A smile is reassuring to the child.

   3. Use techniques that often put the child at ease:
      - Tell a brief story.
      - Explain the examination in simple terms, demonstrating on yourself or a toy animal.
      - Let the child (carefully) play with the stethoscope and otoscope to gain familiarity with them.

   4. Since the parent is the chief source of comfort for the child, let the child stay near to the parent.
      - Often, much of the examination can be performed while the child sits on the parent's lap or stands next to the parent.

   5. Touch the child with a gentle but confident manner. Children are extremely sensitive to the manner of the clinician and, if provoked, they will frequently resist or cry.
      - For this reason, a little extra time in putting the child at ease can ultimately speed the examination rather than slow it.

- A gentle but professional manner is also more reassuring to the parents than an examination done with haste.

6. Speak to the child with kindness but authority, telling the child "I want you to . . ." rather than "Will you please . . ."

7. Perform the first portion of the examination with the child upright, since the supine position is more vulnerable and anxiety provoking.
   - Similarly, remove the underpants last, since this affords the child some security. Children are often more modest than adults.
   - Be prepared to change the order of your examination. Young children often move around; you may need to examine various body parts as they come within reach.

8. Examine, as with adults, from least to most invasive.
   - Examine in the general order: inspection, auscultation, percussion, palpation.
   - Perform any maneuvers last that are likely to result in pain or discomfort. This includes examination of the ears and throat.
   - In a fearful child, start peripherally and move centrally, starting with examination of the feet and moving up to the abdomen.
   - Complete the examination as quickly as possible. Children have a very short attention span and will become more irritable if the examination is prolonged.

III. SPECIFIC AREAS OF EXAMINATION.

A. General Inspection.

1. State of health, activity, posture, facial expression, apparent age, degree of cooperation, interaction between child and parent.
2. Note any congenital anomalies or physical deformities.
3. Note parent's reaction to child's spontaneous behavior. Is parent supportive, punitive, indifferent.

B. Vital Signs: Measure.

1. Temperature: usually tympanic, oral, or rectal.
2. Pulse, measured brachial or apical.
3. Respirations, including crying.
4. Blood pressure (in infants 3 years and older). Use the pediatric cuff.

C. Growth Measurements.

1. Under 3 years of age: recumbent length, body weight, head circumference (optional chest circumference).
2. Over 3 years of age: standing height and weight.
3. These should be plotted on standardized growth charts appropriate to the child's age.
   - Watch for trends of deviation from the established borders of normalcy, but remember to also evaluate the child's growth in comparison to that of other family members. Short stature in children is most often secondary to short stature in parents or first-degree relatives.

D. Skin.

1. Note color, texture, turgor, rashes, macules or other lesions, and hair growth.
2. Pay particular attention to "birthmarks" such as nevus flammeus ("stork-bite") and strawberry hemangiomas. Note their change over time.

E. Head and Neck.

1. Head: Note shape, symmetry, hair, and scalp.
   - When scalp flattening is seen in infants, ask the parent which side the infant sleeps on. The side may need to be changed.
2. Facial motion, symmetry, and visible genetic appearances (such as Down syndrome).

3. Eyes (may be postponed to the end of the examination).
   - Check visual acuity testing appropriate to age, strabismus, and extraocular motion.
     —Pediatric eye charts are available (see Chapter 4, Head and Neck).
     —Infants are at highest risk for undiagnosed strabismus. Note position of the corneal light reflex on each eye. Use the cover test.
   - Check pupillary response to light, ophthalmoscopy (including red reflex and retinal examination).
4. Ears (may be postponed to the end of the examination).
   - External appearance and symmetry.
   - Auditory acuity—roughly tested by whispering to the child or clapping your hands and seeing if the child blinks.
   - Internal examination.
     —May require the child to be restrained.
       • For babies, have the parent grasp both hands and roll the infant to one side. The head will follow, making examination easier.
       • For toddlers, have the child sitting on the examination table or held by the parent. The parent can support the child with one hand and press the child's head to his/her chest with the other, placing the restraining hand above the ear.
       • By 4 years of age, most children allow themselves to be examined.
       • A time-tested technique is to tell the child you can see animals in his or her ear. As you look in, vividly describe the animal you see today. The child will often be fascinated by your narrative.
     —Evaluate the deep canal and eardrum by otoscopy. Cerumen may need to be removed.
       • In infants, pull the pinna directly backward. In older children, pull back and up as for adults.

- Remember that the Valsalva maneuver caused by crying can transiently redden the eardrum. Note the eardrum reflectivity and any bulging, not just its color.
- One of the arts of medicine is the ability to take a mental "flash photo" of the eardrum or pharynx, since the opportunity to visualize these structures in children is often quite brief.

5. Nose.
   - External: shape, deviation.
   - Internal: bleeding or discharge, septum, and turbinate examination.
     —Nosebleeds are common. Note any crusting on the anterior septum, usually from local irritation.

6. Mouth.
   - Examine the lips, teeth (number, position, caries), tongue, cheek, palate. This is a convenient time to ask if the child has yet had a dental visit. The first visit is generally recommended at age 3.
     —Do as much of the examination as possible without the tongueblade. If needed, the child may be restrained.
     —If the child clamps his teeth down on the tongueblade, slide it gently backward until it causes a gag response. When this occurs, quickly examine the mouth and pharynx.

7. Throat (often examined last). Restraint of the small child may be needed.
   - Uvula, tonsils.
   - Attempt to avoid eliciting the gag reflex by:
     —Asking the child to say "Ah..."
       - As with adults, ask the child to "pant like a puppydog," and demonstrate it. This lessens the gag response and often causes the palate to rise and the tongue to lower, opening a view of the pharynx.
     —Examining the tonsils one at a time by pushing the tongue to either side with the tongue blade.

8. Neck.
- Position, lymph node inspection and palpation.
  —Children often have soft, movable 1 cm anterior cervical nodes as residual from their last upper respiratory infection.
- Thyroid gland inspection and palpation.
- Visible veins or muscular swellings.

F. Thorax and Lungs.

1. Inspection.
- Shape and symmetry.
  —Sternal and spinal contours.
- Intercostal retractions or bulging.
  —Respiratory motion is mostly abdominal until ages 6 to 7, when thoracic motion becomes more visible.

2. Palpation: Tactile fremitus is more pronounced than in adults.

3. Percussion: more resonant than adults.

4. Auscultation:
- If the child does not respond to instructions to breathe deeply, demonstrate with a theatrical deep breath. If you repeat this as you reposition your stethoscope, the child will often mimic each breath.
- Remember that breath sounds seem louder since children have a thinner chest wall.
  —Also the breath sounds are more bronchial and the expiratory phase is more prolonged.
- If the child cries during the examination and cannot be soothed, listen at least during inspiration for crackles and wheezes.

G. Heart.

1. Inspection and palpation: the heart is normally higher and more leftward than in the adult. In children under 4 years of age, the apical impulse is in the fourth left intercostal space.
- Also palpate for vibratory thrill.

2. Auscultation.
   - Heart sounds are typically louder in children.
   - Variation in pulse rate is often pronounced with respiration. This is the normal *sinus arrhythmia.*
   - Your auscultation may be divided into two parts: one while the child is sitting on the parent's lap and later while the child is supine on the examination table.
   - Benign murmurs are common. Their typical characteristics are:
     —Heard best in supine position.
     —Systolic in timing.
     —Maximal at left sternal border.
     —Grade 1 or 2 in intensity.
     —Unassociated with other signs of cardiac disease.

H. Abdomen.

1. Inspection.
   - Size and contour (often pot-bellied).
   - Visible veins.
   - Hernias (inguinal, femoral, umbilical).
     —Umbilical hernias are common and often spontaneously resolve by 3 years of age (or later in African-American children).

2. Auscultation for bowel sounds.

3. Percussion for liver or spleen enlargement.

4. Palpation for masses, tenderness, or rigidity.
   - Children are often quite ticklish. Palpate gently at first, but deeply later, if possible:
     —Feel in particular for kidney size.
     —Under 4 years of age, the liver edge is often palpable 1 or 2 cm below the right costal margin.
     —Flex the knees if necessary to relax the abdomen.

I. Male Genitalia.
1. Note circumcision, meatal position and opening, size and location of testes, sexual maturity rating (see Appendix A).

J. Female Genitalia.
1. Note perineal hygiene, vaginal opening, and any discharge.

2. Assess sexual maturity rating (see Appendix A).

K. Rectum and Anus.
1. Note inflammation or skin lesions.

2. Rectal examination, if needed, is performed with the little finger, well-lubricated, and inserted slowly. The parent needs to be near the child for reassurance.
   - Inspect stool and check for occult blood.

L. Musculoskeletal.
1. Note obvious deformities, genu varum (knock-knees, common from ages 2 to 7), gait, paralysis, spinal curvatures (kyphosis, lordosis, scoliosis).
   - Watch in particular for limp, tibial torsion, and pes planus.

2. Note joint swelling and any tibial torsion.

M. Neurologic.
1. For older children, the techniques are similar to adult examination. Adjust parameters of mental status examination for the child's level of intellectual capacity. The neurologic examination of the infant is beyond the scope of this book.

15 Approach to the Elderly Patient

I. MEDICAL HISTORY.

A. The Geriatric Assessment Includes Far More than the Routine History and Physical Examination.

1. Because of the volume of information required for a geriatric assessment, consider breaking the encounter into two 1-hour visits, or use extensive questionnaires completed before the patient's visit.
   - Many healthy "well elderly" do not require in-depth assessment and require a much briefer encounter.
2. The medical history differs from a younger patient and is divided into the following:

B. History of Current Problems.

1. A listing of the patient's and caregiver's major concerns.
2. Since elderly patients often have multiple pathologic conditions, many may be present simultaneously.
   - Obtain a recent and interval history for each problem.
   - Many elderly patients do not have a single "chief complaint."

C. Review of Systems.

1. Under-reporting of illness is common in elderly patients.
2. Hidden illness must be elicited by direct questioning, since important symptoms may not be mentioned out of fear, ignorance, or minimizing behavior.
   - Include dementia, depression, falls, incontinence, problems with sleep, and weight loss.

D. Past Medical History: old records are very helpful for comparison and as background information.

E. Family History, more for its effect on patient's attitude toward a disease than to his/her risk of contracting it.

F. The Medication History.

1. Best elicited with the "paper bag test." Ask the patient to bring in *all* medicines and supplements used.
   - This includes vitamins, laxatives, sleeping pills, herbal medicines, and cold preparations.

2. Place all medications on the exam room desk and ask how often and for what reason each medication is taken.
- Use this as a prompt for past medical history that may have gone unmentioned.

3. You will often be surprised at the degree of polypharmacy that is occurring and the risk of multiple drug interactions.

G. Nutritional Status and Needs.
1. This includes a typical day's diet history, pattern of weight in recent years, and shopping/food preparation habits.

2. Access to meals: who prepares them? Is it through an elder daycare center, "meals on wheels," family members, or the patient?

H. Patient Profile and Social History.
1. This includes current or previous occupation, hobbies, and interests, past or present alcohol or tobacco use.

2. Assessed most easily by eliciting an average patient day. Ask "What is your average day like?"
- This helps to assess the degree of disability or dysfunction, and how it affects the patient's lifestyle.

I. Health Promotion/Disease Prevention.
1. Mammography and Pap test; date performed and last result.

2. Immunization history.
- Elderly patients are usually candidates for influenza and pneumonia vaccination.
- Tetanus booster may be out of date.
- Residents of long-term care facilities are also candidates for yearly tuberculosis skin test screening.

3. Seat belt use.

4. Recent laboratory testing or imaging studies.

II. ELDER-SPECIFIC HISTORY. Besides the routine medical history, the geriatric history includes:

A. Assessment of Function, Including:

1. Activities of daily living, needed for basic self-care: (bathing, dressing, toileting, transferring, continence, and feeding).

2. Instrumental activities of daily living, needed for independent living: (includes ability to travel beyond walking distance [driving or use of public transportation], ability to go shopping, prepare own meals, do housework, do laundry, use telephone, self-administer medications, and manage finances).

3. Use of assistive devices.
   - This includes a hearing aid, glasses, dentures, cane, walker, or wheelchair.
   - Inspect the device. Was it prescribed for the patient or given/left by a relative? Is it in working order?

B. Assessment of Environment.

1. Patient's living situation and physical layout. Does the home pose dangers such as steep stairs, high-walled bathtub, etc?
   - Also consider the presence of rugs (patient can slip and fall), thresholds (patient can bump into or miss the step), heating and cooling, proximity of laundry facilities, and neighborhood crime.
   - Are there fixed assistive devices in the home, such as raised toilet seats, tub benches, etc?

C. Assessment of Support Structure.

1. The patient's network of friends and relatives.
   - The extent of social relationships is a powerful predictor of functional status and mortality.
   - Assess involvement with church, temple, etc; other organizations; and senior centers.

2. Caregiver's status, including family situation and availability. This area includes caregiver stress and potential burnout.

3. Contingency plans.
   - Who can help, and where can the patient go if illness or decline in function occurs. Such planning may not have been addressed before.

4. Community services currently provided (and desired).

5. Access to emergency medical response (EMS) system. How does the patient or family reach an ambulance?

D. Advance Directives.

1. An often overlooked area; a *living will* or *durable power of attorney for health care* assist the patient, the family, and the physician in following the patient's wishes in case of a catastrophic illness.

2. If not completed, encourage the patient to complete these documents.
   - A simple way to ask is "Who would you want to make decisions for you if you were unable?"

3. If the patient has lost decision-making ability, other family members will often have taken jurisdiction, sometimes without formal paperwork. Encourage the formalization of this arrangement. Hidden in this problem are often issues of control and authority among family members.

III. PHYSICAL EXAMINATION. This section contains useful tips, not thorough technique. It is intended to heighten your suspicion of certain problems as you perform your examination.

A. Vital Signs.

1. Height and weight; useful for following patient over time. Correlate loss of height with any thoracic kyphosis, a warning sign of osteoporosis.

2. Temperature; elderly patients are often normally hypothermic. These patients can have a "normal" temperature during severe infections.

3. Respiratory rate; tachypnea is a reliable sign of lower respiratory infection, particularly with a rate exceeding 24 breaths per minute.

4. Pulse; useful for arrhythmias, common in the elderly. Remember that premature beats will often *not* transmit to the radial pulse, and will be perceived as skipped beats.

5. Blood pressure; check for postural (orthostatic) changes in blood pressure.
   - Check standing blood pressure after the patient has been supine for 10 minutes. Check immediately and after 3 minutes. Orthostatic hypotension is defined as a 20 mmHg drop in systolic pressure, or any drop accompanied by symptoms. Have the patient lie down immediately if symptomatic.

B. Skin.

1. Aging skin also often has a variety of benign skin lesions such as seborrheic keratoses, capillary angiomas, and senile lentigos.

2. Pay particular attention to sun-exposed areas for premalignant lesions, such as actinic keratoses, and malignant lesions, such as basal cell or squamous cell carcinoma, or melanoma.

3. If the patient is not ambulatory, inspect for pressure sores, particularly on the heels, malleoli, sacral area, and ischial tuberosities.

4. Watch for ecchymoses. They may be due to fragile skin, but raise suspicion of falls or elder abuse.

5. Examine the toenails. Thickening or longitudinal ridging is common "nail dystrophy." Differentiate this from onychomycosis, with yellow-green crumbly nails, often only on the halluces.

C. **Head and Neck.**
   1. Head.
      ▪ Palpate temporal arteries if history of headache or local tenderness is present. Tenderness or thickening occurs with temporal arteritis.

   2. Eyes.
      ▪ Check visual acuity with a wall-mounted or pocket Snellen chart. If using the pocket Snellen chart, remember that older patients often have presbyopia and need to use reading glasses for near vision.
      ▪ Check for cataracts; they are *extremely* common in this age group.
      ▪ If the fundi can be seen, check for macular degeneration, also common. This will show itself with yellow spots (drusen) near the macula and/or discoloration in the macular region.
      ▪ Note the lower eyelids for outward (ectropion) or inward (entropion) deviation. This may be associated with dryness of the eyes.
      ▪ A corneal arcus is common and has no significance in this age group. Pupil size may be smaller, although symmetrically so. Extraocular motion often shows a normal impairment in upward gaze.

   3. Ears.
      ▪ Screen for hearing loss with whispered voice bilaterally. Hearing loss in the elderly, known as presbycusis, is *quite* common in this age group.
      ▪ Inspect ear canals; cerumen impaction is common. Briefly remove any hearing aid earpiece to access the canals.
      ▪ If the patient is hard of hearing, speak slowly and clearly to the patient in a louder than usual voice, allowing him/her to see your lips as you speak.

   4. Mouth.
- Pay close attention to gum or dental problems, which increase significantly in the elderly population. Note eroded (ground-down) teeth and gum recession or inflammation.
- If dentures are present, examine the oral mucosa with dentures removed.
  - Check the dentures for fit. Are they loose when in place? Dentures are expensive and seldom are changed.
- Inspect for oral premalignant or malignant lesions, including the sides and bottom of the tongue.

   5. Neck.
- Auscultate for carotid bruits, which are associated with significant stenosis in about half the cases.
- Examine the thyroid for goiter or nodules. Thyroid disease is "the great mimicker" in the elderly and presents with a variety of manifestations.
- Cervical lymph nodes are often smaller, softer, and more difficult to palpate.

D. Breasts.
   1. The incidence of breast cancer rises steadily with advancing age. Perform a thorough examination, which is often easier since breast tissue is usually softer in this age group.

E. Heart.
   1. Sclerosis of aortic valve leaflets is common and causes a soft (grade 2/6) ejection type murmur, loudest at the base, sometimes radiating to the apex. This does not impair blood flow. True aortic stenosis, however, is more likely when other signs are present, such as a louder murmur, diminution of S_2, and dampening of the carotid upstroke.

   2. Calcification of the mitral valves can also occur, usually causing mitral regurgitation. This is pathologic and causes physiologic consequences to the heart.

   3. Loss of peripheral pulses, particularly pedal, may be considered normal as long as intermittent claudication and signs of peripheral vascular disease are absent.

F. Chest and Lungs.
1. Deformities of kyphosis or scoliosis may decrease tidal volume and amplitude of breath sounds.
2. If the patient is bedridden or hospitalized in bed, remember that the dependent portions of lung will normally produce showers of crackles that clear with a few deep breaths.
3. Frail, elderly patients may be unable to sit up and lean forward by themselves. To auscultate the posterior lung fields, either obtain the assistance of nursing staff or have the patient turn his/her upper body to each side, exposing half of the posterior chest at a time.

G. Abdomen.
1. Laxity of the abdominal wall muscles often causes a "potbelly."
2. An abdominal mass may present with no symptoms. Conversely, constipation can present with a fecal mass that resembles a malignancy. Reexamination in a few days can help to differentiate after the fecal mass has passed spontaneously with the use of enemas and/or suppositories.
3. Routinely percuss the bladder, since asymptomatic urinary retention is common in both elderly men and women.
4. Palpate for an aortic aneurysm, usually demonstrating a width greater than 3 cm.
5. Just as the elderly patient mounts less of a white cell and fever response to infection, the abdominal examination may show less signs of peritonitis, with diminished involuntary guarding or rebound tenderness.
6. Note any urine leakage or fecal soiling on underwear, which are signs of incontinence.

H. Male Genitalia.
1. Pubic hair may become scanty, and the testes hang more loosely in the scrotum.
2. Palpate routinely for inguinal or femoral hernias.

3. The prostate gland often enlarges in elderly men. Pay particular attention to the presence of any prostate nodules. When performing the rectal examination in either sex, remember that the risk of colorectal cancer is highest in this age group. Probe as high as possible into the rectal vault for a mass or induration of the rectal wall.

I. Female Genitalia.

1. Pubic hair becomes more sparse in the elderly woman. Note any vulvar lesions.
2. As estrogen levels decline, vaginal mucosa becomes drier and less elastic. The uterus and ovaries shrink in size and become more difficult to palpate.
3. Because the vaginal canal also shortens, be sure to use a small speculum and adequate water or lubricant jelly. The cervix is often small and atrophic. You may be limited to inserting one finger for the bimanual examination, and you will not be able to enter as deeply.
   - Ask about incontinence if you have not asked before. Check for stress incontinence as the patient coughs; watch for a spurt of urine.
   - Check for cystocele and rectocele as you insert and remove the speculum.
   - Check for laxity of the pelvic floor musculature by having the patient attempt to "tighten" around your fingers inserted into the vagina.
4. If the patient cannot comfortably assume the lithotomy position, the pelvic examination can be performed in the left lateral position, either with the legs drawn up, or with the upper leg lifted with the aid of an assistant.

J. Musculoskeletal.

1. Assess for signs of osteoarthritis in fingers, neck, hips, and knees. Pain from these are sometimes so long-standing the patient may not mention it.

2. Screen for functional loss.
   - For upper extremities, have the patient touch his/her hands to the back of the head. This tests shoulder abduction and external rotation, along with shoulder girdle muscle strength. Have the patient touch the small of the back to test internal rotation.
   - For lower extremities, use the timed "Up and Go" test,[1] where the patient rises from a chair, walks 3 meters, turns, walks back, and sits down again.
3. Follow with complete joint examination when joint pain is present (see Chapter 11, Musculoskeletal Examination).

K. Neurologic Examination.

1. Mental status. Any suspicion of impaired mental status should lead to some form of screening. One such screening tool is the Mini-Mental State Examination (see Appendix B).
   - Always consider depression in the differential diagnosis of altered mental status.
   - The Short Form Geriatric Depression Scale[2] is an easy to answer "yes/no" format that has been found to be a reliable indicator for depression even in patients with medical illness or mild dementia.
2. Cranial nerves: tested as part of routine examination.
3. Reflexes. Most elderly patients have deep tendon responses, but they are more difficult to elicit. Achilles tendon responses are often diminished. Check them carefully.
4. Motor exam. Check for tremor, both of the hands (at rest and in motion) and of the head. Check resting motor tone. Strength, gait, and balance are screened for during the "Up and Go" test.
5. Sensory exam. Vibratory sensation of the toes is typically lost in some elderly patients. However, position sense usually remains intact in healthy patients, and travels in the same posterior column location.

1. Mathias S, Nayak USL, Issacs B: The "get up and go" test; a simple clinical test of balance in old people, *Arch Phys Med Rhabil* 429-434, 1986.
2. Sheikh JI, Yesavage JA: Geriatric depression scale: recent evidence and development of a shorter version, *Clin Gerontol* 5:165-172, 1986.

I. FEMALES.

A. Two Criteria.

1. Pubic hair character and distribution.
   - Stage 1: preadolescent, no pubic hair except for fine vellus hair, such as seen on the arms or abdomen.
   - Stage 2: presence of early pubic hair, fine and only slightly curly, along the labia (usually ages 11 to 12).
   - Stage 3: darker, coarser, curlier hair covering the central area of the mons pubis (usually ages 12 to 13).
   - Stage 4: adult type in coarseness and curliness, nearly complete distribution but excluding the inner thighs (usually ages 13 to 14).
   - Stage 5: same as in stage 4 with extension onto the inner thighs.
     —Additional notes:
     - In the adult, the pubic hair appears roughly as an inverted triangle.
     - The base reaches the top of the mons pubis.
     - The apex extends to the labia.
     - In some young women with familial hirsutism, the hair may extend up the abdomen to the umbilicus, resembling the male hair distribution.
     - In the elderly, pubic hair is thin, sparse, and gray.

2. Breast development.
   - Stage 1: preadolescent, elevation only of nipple.
   - Stage 2: presence of breast bud and increased diameter of areola.
   - Stage 3: further elevation and enlargement of breast and areola, with continuous contour from breast to areola.
   - Stage 4: elevation of the nipple and areola to form a discrete mound at the tip of the breast.

- Stage 5: adult stage with breast at full size, projection of nipple only, with the areola receded back to normal breast contour. In some normal cases, the areola lingers as a secondary mound.

B. During the Examination, Note any:

1. Increase in prominence of labia majora.

2. Enlargement of the labia minora.

3. Increase in size of the clitoris.

4. Increase in elasticity of vaginal walls.

5. Enlargement of vagina and ovaries.

C. The Stages of Development Usually Occur Between the Ages of 12 and 16.

II. MALES.

A. Three Criteria.

1. Pubic hair character and distribution.
   - Stage 1: preadolescent, no pubic hair except for fine body hair, such as seen on the abdomen.
   - Stage 2: sparse growth of thin, slightly pigmented, and curly hair at the base of the penis.
   - Stage 3: darker hair that is curlier and coarser, extending onto the symphysis pubis.
   - Stage 4: adult type in coarseness and curliness, nearly complete distribution, but excluding the inner thighs.
   - Stage 5: same as in stage 4 with full growth and extension onto the inner thighs.

2. Penile growth.
   - Stage 1: same size and proportional growth as in childhood.
   - Stage 2: slight enlargement.
   - Stage 3: elongation, slight increase in diameter.
   - Stage 4: further enlargement and elongation with development of the glans penis.
   - Stage 5: adult appearance.

3. Growth of the testes and scrotum.
   - Stage 1: same size and proportional growth as in childhood.
   - Stage 2: slight enlargement, reddening of scrotal skin and more prominence of skin texture.
   - Stage 3: continued enlargement.
   - Stage 4: continued enlargement with darkening of skin pigmentation of the scrotal skin.
   - Stage 5: adult appearance.

B. **In General,** if a boy's testes have increased in size to 2.5 cm or more, or if his pubic hair has reached stage 2, he can be reassured that sexual development has begun.
   1. In the adult male, the pubic hair rises in the midline toward the umbilicus.

   2. The time of onset of adult sexual characteristics is extremely variable.
      - In general, the stages of development usually occur between the ages of 12 and 16, with penile growth slightly delayed behind pubic hair and scrotal maturation.

Adapted from Tanner JM: *Growth of adolescents,* ed 2, Oxford, England, 1962, Blackwell Scientific Publications.

B Mini-Mental State Examination

Used to quickly assess dementia and its change over time. Each correct reply is assigned a score of "1." A normal score is between 24 and the maximum score of 30. The test is divided into five sections:

I. ORIENTATION (One point per question, maximum score is 10.)
A. Time.
1. What is today's date?
2. What is the year?
3. What is the month?
4. What day is today? (e.g., Monday)
5. Can you also tell me what season it is?

B. Place.
1. Can you tell me the name of this hospital (clinic)?
2. What floor are we on?
3. What town or city are we in?
4. What county are we in?
5. What state are we in?

II. IMMEDIATE RECALL (One point per word, maximum score is 3.)
A. Ask the Patient if You May Test His/Her Memory.
Then say "ball," "flag," and "tree" clearly and slowly, about one second for each.

B. After You Have Said all Three, Ask Him/Her to Repeat Them.
1. This first repetition back by the patient determines his/her score (0 to 3).
2. If the patient fails to repeat all three, repeat the three words to the patient and retest, up to six more tries.
3. If the patient is not eventually able to learn all three words, recall cannot be meaningfully tested.

III. ATTENTION AND CALCULATION (Maximum score is 5.) There are two methods:

A. Ask the Patient to Begin with 100 and Count Backwards by 7. Stop after five subtractions (93, 86, 79, 65). Score the total number of correct answers, one point for each.

B. If the Patient Cannot or Will Not Perform as Above, Ask Him/Her to Spell the Word "World" Backwards. The score is the number of letters in correct order.

   1. For example, "dlrow" is a score of 5, dlorw is a score of 3.

IV. RECALL (Maximum score of 3.)

A. Ask the Patient to Recall the Three Words You Previously Asked Him/Her to Remember. Score one point for each word correctly recalled.

V. LANGUAGE (Maximum score is 9.)

A. Naming (2 points).

   1. Show the patient a wrist watch and ask him/her what it is.

   2. Repeat for a pencil.

B. Repetition (1 point).

   1. Ask the subject to repeat, "No ifs, ands, or buts."

C. Three-Stage Command (3 points).

   1. Give the patient a blank piece of paper and say:
   - "Take the paper in your right hand."
   - "Fold it in half."
   - "Put it on the floor."

   2. Score one point for each of the three steps performed successfully.

D. Reading (1 point).
  1. On a blank piece of paper, print the words "Close your eyes" in letters large enough for the patient to see clearly.

  2. Ask him/her to read it and do what it says.

  3. Score 1 point only if he/she actually closes his/her eyes.

E. Writing (1 point).
  1. Give the patient a blank piece of paper and ask him/her to write a sentence. It is to be written spontaneously.

  2. It must contain a subject and a verb, and be sensible.

  3. Correct grammar and punctuation are not necessary.

F. Copying (1 point).
  1. On a clean piece of paper, draw intersecting pentagons, each side about one inch.

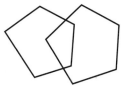

  2. Ask the patient to copy it exactly as it is.

  3. All ten angles must be present and two must intersect to score 1 point. Tremor and rotation are ignored.

Adapted from Folstein MF, Folstein SE, McHugh PR: "Mini-Mental State": a practical method for grading the cognitive state of patients for the clinician, *J Psychiatr Res* 12:196-198, 1975.

Index

A